Effects of Ionizing Radiation in Cancer Radiotherapy

Effects of Ionizing Radiation in Cancer Radiotherapy

Guest Editor
François Chevalier

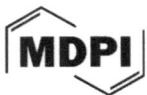

Basel • Beijing • Wuhan • Barcelona • Belgrade • Novi Sad • Cluj • Manchester

Guest Editor
François Chevalier
CIMAP laboratory
Caen Normandy
Caen
France

Editorial Office
MDPI AG
Grosspeteranlage 5
4052 Basel, Switzerland

This is a reprint of the Special Issue, published open access by the journal *International Journal of Molecular Sciences* (ISSN 1422-0067), freely accessible at: www.mdpi.com/journal/ijms/special_issues/nte.

For citation purposes, cite each article independently as indicated on the article page online and using the guide below:

Lastname, A.A.; Lastname, B.B. Article Title. *Journal Name* **Year**, *Volume Number*, Page Range.

ISBN 978-3-7258-3386-3 (Hbk)
ISBN 978-3-7258-3385-6 (PDF)
https://doi.org/10.3390/books978-3-7258-3385-6

Cover image courtesy of Francois Chevalier

© 2025 by the authors. Articles in this book are Open Access and distributed under the Creative Commons Attribution (CC BY) license. The book as a whole is distributed by MDPI under the terms and conditions of the Creative Commons Attribution-NonCommercial-NoDerivs (CC BY-NC-ND) license (https://creativecommons.org/licenses/by-nc-nd/4.0/).

Contents

About the Editor vii

Preface ix

Mihaela Tudor, Antoine Gilbert, Charlotte Lepleux, Mihaela Temelie, Sonia Hem and Jean Armengaud et al.
A Proteomic Study Suggests Stress Granules as New Potential Actors in Radiation-Induced Bystander Effects
Reprinted from: *Int. J. Mol. Sci.* **2021**, 22, 7957, https://doi.org/10.3390/ijms22157957 1

Maria Grazia Andreassi, Nadia Haddy, Mats Harms-Ringdahl, Jonica Campolo, Andrea Borghini and François Chevalier et al.
A Longitudinal Study of Individual Radiation Responses in Pediatric Patients Treated with Proton and Photon Radiotherapy, and Interventional Cardiology: Rationale and Research Protocol of the HARMONIC Project
Reprinted from: *Int. J. Mol. Sci.* **2023**, 24, 8416, https://doi.org/10.3390/ijms24098416 21

Ilona Barbara Csordás, Eric Andreas Rutten, Tünde Szatmári, Prabal Subedi, Lourdes Cruz-Garcia and Dávid Kis et al.
The miRNA Content of Bone Marrow-Derived Extracellular Vesicles Contributes to Protein Pathway Alterations Involved in Ionising Radiation-Induced Bystander Responses
Reprinted from: *Int. J. Mol. Sci.* **2023**, 24, 8607, https://doi.org/10.3390/ijms24108607 34

Rim Jenni, Asma Chikhaoui, Imen Nabouli, Anissa Zaouak, Fatma Khanchel and Houda Hammami-Ghorbel et al.
Differential Expression of ATM, NF-KB, PINK1 and Foxo3a in Radiation-Induced Basal Cell Carcinoma
Reprinted from: *Int. J. Mol. Sci.* **2023**, 24, 7181, https://doi.org/10.3390/ijms24087181 59

Radhia M'Kacher, Bruno Colicchio, Steffen Junker, Elie El Maalouf, Leonhard Heidingsfelder and Andreas Plesch et al.
High Resolution and Automatable Cytogenetic Biodosimetry Using In Situ Telomere and Centromere Hybridization for the Accurate Detection of DNA Damage: An Overview
Reprinted from: *Int. J. Mol. Sci.* **2023**, 24, 5699, https://doi.org/10.3390/ijms24065699 77

Margarita Pustovalova, Philipp Malakhov, Anastasia Guryanova, Maxim Sorokin, Maria Suntsova and Anton Buzdin et al.
Transcriptome-Based Traits of Radioresistant Sublines of Non-Small Cell Lung Cancer Cells
Reprinted from: *Int. J. Mol. Sci.* **2023**, 24, 3042, https://doi.org/10.3390/ijms24033042 97

Lina Alhaddad, Zain Nofal, Margarita Pustovalova, Andreyan N. Osipov and Sergey Leonov
Long-Term Cultured Human Glioblastoma Multiforme Cells Demonstrate Increased Radiosensitivity and Senescence-Secretory Phenotype in Response to Irradiation
Reprinted from: *Int. J. Mol. Sci.* **2023**, 24, 2002, https://doi.org/10.3390/ijms24032002 114

Maria P. Souli, Zacharenia Nikitaki, Monika Puchalska, Kateřina Pachnerová Brabcová, Ellas Spyratou and Panagiotis Kote et al.
Clustered DNA Damage Patterns after Proton Therapy Beam Irradiation Using Plasmid DNA
Reprinted from: *Int. J. Mol. Sci.* **2022**, 23, 15606, https://doi.org/10.3390/ijms232415606 127

Lina Alhaddad, Andreyan N. Osipov and Sergey Leonov
The Molecular and Cellular Strategies of Glioblastoma and Non-Small-Cell Lung Cancer Cells Conferring Radioresistance
Reprinted from: *Int. J. Mol. Sci.* **2022**, 23, 13577, https://doi.org/10.3390/ijms232113577 . . . . . **148**

Mateusz Smolarz, Łukasz Skoczylas, Marta Gawin, Monika Krzyżowska, Monika Pietrowska and Piotr Widłak
Radiation-Induced Bystander Effect Mediated by Exosomes Involves the Replication Stress in Recipient Cells
Reprinted from: *Int. J. Mol. Sci.* **2022**, 23, 4169, https://doi.org/10.3390/ijms23084169 . . . . . . **191**

About the Editor

François Chevalier

Dr. François Chevalier, PhD, HDR, with a background in protein chemistry and molecular biology, received his doctoral degree in biochemistry in 2001 (INRA, Nantes, France) for the biochemical characterization of glycated proteins. He completed a 5-year post-doctoral research position in Montpellier (INRA, France) with a special focus on the global analysis of proteins using two-dimensional electrophoresis and mass spectrometry. Following a research position in Cork (UCC, Ireland) with a study of protein quality using proteomics tools, he is currently employed in CEA (DRF-IRAMIS-Cimap in Caen) as research director and team leader in radiation biology in the ARIA group (Applications in Radiobiology with Accelerated Ions).

Dr. François Chevalier is specialized in radiation-biology of radioresistant cancer cells, the hypoxic micro-environment, and bystander effects in the context of hadrontherapy.

He has published more than 70 scientific and technical papers in peer-reviewed journals.

Preface

Dear Colleagues,

For a long time, it was widely accepted that the biological effects of ionizing radiation such as cell death, DNA damage, and mutagenesis result from the direct ionization of cell structures, particularly DNA, or from indirect damage through reactive oxygen species produced by the radiolysis of water. This "targeted effect" (TE) model has been questioned by numerous observations, in which cells, that were not directly irradiated, exhibited responses similar to those of the directly irradiated cells. Therefore, it is nowadays accepted that the detrimental effects of ionizing radiation are not restricted only to the irradiated cells, but also to non-irradiated adjacent or distant cells.

The non-targeted effects (NTEs) of ionizing radiation, which include genomic instability, radiation-induced bystander effects, and abscopal effects, are defined as the occurrence of biological effects in non-irradiated cells because of the irradiation of other cells in the population. In opposition with TE, that display a linear dose–response, NTEs exhibit a non-linear dose–response, with a marked effect at low doses of radiation. The related cellular and molecular mechanisms of NTEs are still not completely understood, as they are mainly dependent on the cell type and the radiation quality. It is now widely admitted that in specific conditions, irradiated cells produce stress factors, which affect non-irradiated cells in the close environment (bystander effect) or at distance (abscopal effect). The cellular response, observed in non-irradiated cells, can be very similar to the response of irradiated cells, with a modulated intensity. NTEs involve the secretion or the release by irradiated cells of a broad range of stress factors, from cytokines and specifically secreted molecules to reactive oxygen species or oxidized cellular wastes. In the case of communication between neighborhood cells, the stress factors can disseminate through gap junctions, or in the case of distance communication, through small vesicles containing various embedded molecules. NTEs are commonly studied as low-dose radiation effects in radioprotection, in association with genomic instability, mutation induction, and secondary cancer risk.

In a radiotherapy context, TE and NTE can be involved at the same time and, in the case of NTE, it could present several risks of complications when the irradiated area is very close to a sensitive organ. On the other hand, NTEs could increase the biological effect of the radiotherapy on distant non-irradiated cancer cells (such as metastases) with immune-associated effects (abscopal effect) or on non-irradiated cancer cells adjacent to cancer cells specifically targeted with radioactive antibodies (positive bystander effect).

I am pleased to share with you this Special Issue on the "Targeted and non-targeted effects of ionizing radiation in the context of cancer radiotherapy".

François Chevalier
Guest Editor

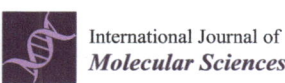 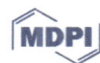

Article

A Proteomic Study Suggests Stress Granules as New Potential Actors in Radiation-Induced Bystander Effects

Mihaela Tudor [1,2], Antoine Gilbert [3], Charlotte Lepleux [3], Mihaela Temelie [1], Sonia Hem [4], Jean Armengaud [5], Emilie Brotin [6], Siamak Haghdoost [3], Diana Savu [1] and François Chevalier [3,*]

[1] Department of Life and Environmental Physics, HoriaHulubei National Institute of Physics and Nuclear Engineering, 077125 Magurele, Romania; mihaela.tudor@nipne.ro (M.T.); mihaela.temelie@nipne.ro (M.T.); dsavu@nipne.ro (D.S.)
[2] Faculty of Biology, University of Bucharest, 050095 Bucharest, Romania
[3] UMR6252 CIMAP, Team Applications in Radiobiology with Accelerated Ions, CEA-CNRS-ENSICAEN-Université de Caen Normandie, 14000 Caen, France; antoine.gilbert@ganil.fr (A.G.); charlotte.lepleux@gmail.com (C.L.); siamak.haghdoost@ganil.fr (S.H.)
[4] BPMP, Montpellier University, CNRS, INRAE, Institut Agro, 34000 Montpellier, France; sonia.hem@supagro.inra.fr
[5] Université Paris-Saclay, CEA, INRAE, Département Médicaments et Technologies pour la Santé (DMTS), SPI, 30200 Bagnols-sur-Cèze, France; jean.armengaud@cea.fr
[6] ImpedanCELL Platform, Federative Structure 4206 ICORE, NormandieUniv, UNICAEN, Inserm U1086 ANTICIPE, Biology and Innovative Therapeutics for Ovarian Cancers Group (BioTICLA), Comprehensive Cancer Center F. Baclesse, 14000 Caen, France; e.brotin@baclesse.unicancer.fr
* Correspondence: chevalier@ganil.fr; Tel.: +33-(0)231-454-564

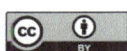

Citation: Tudor, M.; Gilbert, A.; Lepleux, C.; Temelie, M.; Hem, S.; Armengaud, J.; Brotin, E.; Haghdoost, S.; Savu, D.; Chevalier, F. A Proteomic Study Suggests Stress Granules as New Potential Actors in Radiation-Induced Bystander Effects. *Int. J. Mol. Sci.* **2021**, *22*, 7957. https://doi.org/10.3390/ijms22157957

Academic Editor: Sabrina Angelini

Received: 24 June 2021
Accepted: 20 July 2021
Published: 26 July 2021

Publisher's Note: MDPI stays neutral with regard to jurisdictional claims in published maps and institutional affiliations.

Copyright: © 2021 by the authors. Licensee MDPI, Basel, Switzerland. This article is an open access article distributed under the terms and conditions of the Creative Commons Attribution (CC BY) license (https://creativecommons.org/licenses/by/4.0/).

Abstract: Besides the direct effects of radiations, indirect effects are observed within the surrounding non-irradiated area; irradiated cells relay stress signals in this close proximity, inducing the so-called radiation-induced bystander effect. These signals received by neighboring unirradiated cells induce specific responses similar with those of direct irradiated cells. To understand the cellular response of bystander cells, we performed a 2D gel-based proteomic study of the chondrocytes receiving the conditioned medium of low-dose irradiated chondrosarcoma cells. The conditioned medium was directly analyzed by mass spectrometry in order to identify candidate bystander factors involved in the signal transmission. The proteomic analysis of the bystander chondrocytes highlighted 20 proteins spots that were significantly modified at low dose, implicating several cellular mechanisms, such as oxidative stress responses, cellular motility, and exosomes pathways. In addition, the secretomic analysis revealed that the abundance of 40 proteins in the conditioned medium of 0.1 Gy irradiated chondrosarcoma cells was significantly modified, as compared with the conditioned medium of non-irradiated cells. A large cluster of proteins involved in stress granules and several proteins involved in the cellular response to DNA damage stimuli were increased in the 0.1 Gy condition. Several of these candidates and cellular mechanisms were confirmed by functional analysis, such as 8-oxodG quantification, western blot, and wound-healing migration tests. Taken together, these results shed new lights on the complexity of the radiation-induced bystander effects and the large variety of the cellular and molecular mechanisms involved, including the identification of a new potential actor, namely the stress granules.

Keywords: chondrosarcoma; bystander signaling; proteomic analysis; secretome; stress granules

1. Introduction

Healthy normal tissues protection and patient recovery without sequelæ are key factors in modern cancer radiation therapy (RT). Certainly, radiation-induced side effects raise some concern due to the subsequent growth in morbidity among paediatric and adult patients. Models used in RT were initially developed from data collected after photon radiation. Emerging protocols of RT with protons or heavier particle, such as carbon ions in advanced medical facilities, have widely changed the way of thinking about local tumor control and the impact on healthy tissues [1,2]. Particle therapy (hadrontherapy) with protons has the advantage of a minimal exit dose after energy deposition in the target volume, and hence better sparing of critical structures in the vicinity of the tumor. Moreover, RT with carbon ions represents an exciting radiation modality, which combines the physical advantages of protons, excepting for an exit fragmentation tail, with higher radiobiological effectiveness [3]. Carbon ion therapy is expected to diminish the radiation morbidity rate. However, the multitude of combinations of radiation quality (linear energy transfer, energy, dose rate, dose, etc.) and tissue biological status (cell culture conditions, genetic background, etc.) does not ease the building of a relevant model for healthy tissue or tumor exposure during RT.

Irradiated cells may release signals which can induce biological alterations of neighboring non-irradiated cells termed the "radiation-induced bystander effects" (RIBE) [4,5]. There is no concord on a precise designation of RIBE, which involves distinct signal-mediated effects within or outside the irradiated volume [6]. Several cellular mechanisms have been suggested to be involved in the transmission of bystander signals by irradiated cells, including the secretion of soluble factors in the extracellular matrix, or the direct communication via gap junctions [7]. This phenomenon was observed in vivo in a context of major local inflammation, linked with a global imbalance of oxidative metabolism that makes its analysis challenging using in vitro model systems [8].

Several studies have aimed to identify the mechanisms of the radiation-induced bystander effect using proteomic tools. The protein composition of exosomes secreted by irradiated UM-SCC6 (human head-and-neck cancer cells) was investigated by direct mass spectrometry analysis [9], and showed a large number of proteins modulated (425 up-regulated and 47 down-regulated), belonging to different cellular processes, including the response to radiation, the metabolism of radical oxygen species and the DNA repair. Several soluble factors secreted from irradiated WEHI 164 (mouse fibrosarcoma cell line) were identified with a proteomic approach [10], including heat shock cognate, annexin A1, angiopoietin-2, and stress-induced phosphoprotein 1. The same proteomic approach was used to study a bystander communication between irradiated and non-irradiated fish [11]. In bystander fish, several modulated proteins were similar to those induced in irradiated fish, including hemoglobin subunit beta and hyperosmotic glycine-rich protein.

In one of our previous studies, we used a medium transfer approach to study RIBE [12]. Chondrosarcoma cells were irradiated with X-rays or C-ions (0.05 to 8 Gy) and then the supernatant, containing the signals emitted by irradiated cells, was transferred into flasks with non-irradiated chondrocytes. We use different technical strategies, such as clonogenic assay, multiplex ELISA analysis of conditioned medium, and flow cytometry for cell cycle analysis of direct irradiated and bystander cells. Our results showed a significant reduction in chondrocyte survival after transfer of the conditioned medium from chondrosarcoma cells irradiated with low doses (0.05 and 0.01 Gy) of X-rays and C-ions. By diluting this medium, the phenomenon decreased proportionally, confirming the presence of bystander factors. Some of these factors were partially observed using multiplex analysis of cell cytokines. Taken together, these results showed the capacity of chondrosarcoma cells to secrete bystander signals, particularly at a low irradiation dose, and the capacity of chondrocyte cells to receive these signals [12].

The goal of this study was to better understand the intercellular communication between the irradiated chondrosarcoma cells and the bystander chondrocytes using proteomics [5]. These approaches allowed us to propose new bystander candidates and cellular responses potentially involved in these non-targeted effects. Some of these results were presented at the 45th Annual Meeting of the European Radiation Research Society in Lund, Sweden [13].

2. Results

2.1. Secretome Analysis of the Conditioned Medium of Low Doses Irradiated Chondrosarcoma Cells

The dataset acquired on the 12 samples comprises 1,338,540 high-resolution MS/MS spectra. First, as we expected, the presence of contaminants due to fetal calf serum, an interpretation of the MS/MS spectra dataset against the "Bostaurus" theoretical annotated genome was performed, prior to interrogating the "Homo sapiens" theoretical coding sequences.

A total of 357,084 MS/MS spectra were interpreted in this first search round. We identified a large number of bovine serum proteins: 889 were validated with at least two peptides of different sequences. The most abundant proteins were: serum albumin with a 21,209 spectral count (i.e., 6% of the total), but this ratio is by far lower than for a serum analysis which shows that the washes were effective but far to be sufficiently exhaustive to remove all traces of bovine proteins. It is interesting to note the BSA rate for each sample: around 2% for the six samples (3 samples 0 Gy and 3 samples 0.1 Gy) with x10 PBS washes to 10–12% for the other samples with x5 PBS washes, showing the necessity to extensively wash the cells prior to incubation and extraction of the secreted proteins.

In a second search round, we analyzed the yet unassigned MS/MS spectra against the SwissProt human database. In this case, a total of 547,589 MS/MS spectra were unambiguously assigned to peptide sequences. With this dataset, we validated 1522 additional proteins identified with at least two distinct peptides. So, we observed a greater number of proteins compared to the "Bostaurus" request. This double round interpretation confirmed that we had more than just serum proteins in these samples, and certified the presence of the human proteins.

A comparison was then carried out in order to identify the overabundant proteins in the irradiated comparison (0.1 Gy) versus control condition (three biological replicates x two analytical replicates) following the "PatternLab for proteomics" procedure. Considering the condition with 10X PBS washes, a total of 87 groups of proteins were found significantly modulated (p-value ≤ 0.05 and fold change $\geq 1.5\times$), with a total of 55 more abundant and 32 less abundant proteins. From these protein groups, several accessions associated with bovine origin were removed and, finally, 40 were associated with a known human accession. The abundance of 24 proteins were increased while 16 were decreased in the conditioned medium of irradiated cells (Table 1).

We focused on proteins specifically which significantly increased in the conditioned medium of low-dose irradiated cells. Polyadenylate-binding protein 1 (P11940) was over-secreted 23.8 times in the conditioned medium of SW1353 cells irradiated with 0.1 Gy X-rays when compared with the conditioned medium of non-irradiated SW1353 cells. It is interesting to note that several ribosomal proteins increased in the conditioned medium of low-dose irradiated cells (60S ribosomal protein L34; 60S ribosomal protein L7a; 60S ribosomal protein L8; 40S ribosomal protein S2; 40S ribosomal protein S6; Ubiquitin-40S ribosomal protein S27a).

Several other proteins were identified, in relation with the oxidative response and red/ox status (Acetyl-CoA acetyltransferase; Transmembrane protein 189), cadherin binding (Septin-7), cell migration (Profilin-2) or the response to DNA damage stimulus (E3 ubiquitin-protein ligase RBBP6). Several of these proteins were reported to be involved in extracellular exosomes (glyoxalase domain-containing protein 4; protein HSPD1; S-methyl-5′-thioadenosine phosphorylase; Endoplasmic reticulum aminopeptidase 1).

Table 1. List of 40 modulated proteins (24 up-regulated and 16 down-regulated) in the conditioned medium of low-dose irradiated chondrosarcoma cells, as compared with non-irradiated chondrosarcoma cells.

Accession	Name	pI	Mass (Da)	Tfold *	p-Value
P11940	Polyadenylate-binding protein 1	9.85	106.299	23.83	0.0264
P24752	Acetyl-CoAacetyltransferase, mitochondrial	8.39	58.871	4.00	0.0051
A5PLL7	Transmembraneprotein 189	9.07	107.703	3.33	0.0278
P08243	Asparagine synthetase [glutamine-hydrolyzing]	6.86	67.256	3.17	0.0155
P35080	Profilin-2	8.87	77.777	2.86	0.0423
P49207	60S ribosomal protein L34	10.64	21.824	2.50	0.0011
Q9HC38	Glyoxalase domain-containing protein 4	7.94	68.961	2.11	0.0191
P62424	60S ribosomal protein L7a	10.54	33.547	2.00	0.0150
P62753	40S ribosomal protein S6	10.74	31.799	2.00	0.0064
Q16181	Septin-7	8.97	244.012	2.00	0.0076
P27361	Mitogen-activated protein kinase 3	9.14	69.163	2.00	0.0250
O60763	General vesicular transport factor p115	5.88	159.184	1.91	0.0191
P62979	Ubiquitin-40S ribosomal protein S27a	9.64	19.523	1.84	0.0356
Q53SE2	Uncharacterized protein HSPD1	8.32	70.924	1.83	0.0186
P62917	60S ribosomal protein L8	11.15	32.789	1.79	0.0017
Q9NQR4	Omega-amidase NIT2	6.73	47.093	1.75	0.0335
P15880	40S ribosomal protein S2	10.37	34.399	1.67	0.0156
O75367	Core histone macro-H2A.1	9.75	68.531	1.67	0.0379
Q13126	S-methyl-5′-thioadenosine phosphorylase	9.17	186.699	1.64	0.0031
Q96D15	Reticulocalbin-3	5.05	46.220	1.64	0.0047
Q7Z6E9	E3 ubiquitin-protein ligase RBBP6	9.65	98.855	1.58	0.0385
O00370	LINE-1 retrotransposable element ORF2 protein	9.51	5.633.488	1.57	0.0179
Q9NZ08	Endoplasmic reticulum aminopeptidase 1	9.00	202.092	1.50	0.0219
P22087	rRNA 2′-O-methyltransferase fibrillarin	10.19	41.124	1.50	0.0219
O15145	Actin-related protein 2/3 complex subunit 3	9.60	28.754	−1.67	0.0379
Q13257	Mitotic spindle assembly checkpoint protein MAD2A	6.30	55.269	−1.67	0.0250
O15498	Synaptobrevin homolog YKT6	8.79	96.462	−1.90	0.0171
Q9UJS0	Calcium-binding mitochondrial carrier protein Aralar2	9.33	119.145	−2.00	0.0011
Q00325	Phosphate carrier protein, mitochondrial	9.34	63.151	−2.00	0.0409
Q8WXF1	Paraspeckle component 1	8.96	74.454	−2.08	0.0003
P10155	60 kDa SS-A/Ro ribonucleoprotein	9.63	350.653	−2.10	0.0160
Q5JXB2	Putative ubiquitin-conjugating enzyme E2 N-like	9.15	95.474	−2.11	0.0030
P53004	Biliverdin reductase A	6.47	41.158	−2.18	0.0405
Q9Y230	RuvB-like 2	5.40	54.097	−2.24	0.0169
O75153	Clustered mitochondria protein homolog	6.34	190.902	−2.29	0.0427
Q9HD20	Manganese-transporting ATPase 13A1	9.48	70.012	−2.50	0.0029
P18754	Regulator of chromosome condensation	5.79	42.947	−2.67	0.0108
Q09328	Alpha-1,6-mannosylglycoprotein 6-beta-N-acetylglucosaminyl transferase A	9.09	255.616	−2.75	0.0003
Q14195	Dihydropyrimidinase-related protein 3	8.69	171.819	−2.85	0.0245
P13645	Keratin, type I cytoskeletal 10	6.00	75.115	−2.87	0.0138

* Tfold is positive for accessions up regulated in the conditioned medium of irradiated cells, and negative for accessions down regulated in the conditioned medium of irradiated cells.

Forty proteins were statistically modulated in the conditioned medium of chondrosarcoma cells irradiated at a low dose (0.1 Gy), when compared with non-irradiated cells; twenty-four proteins were statistically highly expressed. Some of them were involved in key metabolic pathways and were suspected to participate in radiation-induced bystander signaling. These accessions were analyzed according to potential interaction networks with a STRING functional enrichment analysis (Figure 1). A clear and dense cluster can be observed in the middle of the string network, and the accessions all rely on the ribonucleosome compartment (GO:1990904) and the cytoplasmic stress granules (GO:0010494).

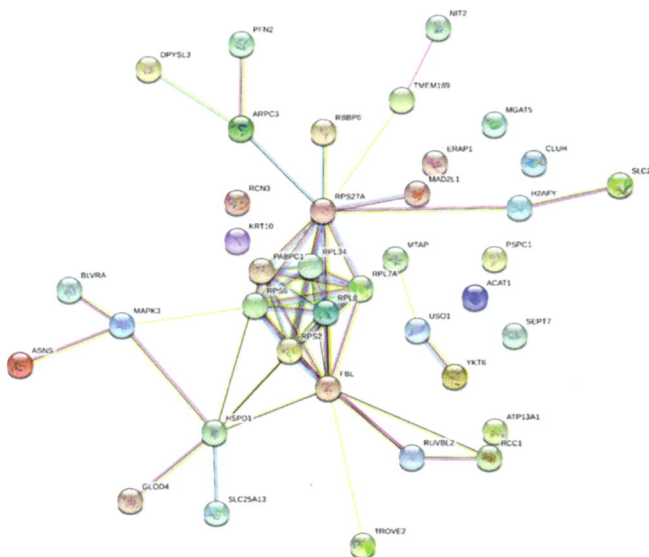

Figure 1. Bystander secretome network. Protein–protein interaction network constructed with protein accession from the list of 40 modulated proteins (24 up-regulated and 16 down-regulated) in the medium-conditioned/secretomic analysis. The network was constructed on STRING database.

2.2. Quantification of 8-oxoG in the Conditioned Medium of Low Doses Irradiated Chondrosarcoma Cells

To further study the potential impact of oxidative stress on irradiated cells and their corresponding conditioned medium, a quantification of 8-OXO dG was performed in the conditioned media of SW1353 cells irradiated at different doses (Figure 2). A significant increase in 8-OXO dG concentration was observed in the conditioned media of samples irradiated with 0.1 Gy when compared with non-irradiated samples. The tendency of these 8-OXO dG concentration showed a maximum with 0.1 Gy (about 1.4 ng/mL) and then a decrease with doses of 0.2 and 0.5 Gy to reach the basal level observed with non-irradiated samples (about 0.8 ng/mL).

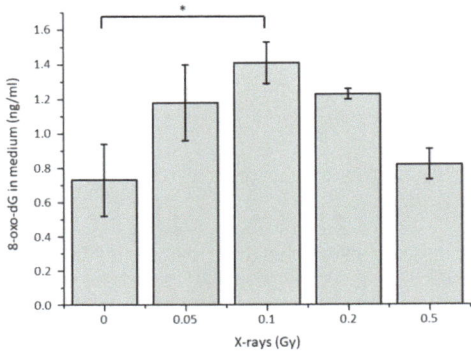

Figure 2. Quantification of 8-oxo-dG in the conditioned medium of chondrosarcoma cells irradiated with different doses of X-rays. (* = $p < 0.05$).

2.3. Whole-Cell Proteome Variations of Chondrocytes in Responses to the Conditioned Medium of Low Doses Irradiated Chondrosarcoma Cells

Quantitative changes in proteins were analyzed by comparing the proteomic map of bystander chondrocytes receiving the conditioned medium of low-dose irradiated chondrosarcoma cells or non-irradiated chondrosarcoma cells (control). A total of 1085 proteins were detected on silver-stained 2D-PAGE gels performed with 250 µg proteins per gel. To analyze the bystander-responsive proteins, significant differences in spot volume (from 25% variation) between control and "treated" samples were assessed and protein spots displaying significant up- or down-expression were regarded as candidates and submitted to MS analysis for identification after trypsin proteolysis.

On the whole, 18 spots, representing 1.6% of all spots on the experiment (Figure 3), showed significant variations ($p < 0.05$); green spots and red spots were over-expressed and under-expressed in the bystander condition, respectively (i.e., cells receiving medium from 0.1 Gy irradiated chondrosarcoma cells). Following a mass spectrometry analysis, 9 proteins were identified as increased (green) and 11 proteins were identified as decreased (red) in the treated sample compared to the control condition (Table 2). Proteins involved in cell-junction and adhesion (Actin, Desmoplakin) as well as cell migration (Microtube-associated protein RP, Tropomyosin alpha-1 chain, CAP-G protein) were identified and differentially modulated. In addition, several proteins participating in protein secretion and an interleukin signaling pathway (cyclophilin A, PSME1, 60S acidic ribosomal protein P0, Hspa9, 26S proteasome regulatory subunit 7) were observed too. It was also interesting to notice the implication of thioredoxin (involved in cell redox homeostasis; 27% increased) and several proteins related to exosome formation (Keratin type II and eukaryotic translation initiation factor 3 subunit I).

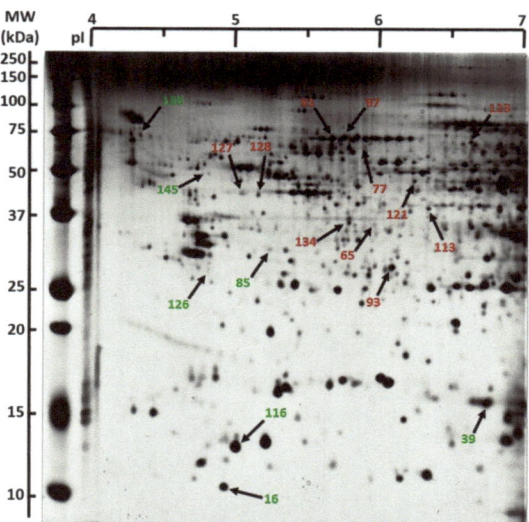

Figure 3. Proteome changes following bystander effect. Whole cell extracts from T/C-28A2 bystander cells receiving the conditioned medium of (1) low-dose irradiated chondrosarcoma cells or (2) non-irradiated chondrosarcoma cells were analyzed and compared by 2DE. One representative gel of (1) is shown. A total of 250 micrograms proteins were separated using 18-cm pH 4-7 pI range strips for the first dimension, and 12% acrylamide gels for the second dimension. Differentially expressed spots were delineated either in green (induced in (1) cells) or in red (repressed in (1) cells).

Table 2. List of 20 modulated proteins in the proteome of bystander cells receiving the conditioned medium of low-dose irradiated chondrosarcoma cells, as compared with bystander cells receiving the conditioned medium non-irradiated chondrosarcoma cells.

Spot Number	Fold	pI *	MW *	Accession	Names	HighestMean	GO—Biological Process
16	1.31	4.79	20	P60709	Actin	Bystander 0.1 Gy	Cell junction assembly
39	1.62	6.69	26	P62937	Cyclophilin A	Bystander 0.1 Gy	positive regulation of protein secretion; interleukin-12-mediated signaling pathway
85	1.38	5.11	63	Q15691	Microtubule-associated protein RP	Bystander 0.1 Gy	cell migration
93	1.31	5.99	57	Q06323	PSME1	Bystander 0.1 Gy	interleukin-1-mediated signaling pathway; tumor necrosis factor-mediated signaling pathway
116	1.27	4.87	23	P15924	Desmoplakin	Bystander 0.1 Gy	adherent junction organization; cell-cell adhesion
116				P10599	Thioredoxin		cell redox homeostasis;
126	1.63	4.67	56	P09493	Tropomyosin alpha-1 chain	Bystander 0.1 Gy	negative regulation of cell migration
138	1.98	4.18	145	P04264	Keratin, type II	Bystander 0.1 Gy	Extracellular exosome
145	1.47	4.67	98	Q9BTY7	Protein HGH1 homolog	Bystander 0.1 Gy	unknown (interact with Peptidyl-prolyl cis-trans isomerase and Heat shock protein 90)
65	1.81	5.86	72	P06733	Alpha-enolase	Bystander 0 Gy	negative regulation of cell growth
65				P05388	60S acidic ribosomal protein P0		interleukin-12-mediated signaling pathway
77	1.56	5.79	130	P01876	IGHA1 protein	Bystander 0 Gy	Extracellular exosome
91	1.29	5.63	140	P11142	HSC 70 protein	Bystander 0 Gy	cytokine-mediated signaling pathway
97	1.32	5.64	141	P38646	Hspa9	Bystander 0 Gy	interleukin-12-mediated signaling pathway
113	1.27	6.25	79	P40121	CAP-G protein	Bystander 0 Gy	Protein motility
121	1.47	6.15	94	P35998	26S proteasome regulatory subunit 7	Bystander 0 Gy	interleukin-1-mediated signaling pathway
123	1.31	6.56	136	P49368	T-complex protein 1 subunit gamma	Bystander 0 Gy	Extracellular exosome
127	1.31	4.91	87	P60709	Actin	Bystander 0 Gy	Cell junction assembly
128	1.36	5.03	87	Q16186	Proteasomal ubiquitin receptor ADRM1	Bystander 0 Gy	Proteasome complex
134	1.26	5.68	73	Q13347	Eukaryotic translation initiation factor 3 subunit I	Bystander 0 Gy	Extracellular exosome

*: pI (iso-electric point) and MW (kDa) according to the 2D gel location. There were 9 up-regulated (highest mean with Bystander 0.1 Gy) and 11 down-regulated (highest mean with Bystander 0 Gy).

Using this list of altered proteins (Table 2), we analyzed the corresponding accessions according to potential interaction networks with a STRING functional enrichment analysis (Figure 4), as previously performed in the case of the secretomic analysis. Again, a dense cluster with several accessions linked together many times (PPIA, TXN, HSPA9, ENO1, HSPA8, RPLP0, CCT3) could be observed. According to this analysis, several accessions associated with interleukin signaling pathways and extracellular exosomes were observed (Table 2).

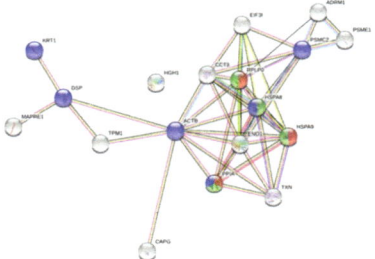

Figure 4. Bystander whole-cell proteome network. Protein–protein interaction network constructed with protein accession from the list of 20 modulated proteins (9 up-regulated and 11 down-regulated) in the bystander proteomic analysis. The network was constructed on STRING database.

2.4. Quantification and Validation of Proteomic Biomarkers

To validate the results of the 2D-gel analysis, the abundances of several proteins were assayed with specific antibodies using protein extracts from samples already used in 2D-GELs selected on the basis of biological functions and fold changes. An equivalent amount of proteins from each sample were loaded, and loading controls (alpha-tubulin and GAPDH) were used in addition. As shown in Figure 5, the expression levels for cyclophilin A, thioredoxin, alpha-enolase, RPLP0, HSC70, HSPA9, and CCT3 were analyzed and quantified by western blotting. The seven proteins displayed a coherent modulation when compared with the 2D-gel proteomic analysis. As an example, in the case of cyclophilin A, a fold change of +1.62 (+62%) was observed by 2D-gel analysis, and an increase of +37% was observed by western blotting when comparing the bystander chondrocytes receiving the conditioned medium of chondrosarcoma cells irradiated at 0.1 Gy with the non-irradiated chondrosarcoma cells (Supplementary Materials). Two proteins (cyclophilin A and thioredoxin) were observed as increased in the condition "0.1 Gy" by western blotting analysis; and five proteins (alpha-enolase, RPLP0, HSC70, HSPA9 and CCT3) were observed as decreased in the condition "0.1 Gy" by western blotting analysis. These proteins appear as good biomarker candidates involved in the cellular response in bystander cells.

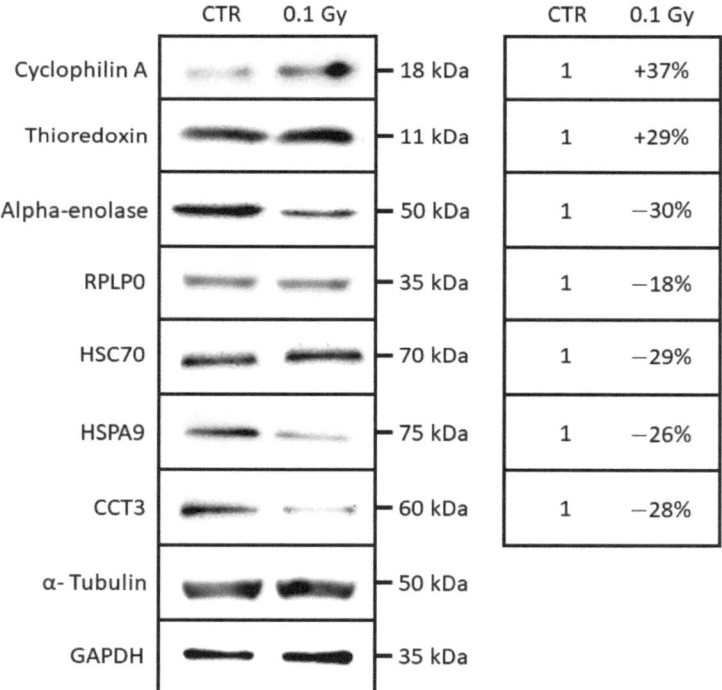

Figure 5. Western blotting analysis of cyclophilin A, thioredoxin, alpha-enolase, RPLP0, HSC70, HSPA9, and CCT3 in a whole-cell extracts from T/C-28A2 bystander cells receiving the conditioned medium of low-dose irradiated chondrosarcoma cells (0.1 Gy) or non-irradiated chondrosarcoma cells (CTR).

2.5. Chondrocyte Motility in Extracellular Matrix Affected by Exogenous Stresses

When taken at 24 h, no difference can be observed on chondrocytes between the conditioned medium of control and 0.1 Gy irradiated chondrosarcoma (Figure 6). On the contrary, when taken at 6 h, a significant difference was observed between the conditioned medium of control and 0.1 Gy irradiated chondrosarcoma. Indeed, chondrocyte motility significantly increased from the time points 5 h to 13 h using the conditioned medium of chondrosarcoma irradiated with 0.1 Gy.

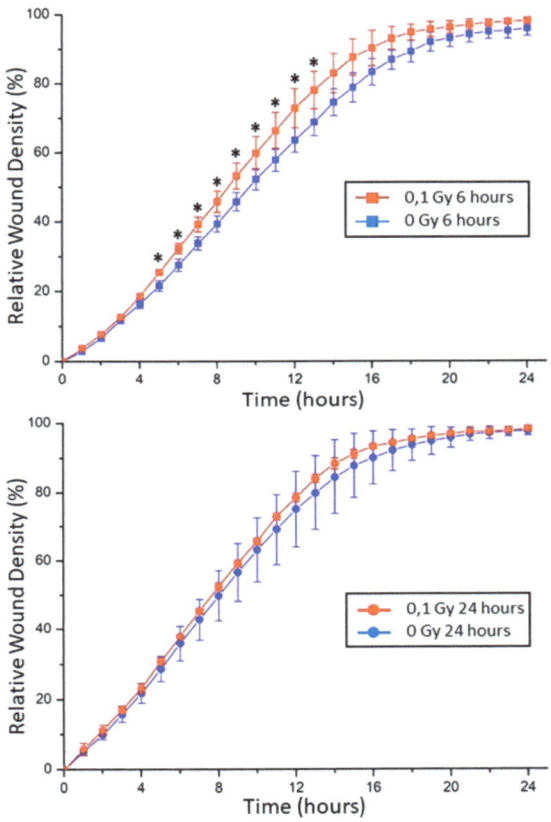

Figure 6. The conditioned medium of low-dose irradiated chondrosarcoma cells transiently increased the motility of T/C-28A2 bystander cells. Wound-healing assay showed the ability of cell migration in each group at 6 h (**top**) and 24 h (**bottom**) of contact with the conditioned media. ($* = p < 0.05$).

3. Discussion

The aim of the present proteomic work was to highlight: (i) potential new effectors in the radiation-induced bystander effect, using a comparative secretomic analysis of conditioned media, and (ii) the corresponding cellular response in bystander cells, using a comparative gel-based proteomic analysis of bystander cells. This double strategy is pertinent for applications required without a priori analysis of different cellular compartments, within the same cellular system [5].

A highly enriched compartment, in relation with stress granules (SGs), was observed following our secretomic analysis. Stress granules are described to be non-membrane bound cytoplasmic entities, and are formed following a cellular stress to minimize damages and promote cell survival. Many membrane-less organelles exist within the cell cytosol such as SGs and P-bodies. These organelle forms are commonly referred to as bio molecular condensates [14]. The formation of SGs has been suggested to regulate gene expression during stress. These assemblies sequester specific proteins and RNAs during stress, thereby providing a layer of post-transcriptional gene adaptation with the potential to affect directly mRNA levels, protein translation, and cell survival [15]. In addition to mRNA, SGs mainly contain 40S ribosomal subunits, translation initiation factors such as eIF4G, and RNA-binding proteins (RBPs) [16]. Different cellular stresses can promote SGs formation, such as endogenous stress (hypoxia, low nutrients) and environmental stressors (genotoxic drugs, heat shock, oxidants, or radiations) [17,18]. Exposure of cells to low doses of UVC induces the formation of SGs [19]; according to this study, cells were blocked in G1 phase of the cell cycle in order to repair DNA damages induced by UVC irradiation, simultaneously to the accumulation of the SGs in the cytoplasm. Such significant enrichment of stress granule proteins in the conditioned medium of chondrosarcoma cells irradiated with 0.1 Gy of X-rays is completely unexpected for several reasons: (i) SGs were never described to participate to any intercellular communication, nor bystander effects, (ii) SGs were not described to be secreted by cells, specifically (as cell cytokines) or non-specifically (in cell cargo, such as exosomes, or after cell death), (iii) SGs were not described to display any biological activity with the capacity to transmit a cellular stress to other cells, until now, these biomolecular condensates were supposed to act as a protective structure of protein translation machinery [14]. For all these reasons, it is mandatory to take this result carefully, and not to give definitive conclusions before any additional experiments performed with other cell lines.

In addition to SGs-related proteins, several other protein groups were observed with a significant enrichment in the conditioned medium of chondrosarcoma cells irradiated with 0.1 Gy. Several proteins already observed in exosomes were identified (glyoxalase domain-containing protein 4, uncharacterized protein HSPD1, omega-amidase NIT2, S-methyl-5'-thioadenosine phosphorylase, and rRNA 2'-O-methyltransferase fibrillarin). Such proteins, without any direct biological links between them, could be involved in exosome traffic, thus reinforcing the potential role of exosomes in radiation-induced bystander effects. The lack of knowledge regarding several proteins such as HSPD1 highlights the difficulty to understand and characterize such a complex multi-parameter effect and calls for new experiments aimed at deciphering their functions.

In addition to these unknown potential bystander effectors, several well-known cellular pathways were also observed. Proteins related to oxidative stress were also observed in the conditioned medium of chondrosarcoma cells irradiated with 0.1 Gy. The mitochondrial acetyl-CoA acetyltransferase was observed amongst the most increased protein abundances (in position two in our list), with a four times fold increase as compared with the conditioned medium of non-irradiated chondrosarcoma cells (Table 1). This enzyme is involved in the acetyl-CoA biosynthetic process (GO:0006085) and exerts a central function in the last step of the mitochondrial beta-oxidation pathway, an aerobic process breaking down fatty acids into acetyl-CoA [20]. Its activity is reversible and it can also catalyze the condensation of two acetyl-CoA molecules into aceto-acetyl-CoA [21].

Moreover, the transmembrane protein 189 increased by 3.33 times as compared with the conditioned medium of non-irradiated chondrosarcoma cells. This accession, also named "Plasmanylethanolamine desaturase", is involved in plasmalogen biogenesis in the endoplasmic reticulum, and is involved in antioxidative (GO:0055114) and signaling mechanisms [22]. An increase in the Profilin 2 protein level with a 2.88 factor was observed. This protein involved in the structure of the cytoskeleton could act as a negative regulator of epithelial cell migration (GO:0010633), as described previously [23]. The reticulocalbin-3 protein (increased 1.64 times) can induce similar effects on cell motility [24]; this protein chaperone exerts an anti-fibrotic activity by negatively regulating the secretion of type I and type III collagens (GO:0032964).

The E3 ubiquitin-protein ligase RBBP6, a protein related to DNA damages, was also observed in the conditioned medium of chondrosarcoma cells irradiated with 0.1 Gy (GO:0006974). This protein, known as being possibly involved in assembly of the p53/TP53-MDM2 complex, results in an increase in MDM2-mediated ubiquitination and degradation of p53/TP53 [25,26], perhaps leading to both apoptosis and cell growth (by similarity) playing a role in the transmission of the radiation-induced bystander effect.

We already observed a bystander cellular response in chondrocyte receiving the conditioned medium of chondrosarcoma cells irradiated with 0.1 Gy of X-rays [12], with a reduction in cell survival and an induction of micronuclei. In order to gain insights into the cell mechanisms and the pathways involved in this bystander response, we analyzed the proteome of the cells using a gel-based proteomic strategy.

While shotgun proteomics may give access to a large list of proteins, 2D-gel-based proteomics allows for the identification of matured proteins, such as the proteolytic cleavage of polypeptide chains or post-translational modifications. Thus, this approach is valuable to assess stress-induced modifications, as already demonstrated by several authors [10,11].

Our findings include the accession identified as cyclophilin A (PPIA = P62937), which is described to be positively regulated with protein secretion and involved in the interleukin 12 (IL-12) signaling pathway. We previously observed this accession as increased in the conditioned medium from irradiated breast cancer cells [27]. IL-12 was defined as a cytokine post-translationally regulated and potentially implicated in the radio-induced apoptotic response in mammary tumor cells. IL-12, observed as increased in bystander cells, could be involved in the propagation of the bystander effect throughout non-irradiated cells.

The accession identified as thioredoxin (TXN = P10599), which is described to be involved in the cell redox homeostasis, was found to have increased in bystander cells according to both the proteomic results and the western blot validation. This factor is believed to contribute to the regulation of transcription factors mediating cellular responses to environmental stress, including radiation [28]. In addition, we observed an increase in 8-oxo-dG in the conditioned medium of low-dose irradiated cells, a nucleotide released by the cells when it is oxidized, which is proof of the presence of oxidative stress. These two mechanisms could be linked in a global oxidative stress response, transmitted to bystander cells, and involved in the cellular response to the bystander effect.

Moreover, besides the identified oxidative stress response, a potential change of cellular motility and migration was observed using a wound healing test on non-irradiated cells receiving the conditioned media of irradiated cells. The bystander cells displayed an increased motility (Figure 5), which could be linked with a decrease in alpha-enolase expression. The nuclear form of the protein was previously identified as Myc-binding protein-1 (MBP1); this form plays a role in the negative regulation of cell growth [29]. Consequently, a decrease in MBP1 could induce an increase in cell motility and migration, at least transitively, as observed in this study after 6 h.

Finally, although SGs were significantly observed as enriched according to our secretomic analysis, no SG-related proteins were observed as modulated in the proteome of bystander cells. One explanation could be that both strategies do not analyze the same cell compartment, i.e., the conditioned medium with the secretomic analysis and the cellular proteome with the proteomic analysis. A second explanation is linked with the biochemical capacities of both strategies: with the secretomic analysis, a gel-free mass spectrometry analysis is performed, allowing for low-abundance and hydrophobic proteins/peptides; on the other hand, with the proteomic analysis, only abundant and soluble proteins can be observed. If SGs are involved in the bystander effects, they can be secreted in the conditioned medium, as observed with our secretomic analysis, but maybe a low amount is able to induce a bystander effect on the non-irradiated cells, which cannot be visualized with our proteomic study.

4. Conclusions

Overall, the proteomic analysis underlines the modulation of the abundance of several bystander-related proteins; modulation that was confirmed by western blot and their physiological effects revealed by functional techniques in some instances. The stress granules related to oxidative stress-coping mechanisms were identified for the first time as potential attractive biomarkers of RIBE in the conditioned medium of irradiated cells. The next step of this analysis would be a deep analysis of the role of stress granules in bystander effect transmission, using, for example, cellular models with defects in the stress granules formation processes. In addition, several proteins involved in intercellular signaling, oxidative stress response, and cell motility were also determined in bystander cells in response to such conditioned medium. The results obtained strengthen our previous results concerning the factors involved in the radiation-induced bystander effect at low doses of irradiation, including interleukin.

Taken together, the findings of this study pinpointed the complexity of the mechanisms involved in the radiation-induced bystander effect and the power of a proteomic analysis to bring into light new biomarker candidates of this phenomenon [5].

5. Methods
5.1. Cell Culture

Two cell lines were used during this study, a chondrosarcoma cell line, SW1353 (CLS Cell Lines Service GmbH, Eppelheim, Germany) and a chondrocyte cell line, T/C28-A2 (gift from Prof. Mary B. Goldring, Hospital for Special Surgery, Weill Medical College of Cornell University, New York, NY, USA), as previously described [12]. These cells were cultured in the same culture medium, minimum essential medium Eagle (MEM, M5650, Sigma-Aldrich, Saint-Louis, MI, USA), supplemented with 5% fetal calf serum, 2 mM L-glutamine, and 1% antibiotics (penicillin–streptomycin solution, Sigma-Aldrich). All experiments were performed in humidified atmosphere with 5% CO_2 and physioxia conditions with 2% O_2 at 37 °C, in a Heracell™ 150i Tri-Gas incubator.

The bystander factors, secreted by chondrosarcoma cells, were first evaluated by direct mass spectrometry analysis. The intracellular bystander response in chondrocytes was analyzed using a gel-based strategy.

5.2. Experimental Strategy to Characterize the Bystander Effect induced by Low Doses Irradiated Chondrosarcoma Cells

In order to study the bystander effect between irradiated chondrosarcoma cells (SW1353 cell line) and non-irradiated chondrocytes (T/C28-A2 cell line), we selected a medium-transfer protocol, and we kept the same treatment strategy with all our endpoints (Figure 7). This simplified process allowed us to compare the cell responses of non-irradiated cells, receiving the conditioned medium from irradiated cells.

X-rays irradiations were performed, as previously described [12,30], at room temperature (20 °C) with a tube tension of 225 kV, a copper filter, and an intensity of 1 mA corresponding to a dose rate of 0.2 Gy/min on the Pxi XradSmart 225cX irradiator, dedicated to preclinical research. The dose rate was measured inside flasks with thermoluminescent dosimeters in the irradiation conditions. Thermoluminescent dosimeters were preliminary calibrated on a 15-cm-thick virtual water phantom thanks to reference dose measurements performed with a calibrated ionization chamber following the "American Association of Physicists in Medicine protocol," developed by the Radiation Therapy Committee Task Group 61, for reference dosimetry of low- and medium-energy X-rays for radiotherapy and radiobiology. The dose rate was finally corrected from the used tube current.

Immediately after irradiation with 0.1 Gy of X-rays, chondrosarcoma cells were cultured with fresh medium. After the incubation period, the conditioned medium was removed from the cells and centrifuged to discard detached cells and cell's debris.

Then, this conditioned medium was directly analyzed (using three independent biological replicates), or used on non-irradiated chondrocytes to study a potential bystander effect (Figure 7).

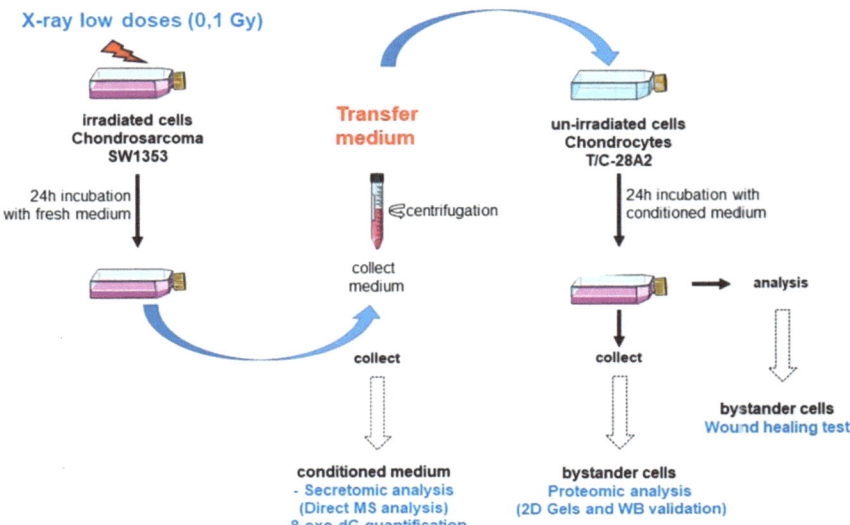

Figure 7. Schematic representation of experiments followed for the medium transfer protocols. Chondrosarcoma cells (SW1353 cell line) were irradiated at confluence in T25 flasks with X-rays or sham irradiated. Immediately after irradiation, the medium was changed with fresh new medium and incubated for 24 h. Then, the conditioned medium was centrifuged and collected. This conditioned medium (three independent biological replicates) was then analyzed for proteomic composition (secretomic analysis by direct MS analysis) or 8-oxo-dG quantification; or transferred to non-irradiated chondrocytes (T/C-28A2 cell line) for 24 h in T25 flasks with the same cell density. Then, cells were collected for proteomic composition (2D gel comparison and WB validation) or woundhealing test.

5.3. Preparation of Conditioned Medium and Shotgun Proteomics Analysis

In the case of the secretome analysis, just before irradiation with X-rays, the complete medium was removed from the flasks and the cell monolayer was extensively washed with PBS. This step was mandatory to reduce the presence in the conditioned medium of bovine serum albumin that could prevent the identification of other proteins. Then, chondrosarcoma cells were irradiated at a low dose (0.1 Gy X-ray) with a serum-free medium. After irradiation, the medium was changed with fresh/serum-free medium and two wash procedures were performed for each irradiation condition and with three independent biological replicates (12 samples). After 24 h, the conditioned medium was removed from the flasks and analyzed by tandem mass spectrometry with technical replicates, thus 24 nanoLC-MS/MS analytical runs.

SW1353 cells were irradiated at confluence and, immediately after irradiation, the monolayer was washed with PBS several times (5× and 10×), and then 3 mL of serum-free medium was added. After 24 h, the conditioned medium was removed from the flasks, centrifuged (2000× g), and stored at −80 °C. These experiments were performed in triplicates. Proteins from the 12 samples (2 irradiations, 0 and 0.1 Gy, 2 washing conditions, i.e., X5 and X10 times with PBS, 3 biological replicates) were first precipitated with TCA. For this, 250 µL of trichloroacetic acid at 50% (w/v) were added to 1 mL of conditioned medium. Precipitated proteins were collected by centrifugation for 15 min at 16,000 g and then dissolved into 30 µL of LDS1X (Invitrogen). The samples were heated at 99 °C for 5 min, briefly centrifuged, and then loaded onto a 4–12% gradient 10-well NuPAGE (Invitrogen) polyacrylamide gel. After a short electrophoresis (5 min), the gel was stained with Coomassie blue safe staining (Invitrogen, Waltham, MA, USA) for 5 min. The polyacrylamide bands corresponding to the whole exoproteomes were sliced and treated with dithiothreitol and iodoacetamide, as recommended [31]. Then, the proteins were subjected to trypsin proteolysis to generate peptides. Each peptide fraction was analyzed twice by nanoLC-MS/MS (analytical duplicates) in data-dependent mode with a Q-Exactive HF (Thermo) mass spectrometer coupled with an Ultimate 3000 chromatography system (Thermo), resulting in 24 runs of high-resolution tandem mass spectrometry. For each peptide fraction, a volume of 10 μL (out of 50 μL) was injected on a nanoscale 500-mm C18 PepMap TM 100 (5 mm × 300 μm I.D., Thermo) column operated, as previously described [32], except that the gradient of acetonitrile (from 4% to 40% of a solution of 80% CH3CN, 20% H20, 0.1% formic acid) was extended to 120 min for deepening the analysis. MS spectra of peptide ions were acquired at a resolution of 60,000. Only peptide ions with 2+ or 3+ charge were selected for fragmentation according to a Top20 method and using a dynamic exclusion of 10 sec. MS/MS spectra of fragment ions were acquired at a resolution of 15,000.

MS/MS spectra were interpreted using the MASCOT search engine, version 2.5.1 (Matrix Science, Boston, MA, USA), with fixed carbamidomethyl modification of cysteines, variable oxidation of methionines, and deamidation of asparagines and glutamines, a maximum of two missed cleavages, mass tolerance of 5 ppm and 0.02 Da on parent ions and secondary ions, respectively. Peptides with a score above the query identity threshold (p value below 0.05) were selected and parsed with the Irma software [33]. Only proteins with at least two different peptides were validated. The decoy search option of Mascot was systematically activated to estimate the FDR (<1%). Abundances of the proteins were evaluated based on their spectral counts.

5.4. Determination of Extracellular 8-oxo-dG in the Conditioned Media

The media were thawed and 1 mL of each sample was used for the determination of 8-oxo-dG using an ELISA-based method (Health Biomarkers, Stockholm, Sweden, AB). Briefly, one ml of cell culture medium was loaded on a solid-phase-extraction column, followed by a washing step and elution of 8-oxo-dG according to protocols provided by the company Health Biomarker Sweden AB, as previously described [34]. The eluates were concentrated by freeze-drying and dissolved in PBS, pH 7.4, to a volume of 1 mL and the clean-up process was repeated once more to purify 8-oxo-dG. Then, the samples were dissolved in PBS, pH 7.4, to a volume of 1 mL. Based on protocol from kit-provider, 90 μL aliquots of samples were mixed with 50 μL of the primary antibody and transferred to 96-well ELISA plates coated with 8-oxo-dG. After overnight incubation at 4 °C, the plates were washed 3 times by washing solution. Next, 140 μL of HRP-conjugated secondary antibody (goat anti-mouse IgG-HRP, Scandinavian Diagnostic Services, Uppsala, Sweden) was added to each well and incubated for 2 h at room temperature. The wells were washed 3 times with the washing solution. Then, 140 μL of tetramethylbenzidine liquid substrate (ICN BiomedicalsInc, Costa Mesa, CA, USA) was added to each well. The samples were incubated for 15 min at room temperature. The reaction was terminated by adding 70 μL of 2 M H_3PO_4 (Merck Millipore, Darmstadt, Germany). The absorbance was read at 450 nm using an automatic ELISA plate reader. All samples were analyzed in triplicate. Standard curves for 8-oxo-dG (from 0.05 up to 10 ng/mL) were established for each plate and the quantity of 8-oxo-dG calculated based on the standard curve and expressed as ng/mL medium.

5.5. Medium-Transfer Protocol from Irradiated Cells to Non-Irradiated Cells

Irradiated SW1353 cells and T/C-28a2 bystander cells were plated in T25 cm^2 flasks at confluence. As previously described [12], immediately after irradiation with X-rays, the medium of irradiated flasks was changed with fresh medium and, after 24 h in contact with irradiated SW1353 cells (to allow the bystander factors to be released), this medium was collected (Figure 7). The condition medium was then centrifuged (2000 g) and transferred in flasks of the same size (T25 cm^2) containing bystander T/C-28a2 cells at confluence. Bystander cells were kept in contact with the conditioned medium for 24 h and then harvested. The cell pellet was washed with PBS and the dry pellet was kept at 80 °C, until protein extraction.

5.6. Gel-Based Proteomic Study of Bystander Chondrocytes

5.6.1. Chemicals

TRIS base, urea, thiourea, CHAPS, iodoacetamide, TEMED, low-melt agarose, Triton X-100, spermine, phosphatase inhibitor cocktail, and bromophenol blue were obtained from Sigma-Aldrich (St. Louis, MO, USA). The protease inhibitor cocktail (Complete Mini EDTA-free) was from Roche Diagnostics (Mannheim, Germany); IPG buffers, IPG strips (pH 4-7) were purchased from VWR (acrylamide was obtained from Bio-Rad (Hercules, CA, USA); and SDS, glycerol, DTT, and TGS 10X were from Eudomedex (Mundolshein, France). All other reagents were of analytical grade.

5.6.2. Protein Extraction and Solubilisation

Proteins were extracted from TC-28/Ac cells (dry pellet) in a sample buffer containing 7 M urea, 2 M thiourea, 4% CHAPS, 0.05% Triton X100, 65 mM DTT, 40 mM spermine, protease, and phosphatase inhibitor cocktails. This suspension was centrifuged at 28,000 g for 60 min, supernatants were collected, and the protein content was estimated using the Bradford method [35]. Proteins were then precipitated using the 2D clean-up kit (GE Healthcare, Chicago, IL, USA) and the pellet was solubilized with TUC solution (7M urea, 2M thiourea, 4% CHAPS) and quantified with the 2D quant kit (GE Healthcare).

5.6.3. Strip Rehydration with Protein Samples: "Sample In-Gel Rehydration"

A protein sample (250 µg) was mixed with rehydration buffer (RB): 7M urea, 2M thiourea, 4% CHAPS, 0.05% triton X100, 0.5% ampholytes (IPG buffer 4–7 GE) and adjusted to the correct volume to rehydrate 18 cm strip (here, 320 µL). Strips were then placed acrylamide face down in the focusing tray equipped with platinum electrode embedded into the running tray (Protean IEF, Bio-Rad, Hercules, CA, USA) and passively re hydrated at 20°C without electricity for 16 h, and then actively rehydrated at 50 V during 9 h, as previously described [27,35,36]. During protein focalization, small electrode wicks were placed between acrylamide and electrode. These paper wicks (Ref 1654071, Electrode wicks, Bio-Rad, Hercules, CA, USA) were, in advance, soaked with water in order to absorb salts and other contaminant species during active rehydration. The IPG strips were then focused according to the following program: 500 V for 1 h, a linear ramp to 1000 V for 1 h, a linear ramp to 10000 V for 33 KV-1 h, and finally 10000 V for 24 KV-1 h.

5.6.4. IPG Strips Equilibration and Second Dimension

The strips were incubated in the first equilibration solution (50 mM Tris–HCl pH 8.8, 6 M urea, 30% (v/v) glycerol, 2% (w/v) SDS) with 130 mM DTT, and then in the second equilibration solution (50 mM Tris-HCl pH 8.8, 6 M urea, 30% (v/v) glycerol, 2% (w/v) SDS) with 130 mM iodoacetamide.

Strips were then embedded using 1% (w/v) low-melt agarose on the top of the acrylamide gel and trapped using plastic blockers, as described previously [35]. SDS-PAGE was carried out on a 12% acrylamide gel, using the Dodeca Cell electrophoresis unit (Bio-Rad, Hercules, CA, USA).

5.6.5. Gel Staining and Picture Acquisition

Gels were stained with silver nitrate, as previously described, with some modifications. Briefly, gels were first fixed at least 1 h with 30% ethanol and 5% acetic acid; washed 3 times 10 min with water; sensibilized 1 min with 0.02% sodium thiosulfate; washed 2 min with water; stained 30 min with 0.2% silver nitrate and 0.011% formaldehyde; washed 10 s with water; developed 5 min with 85 mM sodium carbonate, 0.00125% sodium thiosulfate and 0.011% formaldehyde; stopped with 0.33 M TRIS and 1.7% acetic acid; and stored with 5% acetic acid with 2% DMSO [37].

Gels were scanned to images right after staining to limit the polychromatic color of spots. Images were acquired with a GS 800 densitometer (Bio-Rad, Hercules, CA, USA).

5.6.6. Image Analysis

Images from stained gels were analyzed using the Samespots software v4.5 (Non-linear Dynamics, UK). Gels were grouped to create a global analysis with all conditions. Spots of each samples were compared between conditions, and spots were numbered with the same detection parameters, as previously described [35]. A multivariate statistical analysis was performed using the statistic mode of the Samespots software (Non-linear Dynamics, UK). Spots with significant differences (modulation of $+/-20\%$ and ANOVA t-test $p < 0.05$) were chosen. Spots of interest were selected for subsequent protein identification by mass spectrometry analysis and were picked up using the corresponding preparative silver stained gels.

5.6.7. Mass Spectrometry Analysis of 2D-Spots

Gel spots 2D were manually cut and prepared, as previously described [38]. The LC-MS/MS experiments were performed using a U3000 NCS nano-high-performance liquid chromatography (Thermo Fisher Scientific Inc, Waltham, MA, USA) system and a Q-Exactive Plus Orbitrap mass spectrometer. Next, 6 µL of peptides were loaded onto a pre-column (Thermo Scientific PepMap 100 C18, 5 µm particle size, 100 Å pore size, 300 µm i.d. × 5 mm length) from the Ultimate 3000 autosampler with 0.05% TFA for 3 min at a flow rate of 10 µL/min. Separation of peptides was performed by reverse-phase chromatography at a flow rate of 300 nL/min on a Thermo Scientific reverse-phase nano column (Thermo Scientific PepMap C18, 2 µm particle size, 100 Å pore size, 75 µm i.d. x 50 cm length). After the 3 min period, the column valve was switched to allow elution of peptides from the pre-column onto the analytical column. Solvent A was water + 0.1% FA and solvent B was 80% ACN, 20% water + 0.1% FA. The linear gradient employed was 4–40% of solvent B in 19 min, then 40–90% of solvent B from 19 to 20 min. The total run time was 35 min including a high organic wash step and re-equilibration step. The nanoHPLC and the spectrometer were coupled by nano-electrospray source. Peptides were transferred to the gaseous phase with positive ion electrospray ionization at 1.7 kV. Mass spectrometry data was processed using the Proteome Discoverer software (Version 1.4.0.288, Thermo Fisher Scientific, Bremen, Germany) and the search engine employed in local was Mascot (version.2.4, Matrix Science, Boston, MA, USA). The mass spectrometry data was searched against SwissProt with taxonomy Homo sapiens (20215) with the following parameters: trypsin as enzyme, 1 missed cleavage allowed, and carbamidomethylation of Cystein were used as fixed modifications, and N-terminal acetylation, deamidation of asparagine and glutamine, Nterminal-pyroglutamylation of glutamine and glutamate, oxidation of methionine were used as variable modifications. Mass tolerance was set to 10 ppm on full scans and 0.02 Da for fragment ions. Proteins were validated once they contained at least two peptides with a p-value < 0.05) and a false discovery rate <1%.

5.7. Western Blotting Analysis

Chondrosarcoma cells (SW1353) were irradiated with a 0.1 Gy dose using the XS-TRAHL XRC 160 machine of IFIN-HH, followed by a media transfer to the chondrocyte (T/C28a2) after 24 h, as previously described [12]. At 24 h, after the media transfer, the bystander cells (T/C-28a2) were washed with PBS. The cell pellet was resuspended with homemade RIPA lysis buffer supplemented with protease inhibitors (Roche) and incubated for 30 min on a cold rack, followed by a 15 min centrifugation at $12,000\times g$ at room temperature. Protein concentration was determined for all samples with a Bradford assay (Thermo Scientific). Laemmli buffer was added to the sample and denatured at 95 °C for 5 min, followed by a 1 min centrifugation at 16,000 xg. Samples were separated on SDS-poly-acrylamide (15%) gel electrophoresis (SDS-PAGE) using a TV100 electrophoresis unit, run at 110 V for about 1 h, followed by transfer on a PVDF membrane using a TV 100 Electroblotter, at 210 mA for 1 h and blocked with Tris-buffered saline with 0.05% Tween 20 (TBS-T) buffer with 5% milk on slow agitation for 1 h. Membranes were incubated overnight at 4 °C on agitation with the following antibodies: anti-HSPA9 (MA1-91639,

Thermo Scientific), anti-HSC70 (PA5-24624, Thermo Scientific), anti-CCT3 (PA5-78953, Thermo Scientific), anti-EN01 (MA5-17627, Thermo Scientific), anti-RPL20 (PA5-89335, Thermo Scientific), anti-cyclophilin A (39-1100, Thermo Scientific), anti-thioredoxin 1 (MA5-14941, Thermo Scientific), anti α-Tubulin (T5168, Sigma-Aldrich) or GAPDH (sc-32233, Santa Cruz Biotechnology), in the concentrations recommended by the manufacturer. Membranes were than washed 3 times with TBS-T for 10 min, followed by an incubation with specific secondary antibody conjugated with horseradish peroxidase for 2 h at room temperature on agitation, covered from light in concentrations of 1:500 (Goat anti-Rabbit IgG (H+L), 32460, Thermo Scientific, Waltham, MA, USA) and 1:1000 (Goat anti-Mouse IgG (H+L) Poly-HRP, 32230, Thermo Scientific). For α-Tubulin, the primary antibody was diluted 1:30,000 and the incubation times were shortened at 30 min. Membranes were washed 3 times with TBS-T for 10 min and then treated with ECL reagent (Thermo Scientific). Development of blots was carried out with a Biospectrum Imaging System (UVP LLC, Upland, CA, USA) using the Vision Works LS software. Image analysis was carried out using the Quantity One (Bio-Rad, Hercules, CA, USA) software. Both irradiated and sham control data were expressed, normalizing the intensity of the protein of interest to the corresponding α-Tubulin or GAPDH band for each sample. Samples were analyzed in triplicates (Sup data WB blots).

5.8. Wound-Healing Assay (IncuCyte® Live-Cell Analysis Systems)

In order to further study the impact of the conditioned medium on chondrocyte motility, a wound-healing test was performed on chondrocytes using the conditioned medium of chondrosarcoma cell X-rays irradiated with 0 Gy (as control) and 0.1 Gy (as treated sample). This conditioned medium was taken from chondrosarcoma cell after 6- and 24-h incubations. Then, chondrocytes motility was followed during 24 h in contact with these conditioned media. A wound-healing assay was applied to evaluate cell migration ability. Next, 1.5×10^4 T/C28a2 cells/well were seeded in 96-well IncuCyte® ImageLock Plates in media. Cells were seeded at a density of 70 to 80%. After 24 h, cells were scratched by IncuCyte® WoundMaker to build an artificial wound. Afterwards, the media was removed, cells were washed two times with PBS, and conditioned media were added on cells. Cells were cultured at 37 °C and 5% CO_2 and monitored using an IncuCyte® S3 (Sartorius). The migrating distance was measured for 24 h. Data were analyzed by the Cell Migration Analysis software module (Sartorius).

5.9. Statistical Analyses

Secretome statistical analysis. Spectral counts for each condition and each protein were normalized as recommended [39]. Abundances of the proteins, based on their normalized spectral counts, were compared according to the PatternLab Tfold comparison [40]. Only proteins with statistical significance (p value below 0.05) and with a Tfold increase or decrease in at least 50% compared to control were considered as differentially abundant. Two-dimensional-gels statistical analysis. Statistical analyzes were carried out following 3 independent experiments, using the t-test function of the Progenesis SameSpots software. Datasets were considered as significantly different when $p < 0.05$ (*). 8-oxo-dG statistical analysis. Statistical analyzes were carried out following 3 independent experiments, using the t-test function of the Excel Software in order to compare the 0 Gy condition to every other condition. Datasets were considered as significantly different when $p < 0.05$ (*). Western blotting statistical analysis. Statistical analyzes were carried out following 4 independent experiments, each made at least in 4 replicates, using the t-test function (= t-test) of the Excel Software in order to compare the 0 and 0.1 Gy condition, after normalization of the 0 Gy condition. Datasets were considered as significantly different when $p < 0.05$ (*). IncuCyte wound-healing migration test statistical analysis. Statistical analyzes were carried out following 2 independent experiments, each made at least in triplicats, using the t-test function (= t-test) of the Excel Software in order to compare each time point of 0 and 0.1 Gy condition. Datasets were considered as significantly different when $p < 0.05$ (*).

5.10. Mass Spectrometry Data

The mass spectrometry proteomics data were deposited to the ProteomeXchange Consortium via the PRIDE [41] partner repository with the dataset identifier PXD024953 and project doi:10.6019/PXD024953 in the case of secretome and PXD025187 in the case of proteome analyses.

In the case of secretome analysis, the reviewers may access this private dataset using reviewer_pxd024953@ebi.ac.uk as Username and iotcSWYp as Password.

In the case of proteome analysis, the reviewers may access this private dataset using reviewer_pxd025187@ebi.ac.uk as Username and imUEHlnL as Password. These data will be automatically accessible after publication.

Supplementary Materials: The following are available online at https://www.mdpi.com/article/10.3390/ijms22157957/s1.

Author Contributions: C.L., F.C. and J.A. performed the direct M.S. analysis of secretome; C.L. and F.C. performed the 2D gels experiments; C.L., F.C. and S.H. (Sonia Hem) performed the proteomic analysis of 2D gel spots; M.T. (Mihaela Tudor), M.T. (Mihaela Temelie) and D.S. performed the western blotting analyses; S.H. (Siamak Haghdoost) performed the 8-oxodG quantification; M.T. (Mihaela Tudor), A.G. and E.B. performed the wound healing tests; M.T. (Mihaela Tudor), A.G., D.S. and F.C. performed the statistical analysis; F.C. and D.S. conceived the study and its design; F.C. drafted the manuscript. All authors have read and agreed to the published version of the manuscript.

Funding: This work was supported by grants from the Region Normandy, the RIN emergence 2015–2018 project IRHEMME (IRradiation du cartilage lors d'une Hadronthérapie: Effets bystander, Modifications structurales et fragmentation de la Matrice Extracellulaire), and the RIN CPIER 2018-2020 HABIONOR European project, co-funded by the Normandy County Council, the French State in the framework of the interregional development Contract "Vallée de la Seine" 2015–2020. (HAdronBIOlogie en NORmandie: Programme de recherché en Radiobiologie pour l'hadronthérapie au centre ARCHADE). This work was also supported by "Agence Nationale de la Recherche," Equipex Rec-Hadron (ANR-10-EQPX-1401); by grants of EDF (Electricité de France), the funding from Life Sciences group of the four-way national agreement CEA-EDF-IRSN-Areva (2016-2018) and the funding from Life Sciences group of the four-way national agreement CEA–EDF–IRSN–FRAMATOME (2019-2021); by the CEA and Normandy region for the PhD funding of CL; by Romanian Ministry of Education and Research, grants numbers PN 19060203/2019, by the French Institute of Romania and the French Ministry of Foreign Affairs–Partenariat Hubert Curien, (PHC BRANCUSI 2019, 43535RF).

Institutional Review Board Statement: Not applicable.

Informed Consent Statement: Not applicable.

Data Availability Statement: Not applicable.

Acknowledgments: We would like to thank the personnel at CIRIL platform (Cimap Caen, France) for C-ion dosimetry and helpful discussion and the GANIL (Caen, France) for providing us the C-ion beam, as well as Jean-Charles Gaillard (Li2D) for his help with the tandem mass spectrometry measurements. The carbon ion experiments were performed according to the projects P1146-H, (F. Chevalier), from the iPAC committee proposal for High Energy beam line on interdisciplinary research at GANIL.

Conflicts of Interest: The authors declare no conflict of interest.

References

1. Durante, M. New Challenges in High-Energy Particle Radiobiology. *Br. J. Radiol.* **2014**, *87*, 20130626. [CrossRef]
2. Noël, G.; Feuvret, L.; Ferrand, R.; Mazeron, J.-J. Treatment with charged particles beams: Hadrontherapy part I: Physical basis and clinical experience of treatment with protons. *Cancer Radiother.* **2003**, *7*, 321–339. [CrossRef]
3. Thariat, J.; Valable, S.; Laurent, C.; Haghdoost, S.; Pérès, E.A.; Bernaudin, M.; Sichel, F.; Lesueur, P.; Césaire, M.; Petit, E.; et al. Hadrontherapy Interactions in Molecular and Cellular Biology. *Int. J. Mol. Sci.* **2020**, *21*, 133. [CrossRef]
4. Mothersill, C.; Seymour, C. Radiation-Induced Bystander Effects: Past History and Future Directions. *Radiat. Res.* **2001**, *155*, 759–767. [CrossRef]

5. Chevalier, F.; Hamdi, D.H.; Saintigny, Y.; Lefaix, J.-L. Proteomic Overview and Perspectives of the Radiation-Induced Bystander Effects. *Mutat. Res./Rev. Mutat. Res.* **2014**, *763*, 280–293. [CrossRef]
6. Blyth, B.J.; Sykes, P.J. Radiation-Induced Bystander Effects: What Are They, and How Relevant Are They to Human Radiation Exposures? *Radiat. Res.* **2011**, *176*, 139–157. [CrossRef] [PubMed]
7. Azzam, E.I.; de Toledo, S.M.; Little, J.B. Stress Signaling from Irradiated to Non-Irradiated Cells. *Curr. Cancer Drug Targets* **2004**, *4*, 53–64. [CrossRef]
8. Prise, K.M.; O'Sullivan, J.M. Radiation-Induced Bystander Signalling in Cancer Therapy. *Nat. Rev. Cancer* **2009**, *9*, 351–360. [CrossRef] [PubMed]
9. Abramowicz, A.; Wojakowska, A.; Marczak, L.; Lysek-Gladysinska, M.; Smolarz, M.; Story, M.D.; Polanska, J.; Widlak, P.; Pietrowska, M. Ionizing Radiation Affects the Composition of the Proteome of Extracellular Vesicles Released by Head-and-Neck Cancer Cells in Vitro. *J. Radiat. Res.* **2019**, *60*, 289–297. [CrossRef]
10. Desai, S.; Srambikkal, N.; Yadav, H.D.; Shetake, N.; Balla, M.M.S.; Kumar, A.; Ray, P.; Ghosh, A.; Pandey, B.N. Molecular Understanding of Growth Inhibitory Effect from Irradiated to Bystander Tumor Cells in Mouse Fibrosarcoma Tumor Model. *PLoS ONE* **2016**, *11*, e0161662. [CrossRef]
11. Smith, R.W.; Moccia, R.D.; Seymour, C.B.; Mothersill, C.E. Irradiation of Rainbow Trout at Early Life Stages Results in a Proteomic Legacy in Adult Gills. Part A; Proteomic Responses in the Irradiated Fish and in Non-Irradiated Bystander Fish. *Environ. Res.* **2018**, *163*, 297–306. [CrossRef] [PubMed]
12. Lepleux, C.; Marie-Brasset, A.; Temelie, M.; Boulanger, M.; Brotin, É.; Goldring, M.B.; Hirtz, C.; Varès, G.; Nakajima, T.; Saintigny, Y.; et al. Bystander Effectors of Chondrosarcoma Cells Irradiated at Different LET Impair Proliferation of Chondrocytes. *J. Cell. Commun. Signal.* **2019**, *13*, 343–356. [CrossRef]
13. Gilbert, A.; Tudor, M.; Lepleux, C.; Rofidal, V.; Hem, S.; Almunia, C.; Armengaud, J.; Brotin, E.; Haghdoost, S.; Savu, D.; et al. Proteomic Analysis of Bystander Effects in Chondrosarcoma Cells. In Proceedings of the ERRS 45th Annual Meeting of the European Radiation Research Society, Lund, Sweden, 13–17 September 2020. p. Poster N°25.
14. Banani, S.F.; Lee, H.O.; Hyman, A.A.; Rosen, M.K. Biomolecular Condensates: Organizers of Cellular Biochemistry. *Nat. Rev. Mol. Cell Biol.* **2017**, *18*, 285–298. [CrossRef]
15. Guzikowski, A.R.; Chen, Y.S.; Zid, B.M. Stress-Induced MRNP Granules: Form and Function of P-Bodies and Stress Granules. *Wiley Interdiscip. Rev. RNA* **2019**, *10*, e1524. [CrossRef]
16. Kedersha, N.; Anderson, P. Mammalian Stress Granules and Processing Bodies. *Methods Enzym.* **2007**, *431*, 61–81. [CrossRef]
17. Kedersha, N.; Ivanov, P.; Anderson, P. Stress Granules and Cell Signaling: More than Just a Passing Phase? *Trends Biochem. Sci.* **2013**, *38*, 494–506. [CrossRef]
18. Mahboubi, H.; Stochaj, U. Cytoplasmic Stress Granules: Dynamic Modulators of Cell Signaling and Disease. *Biochim. Biophys. Acta Mol. Basis Dis.* **2017**, *1863*, 884–895. [CrossRef]
19. Moutaoufik, M.T.; Fatimy, R.E.; Nassour, H.; Gareau, C.; Lang, J.; Tanguay, R.M.; Mazroui, R.; Khandjian, E.W. UVC-Induced Stress Granules in Mammalian Cells. *PLoS ONE* **2014**, *9*, e112742. [CrossRef] [PubMed]
20. Wakazono, A.; Fukao, T.; Yamaguchi, S.; Hori, T.; Orii, T.; Lambert, M.; Mitchell, G.A.; Lee, G.W.; Hashimoto, T. Molecular, Biochemical, and Clinical Characterization of Mitochondrial Acetoacetyl-Coenzyme A Thiolase Deficiency in Two Further Patients. *Hum. Mutat.* **1995**, *5*, 34–42. [CrossRef] [PubMed]
21. Haapalainen, A.M.; Meriläinen, G.; Pirilä, P.L.; Kondo, N.; Fukao, T.; Wierenga, R.K. Crystallographic and Kinetic Studies of Human Mitochondrial Acetoacetyl-CoA Thiolase: The Importance of Potassium and Chloride Ions for Its Structure and Function. *Biochemistry* **2007**, *46*, 4305–4321. [CrossRef]
22. Gallego-García, A.; Monera-Girona, A.J.; Pajares-Martínez, E.; Bastida-Martínez, E.; Pérez-Castaño, R.; Iniesta, A.A.; Fontes, M.; Padmanabhan, S.; Elías-Arnanz, M. A Bacterial Light Response Reveals an Orphan Desaturase for Human Plasmalogen Synthesis. *Science* **2019**, *366*, 128–132. [CrossRef] [PubMed]
23. Mouneimne, G.; Hansen, S.D.; Selfors, L.M.; Petrak, L.; Hickey, M.M.; Gallegos, L.L.; Simpson, K.J.; Lim, J.; Gertler, F.B.; Hartwig, J.H.; et al. Differential Remodeling of Actin Cytoskeleton Architecture by Profilin Isoforms Leads to Distinct Effects on Cell Migration and Invasion. *Cancer Cell* **2012**, *22*, 615–630. [CrossRef] [PubMed]
24. Martínez-Martínez, E.; Ibarrola, J.; Fernández-Celis, A.; Santamaria, E.; Fernández-Irigoyen, J.; Rossignol, P.; Jaisser, F.; López-Andrés, N. Differential Proteomics Identifies Reticulocalbin-3 as a Novel Negative Mediator of Collagen Production in Human Cardiac Fibroblasts. *Sci. Rep.* **2017**, *7*, 12192. [CrossRef]
25. Miotto, B.; Chibi, M.; Xie, P.; Koundrioukoff, S.; Moolman-Smook, H.; Pugh, D.; Debatisse, M.; He, F.; Zhang, L.; Defossez, P.-A. The RBBP6/ZBTB38/MCM10 Axis Regulates DNA Replication and Common Fragile Site Stability. *Cell Rep.* **2014**, *7*, 575–587. [CrossRef]
26. Chibi, M.; Meyer, M.; Skepu, A.; G Rees, D.J.; Moolman-Smook, J.C.; Pugh, D.J.R. RBBP6 Interacts with Multifunctional Protein YB-1 through Its RING Finger Domain, Leading to Ubiquitination and Proteosomal Degradation of YB-1. *J. Mol. Biol.* **2008**, *384*, 908–916. [CrossRef]
27. Chevalier, F.; Depagne, J.; Hem, S.; Chevillard, S.; Bensimon, J.; Bertrand, P.; Lebeau, J. Accumulation of Cyclophilin A Isoforms in Conditioned Medium of Irradiated Breast Cancer Cells. *Proteomics* **2012**, *12*, 1756–1766. [CrossRef] [PubMed]

28. Wei, S.J.; Botero, A.; Hirota, K.; Bradbury, C.M.; Markovina, S.; Laszlo, A.; Spitz, D.R.; Goswami, P.C.; Yodoi, J.; Gius, D. Thioredoxin Nuclear Translocation and Interaction with Redox Factor-1 Activates the Activator Protein-1 Transcription Factor in Response to Ionizing Radiation. *Cancer Res.* **2000**, *60*, 6688–6695.
29. Ghosh, A.K.; Steele, R.; Ray, R.B. Functional Domains of C-Myc Promoter Binding Protein 1 Involved in Transcriptional Repression and Cell Growth Regulation. *Mol. Cell. Biol.* **1999**, *19*, 2880–2886. [CrossRef]
30. Chevalier, F.; Hamdi, D.H.; Lepleux, C.; Temelie, M.; Nicol, A.; Austry, J.B.; Lesueur, P.; Vares, G.; Savu, D.; Nakajima, T.; et al. High LET Radiation Overcomes In Vitro Resistance to X-Rays of Chondrosarcoma Cell Lines. *Technol. Cancer Res. Treat.* **2019**, *18*, 1533033819871309. [CrossRef]
31. Hartmann, E.M.; Allain, F.; Gaillard, J.-C.; Pible, O.; Armengaud, J. Taking the Shortcut for High-Throughput Shotgun Proteomic Analysis of Bacteria. *Methods Mol. Biol.* **2014**, *1197*, 275–285. [CrossRef]
32. Klein, G.; Mathé, C.; Biola-Clier, M.; Devineau, S.; Drouineau, E.; Hatem, E.; Marichal, L.; Alonso, B.; Gaillard, J.-C.; Lagniel, G.; et al. RNA-Binding Proteins Are a Major Target of Silica Nanoparticles in Cell Extracts. *Nanotoxicology* **2016**, *10*, 1555–1564. [CrossRef]
33. Dupierris, V.; Masselon, C.; Court, M.; Kieffer-Jaquinod, S.; Bruley, C. A Toolbox for Validation of Mass Spectrometry Peptides Identification and Generation of Database: IRMa. *Bioinformatics* **2009**, *25*, 1980–1981. [CrossRef] [PubMed]
34. Shakeri Manesh, S.; Sangsuwan, T.; Pour Khavari, A.; Fotouhi, A.; Emami, S.N.; Haghdoost, S. MTH1, an 8-Oxo-2′-Deoxyguanosine Triphosphatase, and MYH, a DNA Glycosylase, Cooperate to Inhibit Mutations Induced by Chronic Exposure to Oxidative Stress of Ionising Radiation. *Mutagenesis* **2017**, *32*, 389–396. [CrossRef]
35. Dépagne, J.; Chevalier, F. Technical Updates to Basic Proteins Focalization Using IPG Strips. *Proteome Sci* **2012**, *10*, 54. [CrossRef]
36. Chevalier, F.; Hirtz, C.; Sommerer, N.; Kelly, A.L. Use of Reducing/Nonreducing Two-Dimensional Electrophoresis for the Study of Disulfide-Mediated Interactions between Proteins in Raw and Heated Bovine Milk. *J. Agric. Food Chem.* **2009**, *57*, 5948–5955. [CrossRef]
37. Chevalier, F.; Centeno, D.; Rofidal, V.; Tauzin, M.; Martin, O.; Sommerer, N.; Rossignol, M. Different Impact of Staining Procedures Using Visible Stains and Fluorescent Dyes for Large-Scale Investigation of Proteomes by MALDI-TOF Mass Spectrometry. *J. Proteome Res.* **2006**, *5*, 512–520. [CrossRef] [PubMed]
38. Saintigny, Y.; Chevalier, F.; Bravard, A.; Dardillac, E.; Laurent, D.; Hem, S.; Dépagne, J.; Radicella, J.P.; Lopez, B.S. A Threshold of Endogenous Stress Is Required to Engage Cellular Response to Protect against Mutagenesis. *Sci. Rep.* **2016**, *6*, 29412. [CrossRef]
39. Liu, H.; Sadygov, R.G.; Yates, J.R. A Model for Random Sampling and Estimation of Relative Protein Abundance in Shotgun Proteomics. *Anal. Chem.* **2004**, *76*, 4193–4201. [CrossRef]
40. Carvalho, P.C.; Fischer, J.S.G.; Chen, E.I.; Yates, J.R.; Barbosa, V.C. PatternLab for Proteomics: A Tool for Differential Shotgun Proteomics. *BMC Bioinform.* **2008**, *9*, 316. [CrossRef]
41. Perez-Riverol, Y.; Csordas, A.; Bai, J.; Bernal-Llinares, M.; Hewapathirana, S.; Kundu, D.J.; Inuganti, A.; Griss, J.; Mayer, G.; Eisenacher, M.; et al. The PRIDE Database and Related Tools and Resources in 2019: Improving Support for Quantification Data. *Nucleic Acids Res.* **2019**, *47*, D442–D450. [CrossRef] [PubMed]

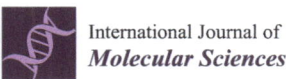

Protocol

A Longitudinal Study of Individual Radiation Responses in Pediatric Patients Treated with Proton and Photon Radiotherapy, and Interventional Cardiology: Rationale and Research Protocol of the HARMONIC Project

Maria Grazia Andreassi [1], Nadia Haddy [2], Mats Harms-Ringdahl [3], Jonica Campolo [4], Andrea Borghini [1], François Chevalier [5,6], Jochen M. Schwenk [7], Brice Fresneau [8,9], Stephanie Bolle [10], Manuel Fuentes [11] and Siamak Haghdoost [3,5,6,*]

1. CNR National Research Council Institute of Clinical Physiology, 56125 Pisa, Italy; andreassi@ifc.cnr.it (M.G.A.); aborghini@ifc.cnr.it (A.B.)
2. Radiation Epidemiology Team, Center for Research in Epidemiology and Population Health, INSERM U1018, Gustave Roussy, Université Paris-Saclay, 94805 Villejuif, France; nadia.haddy@gustaveroussy.fr
3. Department of Molecular Biosciences, The Wenner-Gren Institute, Stockholm University, 10691 Stockholm, Sweden; mats.harms-ringdahl@su.se
4. CNR National Research Council Institute of Clinical Physiology, ASST Grande Ospedale Metropolitano Niguarda, 20162 Milan, Italy; jonica.campolo@cnr.it
5. UMR6252 CIMAP, CEA-CNRS-ENSICAEN-University of Caen Normandy, 14000 Caen, France; francois.chevalier@cea.fr
6. Advanced Resource Center for HADrontherapy in Europe (ARCHADE), 14000 Caen, France
7. Affinity Proteomics, SciLifeLab, School of Engineering Sciences in Chemistry, Biotechnology and Health, KTH—Royal Institute of Technology, 10044 Stockholm, Sweden; jochen.schwenk@scilifelab.se
8. Department of Children and Adolescents Oncology, Gustave Roussy, Université Paris-Saclay, 94805 Villejuif, France; brice.fresneau@gustaveroussy.fr
9. Cancer and Radiation Team, Center for Research in Epidemiology and Population Health, INSERM U1018, Gustave Roussy, Université Paris-Saclay, 94805 Villejuif, France
10. Department of Radiation Therapy, Gustave Roussy, Université Paris-Saclay, 94805 Villejuif, France
11. Department of Medicine and General Service of Cytometry, Proteomics Unit, Cancer Research Centre-IBMCC, CSIC-USAL, IBSAL, Campus Miguel de Unamuno s/n, University of Salamanca-CSIC, 37007 Salamanca, Spain
* Correspondence: siamak.haghdoost@su.se or siamak.haghdoost@unicaen.fr

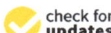

Citation: Andreassi, M.G.; Haddy, N.; Harms-Ringdahl, M.; Campolo, J.; Borghini, A.; Chevalier, F.; Schwenk, J.M.; Fresneau, B.; Bolle, S.; Fuentes, M.; et al. A Longitudinal Study of Individual Radiation Responses in Pediatric Patients Treated with Proton and Photon Radiotherapy, and Interventional Cardiology: Rationale and Research Protocol of the HARMONIC Project. *Int. J. Mol. Sci.* **2023**, *24*, 8416. https://doi.org/10.3390/ijms24098416

Academic Editor: David A. Gewirtz

Received: 15 March 2023
Revised: 1 May 2023
Accepted: 3 May 2023
Published: 8 May 2023

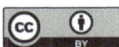

Copyright: © 2023 by the authors. Licensee MDPI, Basel, Switzerland. This article is an open access article distributed under the terms and conditions of the Creative Commons Attribution (CC BY) license (https://creativecommons.org/licenses/by/4.0/).

Abstract: The Health Effects of Cardiac Fluoroscopy and Modern Radiotherapy (photon and proton) in Pediatrics (HARMONIC) is a five-year project funded by the European Commission that aimed to improve the understanding of the long-term ionizing radiation (IR) risks for pediatric patients. In this paper, we provide a detailed overview of the rationale, design, and methods for the biological aspect of the project with objectives to provide a mechanistic understanding of the molecular pathways involved in the IR response and to identify potential predictive biomarkers of individual response involved in long-term health risks. Biological samples will be collected at three time points: before the first exposure, at the end of the exposure, and one year after the exposure. The average whole-body dose, the dose to the target organ, and the dose to some important out-of-field organs will be estimated. State-of-the-art analytical methods will be used to assess the levels of a set of known biomarkers and also explore high-resolution approaches of proteomics and miRNA transcriptomes to provide an integrated assessment. By using bioinformatics and systems biology, biological pathways and novel pathways involved in the response to IR exposure will be deciphered.

Keywords: radiotherapy; ionizing radiation; proton radiotherapy; pediatric oncology; HARMONIC project; congenital heart disease; cardiac catheterization; radiation biomarkers

1. Introduction

The use of ionizing radiation (IR) in medicine represents significant benefits for the medical care of patients. Indeed, IR remains one of the major therapeutic options for cancer treatment [1]. IR is also used for diagnostic and therapeutic imaging, particularly for pediatric patients with congenital or acquired heart disease, who may receive one or more cardiac catheterization procedures as part of their management [2–4]. While benefits for the patients largely outweigh the risk, the potential adverse health effects of exposure to IR are particularly important to be explored in populations of young patients who are more radiosensitive and, nowadays, survive their disease for decades [3,4].

IR is a well-known risk factor for cancer induction, and recent studies support the existence of an excess cancer risk, even at low doses of radiation [5]. Children are especially vulnerable to the oncogenic effects of IR. Moreover, the oncogenic effects of IR require a long latent period (from years to decades) that varies with the type of malignancy; therefore, an infant or child has a longer lifetime risk for developing radiation-induced cancers than an adult. Radiation-induced second malignancies are one of the most serious adverse effects following radiotherapy of primary cancers in childhood cancer [6]. Typically, radiation-induced malignancies develop in normal tissue within radiotherapy fields with a latency period of 5–10 years for hematologic malignancies and 10–60 years for solid tumors [6]. Many clinical studies reported an increased risk for second primary cancer, histopathologically different from the first tumor, in organs inside as well as outside the primary beam [6]. Interestingly, it was reported that leukemias and carcinomas are more often seen in organs receiving low-dose radiation (out-of-field dose), whereas sarcomas are more common in tissues or organ receiving high-dose radiation (in-field doses) [7]. However, the exact mechanism and dose–response relationship for radiation-induced malignancy, for both in-field and out-of-field doses, are not well understood; thus, it is necessary to investigate how radiotherapy, photons, and protons impact carcinogenic risk in childhood cancer management [7]. For instance, the therapeutic use of proton beams has the potential to provide a better depth–dose profile and remarkable reduction in the dose to the adjacent normal tissues compared with photon beams [7]. Additionally, there is growing evidence supporting an increased risk for late adverse non-cancer conditions [8], including cardiac and vascular effects. Thus, late adverse effects of radiotherapy have been observed on large vessels, causing cerebrovascular [9,10] and cardiovascular [11,12] diseases.

Nowadays, there is also evidence for a significant elevation of cancer risk in patients with acquired as well as congenital heart diseases (CHD) in response to repeated radiological exposures [13,14]. However, more data are needed to better define the "malignant price of cardiac care" [15].

The risk estimates of long-term health effects of low doses of IR (cancer and non-cancer) are still incomplete, particularly for pediatric patients. Large patient cohorts, extended follow-up, validated clinical data, and reliable dosimetry for the cohorts are needed to address this challenge. The integration of epidemiological and biological research through panels of biomarkers, together with a mechanistic understanding of the cellular responses to a particular dose and radiation quality, will provide powerful means to improve risk estimates, leading to a better quantification of the magnitude of risks associated with low-dose exposures, e.g., for out-of-field organs.

The Health Effects of Cardiac Fluoroscopy and Modern Radiotherapy in Pediatrics (HARMONIC) is a five-year project funded by the European Commission to improve understanding of the long-term health risks from medical ionizing radiation exposure in children and young patients (https://harmonicproject.eu/, accessed on 4 March 2023). The HARMONIC project uses an integrated approach of conventional epidemiology complemented by non-invasive imaging and molecular epidemiology to assess cancer and non-cancer outcomes in pediatric patients treated with modern radiotherapy techniques (such as proton therapy) for cancer and X-ray-guided interventional catheterization procedures for CHD.

The purpose of the manuscript is to describe the bioanalytical research goals of the HARMONIC project, the rationale, and the study design, including the enrolment, endpoints, and expected results of the study.

The general objective of the bioanalytical studies of the HARMONIC project is to provide a mechanistic understanding of the molecular pathways and the cellular responses that are triggered by the medical applications of IR in pediatric patients.

A mechanistic understanding, together with the identification of biomarkers for individuals at increased risk to develop adverse health effects, has the potential to increase the power of epidemiological studies regarding health effects caused by IR [16–18]. Such biomarkers may be useful in identifying susceptible individuals who are more vulnerable to radiation damage for whom individualized treatment can be considered (by radiation sparing policy or attempts to pharmacologic or dietary radioprotection).

The specific aims are to:
- identify radiation-induced biochemical responses in blood and saliva from pediatric patients exposed to medical IR;
- evaluate dose–response relationships for different radiation qualities and delivery techniques with regards to specific biochemical responses;
- search for pre-existing biomarkers of radiation sensitivity and health effects that may be useful for molecular epidemiological studies to identify patients with a potential higher risk of radiation-induced adverse health effects.

2. Experimental Design

The HARMONIC biological study is a prospective observational study which aims to investigate the biological changes induced by ionizing radiation exposure at various time points before and after exposure. It will focus on specific molecular biomarkers reported as 'early signs' of biological damage and long-term health effects. These include biomarkers of oxidative stress (8-hydroxy-2′-deoxyguanosine) [19–21], protein markers of inflammation (PTX3, IL-6, IL-10, TNF-α, NF-kB, MCP-1, etc.) [22,23], and genetic markers (telomere shortening and mtDNA copy numbers) [24–29].

To decipher significant intracellular pathways and novel potential biomarkers involved in response to the radiation regimes applied, four different approaches will be used multiplexed protein profiling assays on blood plasma [30], reverse-phase protein array (RPPA) on proteins isolated from peripheral blood mononuclear cells [31], miRNA transcriptome on whole blood and saliva [32], and liquid chromatography–mass spectrometry (LC–MS) on saliva.

Finally, we will develop and implement new bioinformatic models to integrate the collected biological, clinical, and dosimetry data. that may be used in epidemiological and clinical approaches to identify patients at higher risk for radiation-induced adverse health effects, not only before starting (by analyzing the sample taken before exposure), but also after finishing the exposure (by analyzing samples taken after exposure). Biomarkers will be studied in both blood and saliva to investigate whether saliva can be used as a non-invasive sample to analyze biomarkers in large-scale molecular epidemiology studies. The overall strategy of the "biology" project is presented in Figure 1.

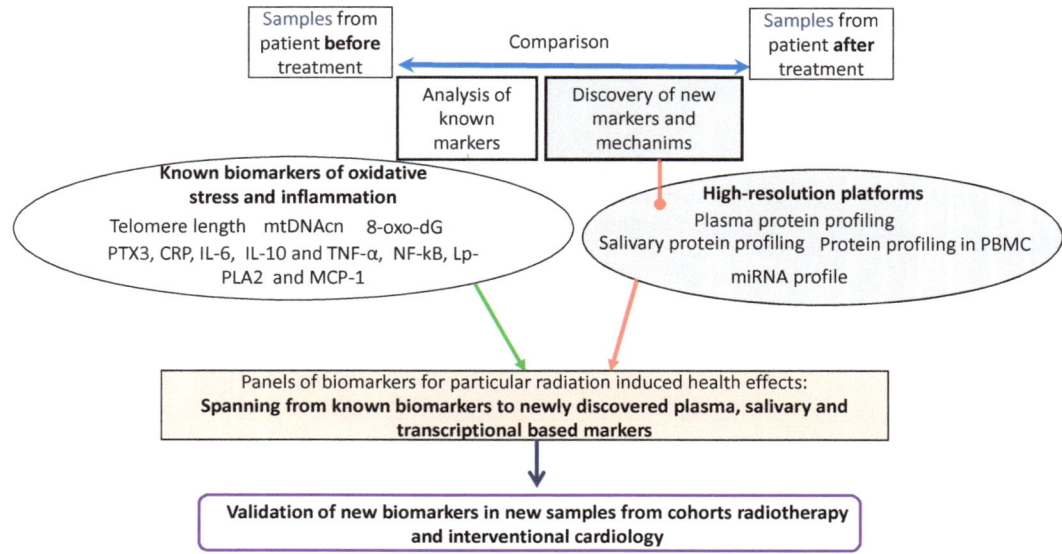

Figure 1. Overall strategy of the planned biological research in the HARMONIC project.

3. Material and Equipment

3.1. Study Population

This exploratory study will include 150 patients: 50 patients treated for cancer with proton therapy, 50 patients with photon therapy, and 50 patients treated with X-ray-guided interventional catheterization procedures for CHD. Specific inclusion and exclusion criteria are listed in Table 1.

Table 1. Inclusion and exclusion criteria.

Radiotherapy	Interventional Cardiology
Inclusion criteria	
<ul><li>Age at diagnosis ≤ 21 years</li><li>Informed consent of parent/guardian as well as child/patient</li><li>Patients treated for: brain tumors (except malignant gliomas); head and neck tumors (e.g., rhabdomyosarcomas and nasopharyngeal carcinoma); Hodgkin's lymphoma</li><li>Patients receiving pulmonary and chest radiation for: Ewing sarcoma; other chest sarcomas; lung metastasis of Wilms and Ewing tumors; other tumors</li><li>Patients receiving craniospinal radiation therapy for: Medulloblastoma or other tumors</li></ul>	<ul><li>Age of patients: 5–22 years</li><li>Patients with congenital heart disease</li><li>Informed consent of parent/guardian as well as child/patient</li></ul>
Exclusion criteria	
<ul><li>Chromosomal abnormalities and/or genetic syndromes</li><li>Absence of informed consent</li></ul>	

Ethics approval has been already obtained in all participating centers. All eligible patients received an information brochure and are invited to participate in the study by the responsible physician. Informed consent is signed by the patient or his/her legal representative before entering the study. Detailed demographic, clinical and treatment data are retrieved by the attending physician and from the patient's medical electronic record. Data protection officers (DPOs) from each organization will be involved to ensure compliance with General Data Protection Regulations (GDPRs).

3.2. Biological Sample Collection

For radiotherapy patients, blood and saliva will be collected at three time points: before radiotherapy; three months after the last fraction (time point for the first follow-up); and one year after completion of the treatment. For X-ray-guided interventional catheterization procedures, biological samples will also be collected at three time points: before intervention; the same day after completion; and one year after completion. Figure 2 summarizes the protocol for the collection, preparation, and storage of biosamples.

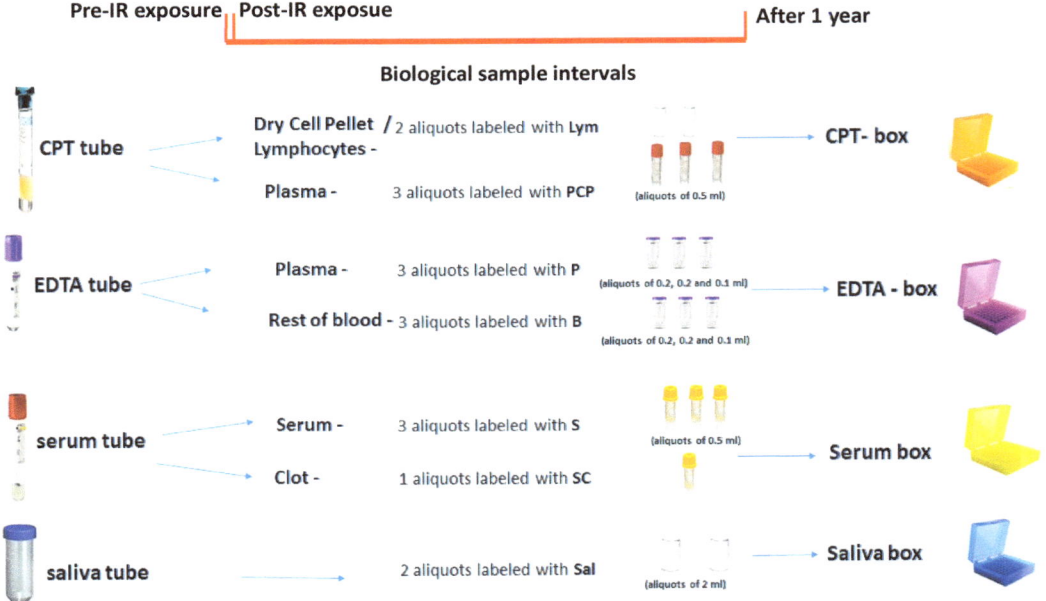

Figure 2. Study design of the Harmonic project and overview of biological sample collection.

Briefly, a maximum of 12 mL blood will be collected at each time point in three different tubes, which are as follows:
- one BD vacutainer® CPT™ tube for the isolation of lymphocytes (~4 mL);
- one vacutainer tube containing EDTA K2 (~4 mL);
- one clot activator serum separation tube (~4 mL).

The samples will be given a unique patient identification number (pseudonymization). Within two hours post collection, tubes with blood samples will be centrifuged according to standard operating procedures (SOPs) prepared by the HARMONIC consortium to obtain lymphocytes, serum, and plasma. To investigate the possible impact of pre-analytical variables, we will record and share information on the study centers, time, and calendar days when the samples are collected. We will also record and share the time that elapses between the blood draw, centrifugation, and first freezing.

Regarding saliva samples, approximately 4–5 mL of saliva will be collected at each time point in a sterile 10 mL plastic tube without any additive. Saliva samples will be divided into two aliquots, 2 mL in each. Aliquots of biological samples from each donor will be immediately stored at −80 °C (Figure 2). The type of tubes, volume, and number of each aliquots are summarized in Figure 2. At specific time points in the project, coded samples will be shipped from a respective clinic on dry ice to a centralized Biobank, where they will be stored at −80 °C until use.

3.3. Biological Measures

The samples will be analyzed by state-of-the-art methods to determine the levels of selected biomarkers. Moreover, the samples will be examined by innovative high-throughput approaches, including analyses of miRNA transcriptomes and proteomics [30–32]. The handling and analytical procedures will follow the respective SOP procedures for all biologic sampling, handling, shipping, and analysis.

4. Detailed Procedure

4.1. 8-Hydroxy-2′-deoxyguanosine (8-oxo-dG) and Markers of Inflammation

The levels of 8-oxo-dG in serum and saliva will be determined using an ELISA method where the samples are essentially purified by Bond Elute columns, as previously described [19,20]. Briefly, 800 µL blood serum or saliva will be purified using a C18 solid phase Bond Elut extraction column. The purified samples will be freeze-dried and reconstituted in PBS. Then, 300 µL of the purified sample will be mixed with 150 µL of primary antibody against 8-oxo-dG and distributed in three wells of a 96-well ELISA plate pre-coated with 8-oxo-dG and then incubated at 37 °C for 120 min. Secondary antibody body will then be added followed by the staining solution in order to quantify the yield of secondary antibodies bounded to primary antibodies in each well using a 96-well automatic ELISA plate reader. Each sample will be analyzed in triplicate. A standard curve for 8-oxo-dG (0.05–10 ng/mL) will be established for each plate and the concentration of 8-oxo-dG in each sample will be calculated based on the standard curve.

4.2. Analysis of Telomere Length (TL) and mtDNA Copy Number (mtDNA-CN)

TL and mtDNA-CN will be measured on DNA extracted from 200 µL of biological samples of blood and saliva samples by real-time PCR (CFX384 Touch™ Real-Time PCR System, Bio-Rad Life Sciences) according to standardized protocols [25,26]. Briefly, TL will be measured in genomic DNA by determining the ratio of a telomere repeat copy number (T) to a single-copy gene (S) and copy number (T/S ratio). The relative telomere length will be calculated using the following formula "T/S ratio = $2-\Delta\Delta Ct$", where ΔCt = Ct telomere − a Ct single-copy gene. The T/S ratio reflects the average length of the telomeres across all leukocytes. For the quantification of mtDNA-CN, the NDI1 gene in the undeleted region for the reference sequence of mtDNA will be used as an internal control (mtNDI1) and human ß-globin gene of genomic DNA (gDNA) will be amplified by PCR in both gDNA and mtDNA. ΔCt values will be calculated from the difference between the Ct for the ß-globin gene and the Ct for the NDI1 gene and used to measure mtDNA-CN relative to gDNA. mtDNA-CN will be calculated using the ($2\Delta Ct$) method (ΔCt = Ct mtNDI1 − CtgDNA).

4.3. miRNA Profiling Analysis

Total RNA will be isolated from 500 µL of blood and saliva samples using a RiboPure™-Blood Kit (ThermoFisher, Waltham, MA, USA) and a miRNeasy Serum/Plasma Kit (QIAGEN, Hilden, Germany), respectively, according to the manufacturer's protocol [32]. The expression profiling of miRNAs will be analyzed using the Illumina MiSeq platform. For each patient, we will carry out a small RNA sequencing experiment to characterize the different miRNA expression profiles in samples for each time point. Prepared libraries will be run on Miseq, and miRNA identification and dysregulated expression analyses will be performed using latest version of iMir software (https://www.labmedmolge.unisa.it/italiano/home/imir, accessed on 5 September 2022), a fully automated workflow for the rapid analysis of high-throughput small RNA-Seq data. Specific dysregulated miRNAs will be further validated using qRT-PCR with sequence-specific TaqMan microRNA assays and a TaqMan Universal PCR Master Mix, as opposed to AmpErase UNG (Thermo

Fisher Scientific, USA), in accordance with the manufacturer's instructions. The miRNA expression levels will be normalized to the U6 small nuclear RNA and calculated using the ΔΔCt method [32]. The target genes from differentially expressed miRNAs will be predicted using DIANA miRPath software (microrna.gr/mirpath, accessed on 5 September 2022). Then, the targets will then be further analyzed for gene ontology (GO) function enrichment terms (geneontology.org/, accessed on 5 September 2022), Kyoto Encyclopedia of Genes Genomes (KEGG) pathway classification (www.genome.jp/kegg/, accessed on 5 September 2022), and Reactome pathway databases (www.reactome.org, accessed on 5 September 2022).

4.4. Plasma Protein Profiling

Briefly, from the literature, a list of 90 protein markers that have previously been identified as potential markers of diseases related to the late effects of radiation exposure, particularly vascular diseases and secondary cancer, will be established. Aliquots of 100 µL plasma will be used for plasma proteome analysis using Olink's affinity proteomics platform. The approach is based on paired antibodies, coupled to unique and partially complementary oligonucleotides, and measured by quantitative real-time PCR. This dual-recognition DNA-coupled method provides high specificity and sensitivity for an analysis of at least 90 proteins in parallel [30]. We plan to analyze the 98 selected proteins in all samples from the three cohorts. Different statistical and computational models for single and multivariate analysis will then be used to identify the modified pathways.

4.5. Reverse-Phase Protein Arrays (RPPAs)

Reverse-phase protein arrays (RPPAs) will allow us to study protein expression levels and the activation status of cell signaling pathways. Isolated peripheral blood mononuclear cells (PBMCs) from blood collected into CPT tubes will be analyzed by customized RPPA (Proteomics Unit. IBSAL. University of Salamanca). To summarize, the cells will be lysed and the protein extract will be serially diluted with a protein lysis buffer, supplemented with proteases and phosphatase inhibitors. Five serial dilutions/sample, ranging from 2000 to 125 µg/mL, and two technical replicates per dilution will be applied on the nitrocellulose microarray membrane. In addition, a few spike-in proteins as RPPAs, such as negative and positive controls, will be included.

The membranes will be incubated with primary antibodies that target proteins of interest or without primary antibodies as negative controls. All primary antibodies for RPPA screening have been previously tested by Western blotting to assess their specificity and selectivity to the targeted protein. RPPA readout is a fluorescent signal correlated to the protein expression level. Samples will be applied on membranes in three technical replicates (spots), and the membranes will then be individually incubated with antibodies targeting one protein of interest, followed by an incubation with a fluorescent dye. Fluorescent signals will be acquired by a microarray scanner at high resolutions and minimal auto-fluorescent background. The NormaCurve method will be used for data quantification and normalization [31]. This method includes a normalization for (i) background fluorescence, (ii) variations in the total amount of spotted protein; and (iii) spatial bias on the membranes. The normalized values will be employed to compare the protein expression levels across samples. Briefly, for each spot, the raw fluorescent signal of the proteins will be corrected with the fluorescent signal of the negative control (signal obtained after incubating an array without the targeted protein antibody). This corrected signal will be divided by the total amount of spotted protein, corresponding to the normalized signal. Finally, the normalized signals of all the proteins will be scaled according to the median for further comparisons and statistical analysis. For each sample, one value will be generated for each targeted protein, and further statistical analysis will be considered.

4.6. Saliva Protein Analysis

The saliva protein concentrations will be determined using a colorimetric protein assay (BCA Protein Assay Kit, Thermo Scientific, Waltham, MA, USA). The proteomic workflow is as follows. The iST-BCT Kit (PreOmics, Martinsried, Germany) will be used to perform a fast, reliable, and reproducible sample preparation on all the patient samples. Fifty microliters of saliva will be used as the starting material (the volume will be adjusted depending on the BCA result). Saliva proteins will be precipitated with 200 µL of ethanol at −20 °C overnight. Samples will then be centrifuged (at 17,000× g for 5 min at 4 °C) and the supernatants will be removed. Salivary protein pellets will be re-suspended, lysed, reduced, and alkylated in 10 min at 95 °C. Proteins will be digested in one hour. Generated peptides will be cleaned before LC-MS injection. Purified tryptic digests will be separated with a predefined 60 SPD method (21 min gradient time and 200 ng peptides) on an Evosep One LC system (Evosep, Odense, Demmark). A fused silica 10 µm ID emitter (Bruker Daltonics, Waltham, MA, USA) is placed inside a nanoelectrospray source (CaptiveSpray source, Bruker Daltonics, Waltham, MA, USA). The emitter is connected to a 8 cm × 150 µm reverse-phase column, packed with 1.5 µm C18 beads. Mobile phases will comprise water and acetonitrile, buffered with 0.1% formic acid. The column will be heated to 40 °C in an oven compartment. LC is coupled online to a TIMS Q-TOF instrument (timsTOF Pro 2, Bruker Daltonics) with a diaPASEF acquisition method. Samples will be acquired using a diaPASEF method, consisting of 12 cycles, including a total of 34 mass width windows (25 Da width, from 350 to 1200 Da) with 2 mobility windows each, leaving a total of 68 windows that cover the ion mobility range (1/K0) from 0.64 to 1.37 V s/cm^2. Saliva proteins will be quantified using a label-free DIA approach with DIA-NN software (https://github.com/vdemichev/diann, accessed on 4 March 2023). DIA-NN version 1.8 will be used first to build an in silico predicted library from the human FASTA database (NextProt 2022-02-25), enabling the 'FASTA digest for library-free search/library generation' and 'Deep learning-based spectra' options, as well as RTs and IMs prediction. The predicted library will be used to analyze the diaPASEF dataset.

4.7. Radiation Doses Data

For each patient, the average whole-body dose or mean/maximum dose and non-target organ (out-of-field organ) doses will be estimated in collaboration with physicists responsible for dosimetry studies in the Harmonic project (https://harmonicproject.eu, accessed on 4 May 2023). Briefly, the strategy for dose estimation will rely on Monte Carlo simulations for CHD patients and on treatment planning systems and analytical models for cancer patients [33]. These strategies were benchmarked against measurements on physical phantoms and reference Monte Carlo simulations [34,35]. As we are analyzing plasma proteins, the total dose to the blood will also be estimated and considered.

4.8. Integrative Analysis of Biological Function and Networks

Integrative data analysis of multiple sets of data types will be performed to construct an interaction network of differentially expressed features (miRNAs and proteins) to elucidate the molecular mechanisms underlying the biological response to IR and to discover new potential biomarkers. In brief, each dataset from the different independent analyses (miRNA transcriptome sequencing and proteomics) will first be analyzed in relation to the available clinical parameters, e.g., age, sex, diagnosis, and background diseases, to identify significantly different features between the baseline and post-IR exposure responses. Then, the radiation-deregulated miRNAs and proteins will be analyzed by an integrative procedure using software, such as ingenuity pathway analysis (Qiagen Bioinformatics; Redwood City, CA, USA; www.qiagen.com/ingenuity, accessed on 5 March 2023), in order to identify the most significantly affected pathways, their components, and associated signaling networks.

4.9. Sample Size and Plan for Statistical Analysis

This study is exploratory as the number of available patients is limited. With the use of data from our previous study on leukocyte telomere length [25], priori power analysis (Spearman's correlation test) requires a sample size of 34 patients to achieve >80% power (alpha = 0.05) and to detect an effect size of 0.5 (G*Power, version 3.1.9.2). We plan to include a target population of 100 patients from each cohort, considering the feasibility aspects of the study, the estimated level of recruitment in each participating clinical site, and a drop-out rate of 50%, aiming for a minimum of 50 participating patients in each cohort. Concerning the statistical plan, a database including clinical (diagnosis, different therapies, CT and MRI images, etc.), dosimetric, and experimental data for each patient will be created in order to perform appropriate statistical analysis. Descriptive data will be presented as frequencies with proportions for categorical variables, and either as means with corresponding SDs or medians with corresponding IQRs for continuous variables depending on the distribution. Statistical tests will include Pearson's x^2 test for frequencies, the Mann–Whitney U test for non-normally distributed continuous variables, and Student's *t*-test for normally distributed variables. Spearman's correlation test will be used to explore the association between variables and radiation doses.

Exploratory analysis, including unsupervised clustering and principal component analysis, will also be performed to stratify patients according to differential protein expression or relative protein abundance. Other soft clustering, dimensionality reduction (e.g., tSNE and UMAP), or unsupervised analyses (e.g., group-based trajectory models) will be conducted to identify groups of individuals that follow similar shifts or trends on protein relative abundance or differential protein expressions over time, considering that all time points will be performed. The differential profiles will be determined based on the data analysis for baseline and each timepoint, as well as changes from baseline values (relative and absolute change).

A mixed-effects model will be used to study the association between different biomarkers at different time points and the dosimetry data (dose, volume, and beam quality). Lastly, the differences in biomarker levels between a follow-up timepoint and baseline will be studied as a function of dosimetric indicators using general linear models, with adjustment for potential confounders (chemotherapy, disease history, medicines, BMI, etc.). Statistical significance for all analyses will be assessed using two-sided tests with an alpha level of 0.05 and adjustment for multiple comparisons.

5. Expected Results

The HARMONIC project addresses a crucial question regarding the health risks for pediatric patients exposed to ionizing radiation from radiotherapy or interventional cardiology (UNSCEAR report 2008) [1–4]. Over the recent years, there has been considerable technological advancements that improve the therapeutic gain of radiotherapy, i.e., maximizing the dose to the tumor while sparing the healthy tissue, [7,36], as well as implementing numerous dose reduction strategies in pediatric interventional cardiology [3,37]. The difficulties associated with cancer and non-cancer risk assessments from pediatric radiation exposure could be partly overcome with precise dose estimation and biochemical studies to better understand the mechanisms that underly the development of disease processes and provide indicators of risk [16–18].

Radiation can induce DNA damage, especially DNA double-strand breaks (DSBs), which are the most lethal type of DNA damage and can result in mutations, chromosomal abnormalities, and the further development of cancer, as well as other severe health effects. However, the full spectra of biological mechanisms underlying the adverse health effects after irradiation are only partly understood. It has been reported that several biological pathways, such as DNA repair, inflammatory response, oxidative stress induction, as well as metabolic changes, are involved in response to IR exposure [17,38]. A multifactorial approach in conjunction with robust high-throughput technologies and integrated computational approaches, such as systems biology, may facilitate the discovery of new pathways and biomarkers for the prediction of long-term adverse health effects of IR exposure [17,38,39].

Accordingly, biological research on the HARMONIC project will investigate the changes induced by medical radiation at the level of specific biomarkers which might be considered 'early signs' of tissue damage before the full development of adverse health effects. The project will focus on changes related to oxidative stress [19,20], inflammation [22,23], as well as nuclear and mitochondrial DNA damage [25,26], in order to identify the long-term health risks [21,24,27–29].

In parallel, the study will also use high-resolution approaches of proteomics and whole miRNA transcriptomes to provide an integrated assessment of bio-molecular responses to pediatric radiation exposure by identifying biological pathways that may underlie the adverse health effects of the exposures.

Of note, this study has a longitudinal design which will allow the shorter-term and longer-term biological response of IR to be compared. To account for the differences between the participants, we will anchor the data of each individual on their own baseline data. This will allow us to measure the treatment effects on an individual level immediately and up to 1 year later.

An additional aspect of this study is the comparison of biomarkers in saliva with those in blood samples. Especially in vulnerable populations, such as children [40,41], saliva offers an attractive non-invasive sampling method that is relatively inexpensive, safe, and easy to use. Saliva could be a valuable alternative as a biological source for human biomonitoring in occupational and environmental medicine [41], but further studies are needed to explore the robustness, reproducibility, and validity of salivary biomarkers in comparison to those analyzed in blood.

As the study includes a cohort of pediatric patients that will be well characterized in terms of dosimetry to "in-field" and "out-of-field" organs [33–35] (https://harmonicproject.eu, accessed on 4 March 2023), it will be possible to investigate dose–response relationships between biomarkers and doses to organs for both radiotherapy and interventional cardiology, as well as a comparison of effects of radiation quality.

The HARMONIC databases will register the individual responses for a defined set of biomarkers and facilitate studies on the mechanisms that underly radiation-induced second/primary cancers, as well as cardiac and vascular damages. A mechanistic understanding, together with biomarkers for individuals at increased risk, has the potential to increase the power of epidemiological studies regarding the health effects of different radiotherapy modalities.

Hence, we believe that a better understanding of the underlying biological and cellular mechanisms will complement the epidemiological approach of the HARMONIC project (https://harmonicproject.eu/, accessed on 4 March 2023). This will provide a unique opportunity to gain better insight into the biological effects of medical radiation doses in pediatric patients.

In summary, the findings of this research project hold the potential to provide mechanistic insight in the molecular and cellular responses involved in the effects of IR of different radiation quality and doses. The HARMONIC project aims to improve the protection of patients and maximize the benefits from medical applications. The final expected output from the biological part of the project will be able to define the predictive biomarkers to be used for molecular epidemiology studies in order to identify patients at higher risk for adverse health effects.

Author Contributions: Writing—original draft and reading review: M.G.A.; reading review and editing: N.H., M.H.-R., J.C., A.B., F.C., J.M.S., B.F., S.B. and M.F.; conceptualization, supervision, and writing—review and editing, S.H. All authors have read and agreed to the published version of the manuscript.

Funding: The HARMONIC project (Health effects of cArdiac fluoRoscopy and MOdeRN radIotherapy in paediatriCs) has received funding from the Euratom research and training program 2014–2018 under grant agreement No 847707.

Institutional Review Board Statement: The study was conducted according to the guidelines of the Declaration of Helsinki and approved by the Local Ethics Committees from the participating centers.

Informed Consent Statement: Written informed consent will be obtained from all patients and their parents involved in the study before the subject undergoes any study procedure.

Data Availability Statement: No new data were created or analyzed in this study. Data sharing is not applicable to this article.

Acknowledgments: Collaborators: HARMONIC CONSORTIUM: Isabelle Thierry-Chef [1,2,3], Christian Bäumer [4], Marie-Odile Bernier [5], Guillaume Boissonnat [6], Lorenzo Brualla [4], Vadim Chumak [7], Jérémie Dabin [8], Inge De Wit [9], Charlotte Demoor-Goldschmidt [10], Marijke De Saint-Hubert [8], Steffen Dreger [11], Agnès Dumas [12], Gaute Døhlen [13], Karin Haustermans [9], Louise Tram Henriksen [14], Morten Høyer [14], Sofie Isebaert [9], Angéla Jackson [12], Andreas Jahnen [15], Neige Journy [12], Kristina Kjaerheim [13], Yasmin Lassen [14], John Maduro [16], Richard McNally [17], Hilde M. Olerud [18], Rodney Ortiz [1,2,3], Eugenio Picano [19], Cécile Ronckers [20], Utheya Salini Thevathas [18], Adelaida Sarukhan [1,2,3], Uwe Schneider [21], Theresa Steinmeier [22], Jacques Balosso [10], Juliette Thariat [10], Beate Timmermann [22,4], Laura Toussaint [14], Camille Vidaud [12], Linda Walsh [21], Martina Wette [22], and Hajo Zeeb [11] ([1] Barcelona Institute for Global Health (ISGlobal), Barcelona, Spain; [2] Universitat Pompeu Fabra (UPF), Barcelona, Spain; [3] CIBER Epidemiología y Salud Pública (CIBERESP), Spain; [4] The West German Proton Therapy Centre Essen (WPE), Essen, Germany; [5] Institut de Radioprotection et de Sûreté Nucléaire (IRSN), France; [6] Commissariat à l'Énergie Atomique & aux Énergies Alternatives (CEA), France; [7] National Research Center for Radiation Medicine (NRCRM), Kyiv, Ukraine; [8] Belgian Nuclear Research Centre (SCK CEN), Belgium; [9] Katholieke Universiteit Leuven (KU Leuven), Leuven, Belgium; [10] Centre Régional François Baclesse (CRFB), Caen, France; [11] Leibniz-Institute for Prevention Research & Epidemiology (BIPS), Bremen, Germany; [12] French National Institute of Health and Medical Research (Inserm), France; [13] Oslo University Hospital (OUS), Oslo, Norway; [14] Aarhus University Hospital (AUH), Aarhus, Denmark; [15] Luxembourg Institute of Science and Technology (LIST), Luxembourg; [16] University Medical Center Groningen (UMCG), Groningen, Netherlands; [17] University of Newcastle upon Tyne (UNEW), Newcastle, United Kingdom; [18] University of South-Eastern Norway (USN), Porsgrunn, Norway; [19] Institute of Clinical Physiology—National Research Council (IFC-CNR), Pisa, Italy; [20] Princess Maxima Center for Pediatric Oncology (PMC), Utrecht, Netherlands; [21] University of Zurich (UZH), Zurich, Switzerland; [22] and University Hospital Essen (UK Essen), Essen, Germany).

Conflicts of Interest: The authors declare no conflict of interest.

Abbreviations

mtDNAcn	mtDNA copy number
8-Oxo-dG	8-hydroxy-2′-deoxyguanosine
IL-6	interleukin-6
IL-10	interleukin-10
TNF-α	tumor necrosis factor-α
MCP-1	monocyte chemoattractant protein-1
NF-kB	nuclear factor kappaB
PBMC	peripheral blood mononuclear cell
PTX3	pentraxin 3
PBMC	peripheral blood mononuclear cells
miRNA	microRNA
Lym	cell pellet/lymphocytes
PCP	plasma from CPT
P	plasma from EDTA
B	rest of blood
S	serum
SC	blood clot
Sal	saliva

References

1. Delaney, G.; Jacob, S.; Featherstone, C.; Barton, M. The role of radiotherapy in cancer treatment: Estimating optimal utilization from a review of evidence-based clinical guidelines. *Cancer* 2005, *104*, 1129–1137. [CrossRef] [PubMed]
2. Brower, C.; Rehani, M.M. Radiation risk issues in recurrent imaging. *Br. J. Radiol.* 2021, *94*, 20210389. [CrossRef] [PubMed]
3. Hill, K.D.; Frush, D.P.; Han, B.K.; Abbott, B.G.; Armstrong, A.K.; DeKemp, R.A.; Glatz, A.C.; Greenberg, S.B.; Herbert, A.S.; Justino, H.; et al. Radiation Safety in Children with Congenital and Acquired Heart Disease: A Scientific Position Statement on Multimodality Dose Optimization from the Image Gently Alliance. *JACC Cardiovasc. Imaging* 2017, *10*, 797–818. [CrossRef] [PubMed]
4. Andreassi, M.G.; Picano, E. Reduction of radiation to children: Our responsibility to change. *Circulation* 2014, *130*, 135–137. [CrossRef]
5. Hauptmann, M.; Daniels, R.D.; Cardis, E.; Cullings, H.M.; Kendall, G.; Laurier, D.; Linet, M.S.; Little, M.P.; Lubin, J.H.; Preston, D.L.; et al. Epidemiological Studies of Low-Dose Ionizing Radiation and Cancer: Summary Bias Assessment and Meta-Analysis. *J. Natl. Cancer Inst. Monogr.* 2020, *2020*, 188–200. [CrossRef]
6. Pettorini, B.L.; Park, Y.S.; Caldarelli, M.; Massimi, L.; Tamburrini, G.; Di Rocco, C. Radiation-induced brain tumours after central nervous system irradiation in childhood: A review. *Childs Nerv. Syst.* 2008, *24*, 793–805. [CrossRef]
7. Zahnreich, S.; Schmidberger, H. Childhood Cancer: Occurrence, Treatment and Risk of Second Primary Malignancies. *Cancers* 2021, *13*, 2607. [CrossRef]
8. Kreuzer, M.; Bouffler, S. Guest editorial: Non-cancer effects of ionizing radiation—Clinical implications, epidemiological and mechanistic evidence and research gaps. *Environ. Int.* 2021, *149*, 106286. [CrossRef]
9. El-Fayech, C.; Haddy, N.; Allodji, R.S.; Veres, C.; Diop, F.; Kahlouche, A.; Llanas, D.; Jackson, A.; Rubino, C.; Guibout, C.; et al. Cerebrovascular Diseases in Childhood Cancer Survivors: Role of the Radiation Dose to Willis Circle Arteries. *Int. J. Radiat. Oncol. Biol. Phys.* 2017, *97*, 278–286. [CrossRef]
10. Haddy, N.; Mousannif, A.; Tukenova, M.; Guibout, C.; Grill, J.; Dhermain, F.; Pacquement, H.; Oberlin, O.; El-Fayech, C.; Rubino, C.; et al. Relationship between the brain radiation dose for the treatment of childhood cancer and the risk of long-term cerebrovascular mortality. *Brain* 2011, *134*, 1362–1372. [CrossRef]
11. Darby, S.C.; Ewertz, M.; McGale, P.; Bennet, A.M.; Blom-Goldman, U.; Bronnum, D.; Correa, C.; Cutter, D.; Gagliardi, G.; Gigante, B.; et al. Risk of ischemic heart disease in women after radiotherapy for breast cancer. *N. Engl. J. Med.* 2013, *368*, 987–998. [CrossRef]
12. Haddy, N.; Diallo, S.; El-Fayech, C.; Schwartz, B.; Pein, F.; Hawkins, M.; Veres, C.; Oberlin, O.; Guibout, C.; Pacquement, H.; et al. Cardiac Diseases Following Childhood Cancer Treatment: Cohort Study. *Circulation* 2016, *133*, 31–38. [CrossRef]
13. Cohen, S.; Liu, A.; Gurvitz, M.; Guo, L.; Therrien, J.; Laprise, C.; Kaufman, J.S.; Abrahamowicz, M.; Marelli, A.J. Exposure to Low-Dose Ionizing Radiation from Cardiac Procedures and Malignancy Risk in Adults with Congenital Heart Disease. *Circulation* 2018, *137*, 1334–1345. [CrossRef]
14. Abalo, K.D.; Malekzadeh-Milani, S.; Hascoet, S.; Dreuil, S.; Feuillet, T.; Cohen, S.; Dauphin, C.; Filippo, S.D.; Douchin, S.; Godart, F.; et al. Exposure to low-dose ionising radiation from cardiac catheterisation and risk of cancer: The COCCINELLE study cohort profile. *BMJ. Open* 2021, *11*, e048576. [CrossRef]
15. Lang, N.N.; Walker, N.L. Adult Congenital Heart Disease and Radiation Exposure: The Malignant Price of Cardiac Care. *Circulation* 2018, *137*, 1346–1348. [CrossRef]
16. Foffa, I.; Cresci, M.; Andreassi, M.G. Health risk and biological effects of cardiac ionising imaging: From epidemiology to genes. *Int. J. Environ. Res. Public Health* 2009, *6*, 1882–1893. [CrossRef]
17. Pernot, E.; Hall, J.; Baatout, S.; Benotmane, M.A.; Blanchardon, E.; Bouffler, S.; El Saghire, H.; Gomolka, M.; Guertler, A.; Harms-Ringdahl, M.; et al. Ionizing radiation biomarkers for potential use in epidemiological studies. *Mutat. Res.* 2012, *751*, 258–286. [CrossRef]
18. Averbeck, D.; Candeias, S.; Chandna, S.; Foray, N.; Friedl, A.A.; Haghdoost, S.; Jeggo, P.A.; Lumniczky, K.; Paris, F.; Quintens, R.; et al. Establishing mechanisms affecting the individual response to ionizing radiation. *Int. J. Radiat. Biol.* 2020, *96*, 297–323. [CrossRef]
19. Haghdoost, S.; Czene, S.; Naslund, I.; Skog, S.; Harms-Ringdahl, M. Extracellular 8-oxo-dG as a sensitive parameter for oxidative stress in vivo and in vitro. *Free Radic. Res.* 2005, *39*, 153–162. [CrossRef]
20. Haghdoost, S.; Svoboda, P.; Naslund, I.; Harms-Ringdahl, M.; Tilikides, A.; Skog, S. Can 8-oxo-dG be used as a predictor for individual radiosensitivity? *Int. J. Radiat. Oncol. Biol. Phys.* 2001, *50*, 405–410. [CrossRef]
21. Valavanidis, A.; Vlachogianni, T.; Fiotakis, C. 8-hydroxy-2′-deoxyguanosine (8-OHdG): A critical biomarker of oxidative stress and carcinogenesis. *J. Environ. Sci. Health C Environ. Carcinog. Ecotoxicol. Rev.* 2009, *27*, 120–139. [CrossRef] [PubMed]
22. Ebrahimian, T.; Le Gallic, C.; Stefani, J.; Dublineau, I.; Yentrapalli, R.; Harms-Ringdahl, M.; Haghdoost, S. Chronic Gamma-Irradiation Induces a Dose-Rate-Dependent Pro-inflammatory Response and Associated Loss of Function in Human Umbilical Vein Endothelial Cells. *Radiat. Res.* 2015, *183*, 447–454. [CrossRef] [PubMed]
23. Halle, M.; Gabrielsen, A.; Paulsson-Berne, G.; Gahm, C.; Agardh, H.E.; Farnebo, F.; Tornvall, P. Sustained inflammation due to nuclear factor-kappa B activation in irradiated human arteries. *J. Am. Coll. Cardiol.* 2010, *55*, 1227–1236. [CrossRef] [PubMed]
24. Ma, H.; Zhou, Z.; Wei, S.; Liu, Z.; Pooley, K.A.; Dunning, A.M.; Svenson, U.; Roos, G.; Hosgood, H.D.; Shen, M.; et al. Shortened telomere length is associated with increased risk of cancer: A meta-analysis. *PLoS ONE* 2011, *6*, e20466. [CrossRef]

25. Vecoli, C.; Borghini, A.; Foffa, I.; Ait-Ali, L.; Picano, E.; Andreassi, M.G. Leukocyte telomere shortening in grown-up patients with congenital heart disease. *Int. J. Cardiol.* **2016**, *204*, 17–22. [CrossRef]
26. Borghini, A.; Vecoli, C.; Piccaluga, E.; Guagliumi, G.; Picano, E.; Andreassi, M.G. Increased mitochondrial DNA 4977-bp deletion in catheterization laboratory workers with long-term low-dose exposure to ionizing radiation. *Eur. J. Prev. Cardiol.* **2019**, *26*, 976–984. [CrossRef]
27. Hu, L.; Yao, X.; Shen, Y. Altered mitochondrial DNA copy number contributes to human cancer risk: Evidence from an updated meta-analysis. *Sci. Rep.* **2016**, *6*, 35859. [CrossRef]
28. Kam, W.W.; Banati, R.B. Effects of ionizing radiation on mitochondria. *Free Radic. Biol. Med.* **2013**, *65*, 607–619. [CrossRef]
29. Campa, D.; Barrdahl, M.; Santoro, A.; Severi, G.; Baglietto, L.; Omichessan, H.; Tumino, R.; Bueno-de-Mesquita, H.B.A.; Peeters, P.H.; Weiderpass, E.; et al. Mitochondrial DNA copy number variation, leukocyte telomere length, and breast cancer risk in the European Prospective Investigation into Cancer and Nutrition (EPIC) study. *Breast Cancer Res.* **2018**, *20*, 29. [CrossRef]
30. Assarsson, E.; Lundberg, M.; Holmquist, G.; Björkesten, J.; Thorsen, S.B.; Ekman, D.; Eriksson, A.; Rennel Dickens, E.; Ohlsson, S.; Edfeldt, G.; et al. Homogenous 96-plex pea immunoassay exhibiting high sensitivity, specificity, and excellent scalability. *PLoS ONE* **2014**, *9*, e95192. [CrossRef]
31. Troncale, S.; Barbet, A.; Coulibaly, L.; Henry, E.; He, B.; Barillot, E.; Dubois, T.; Hupé, P.; de Koning, L. NormaCurve: A SuperCurve-based method that simultaneously quantifies and normalizes reverse phase protein array data. *PLoS ONE* **2012**, *7*, e38686. [CrossRef]
32. Borghini, A.; Vecoli, C.; Mercuri, A.; Carpeggiani, C.; Piccaluga, E.; Guagliumi, G.; Picano, E.; Andreassi, M.G. Low-Dose Exposure to Ionizing Radiation Deregulates the Brain-Specific MicroRNA-134 in Interventional Cardiologists. *Circulation* **2017**, *136*, 2516–2518. [CrossRef]
33. Harbron, R.W.; Thierry-Chef, I.; Pearce, M.S.; Bernier, M.O.; Dreuil, S.; Rage, E.; Andreassi, M.G.; Picano, E.; Dreger, S.; Zeeb, H.; et al. The HARMONIC project: Study design for the assessment of radiation doses and associated cancer risks following cardiac fluoroscopy in childhood. *J. Radiol. Prot.* **2020**, *40*, 1074.
34. De Saint-Hubert, M.; Verbeek, N.; Baumer, C.; Esser, J.; Wulff, J.; Nabha, R.; Van Hoey, O.; Dabin, J.; Stuckmann, F.; Vasi, F.; et al. Validation of a Monte Carlo Framework for Out-of-Field Dose Calculations in Proton Therapy. *Front. Oncol.* **2022**, *12*, 882489. [CrossRef]
35. De Saint-Hubert, M.; Suesselbeck, F.; Vasi, F.; Stuckmann, F.; Rodriguez, M.; Dabin, J.; Timmermann, B.; Thierry-Chef, I.; Schneider, U.; Brualla, L. Experimental Validation of an Analytical Program and a Monte Carlo Simulation for the Computation of the Far Out-of-Field Dose in External Beam Photon Therapy Applied to Pediatric Patients. *Front. Oncol.* **2022**, *12*, 882506. [CrossRef]
36. Ding, G.X.; Alaei, P.; Curran, B.; Flynn, R.; Gossman, M.; Mackie, T.R.; Miften, M.; Morin, R.; Xu, X.G.; Zhu, T.C. Image guidance doses delivered during radiotherapy: Quantification, management, and reduction: Report of the AAPM Therapy Physics Committee Task Group 180. *Med. Phys.* **2018**, *45*, e84–e99. [CrossRef]
37. McFadden, S.L.; Hughes, C.M.; Mooney, R.B.; Winder, R.J. An analysis of radiation dose reduction in paediatric interventional cardiology by altering frame rate and use of the anti-scatter grid. *J. Radiol. Prot.* **2013**, *33*, 433–443. [CrossRef]
38. Reisz, J.A.; Bansal, N.; Qian, J.; Zhao, W.; Furdui, C.M. Effects of ionizing radiation on biological molecules-mechanisms of damage and emerging methods of detection. *Antioxid. Redox. Signal.* **2014**, *21*, 260–292. [CrossRef]
39. Hall, J.; Jeggo, P.A.; West, C.; Gomolka, M.; Quintens, R.; Badie, C.; Laurent, O.; Aerts, A.; Anastasov, N.; Azimzadeh, O.; et al. Ionizing radiation biomarkers in epidemiological studies—An update. *Mutat. Res. Rev. Mutat. Res.* **2017**, *771*, 59–84. [CrossRef]
40. Pfaffe, T.; Cooper-White, J.; Beyerlein, P.; Kostner, K.; Punyadeera, C. Diagnostic potential of saliva: Current state and future applications. *Clin. Chem.* **2011**, *57*, 675–687. [CrossRef]
41. Michalke, B.; Rossbach, B.; Goen, T.; Schaferhenrich, A.; Scherer, G. Saliva as a matrix for human biomonitoring in occupational and environmental medicine. *Int. Arch. Occup. Environ. Health* **2015**, *88*, 1–44. [CrossRef] [PubMed]

Disclaimer/Publisher's Note: The statements, opinions and data contained in all publications are solely those of the individual author(s) and contributor(s) and not of MDPI and/or the editor(s). MDPI and/or the editor(s) disclaim responsibility for any injury to people or property resulting from any ideas, methods, instructions or products referred to in the content.

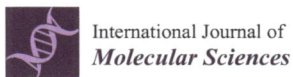

Article

The miRNA Content of Bone Marrow-Derived Extracellular Vesicles Contributes to Protein Pathway Alterations Involved in Ionising Radiation-Induced Bystander Responses

Ilona Barbara Csordás [1,2,†], Eric Andreas Rutten [3,†], Tünde Szatmári [1], Prabal Subedi [4,5], Lourdes Cruz-Garcia [3], Dávid Kis [1,2], Bálint Jezsó [6,7], Christine von Toerne [8], Martina Forgács [1], Géza Sáfrány [1], Soile Tapio [4], Christophe Badie [3] and Katalin Lumniczky [1,*]

1. Unit of Radiation Medicine, Department of Radiobiology and Radiohygiene, National Public Health Centre, 1097 Budapest, Hungary; csordas.ilona@nnk.gov.hu (I.B.C.); szatmari.tunde@nnk.gov.hu (T.S.); kisd@osski.hu (D.K.); forgacs.martina@nnk.gov.hu (M.F.); safrany.geza@nnk.gov.hu (G.S.)
2. Doctoral School of Pathological Sciences, Semmelweis University, 1085 Budapest, Hungary
3. Centre for Radiation, Chemical and Environmental Hazards, UK Health Security Agency, Chilton, Didcot OX11 0RQ, UK; eric.andreasrutten@ukhsa.gov.uk (E.A.R.); lourdes.cruzgarcia@ukhsa.gov.uk (L.C.-G.); christophe.badie@ukhsa.gov.uk (C.B.)
4. Helmholtz Zentrum München, German Research Center for Environmental Health GmbH (HMGU), 80939 München, Germany; psubedi@bfs.de (P.S.)
5. Federal Office for Radiation Protection (BfS), 85764 Oberschleissheim, Germany
6. Doctoral School of Biology, Institute of Biology, Eötvös Loránd University, 1053 Budapest, Hungary; jezso.balint@ttk.elte.hu
7. Research Centre for Natural Sciences, Institute of Enzymology, 1117 Budapest, Hungary
8. Metabolomics and Proteomics Core, Helmholtz Zentrum München, German Research Center for Environmental Health GmbH (HMGU), 80939 München, Germany; vontoerne@helmholtz-muenchen.de
* Correspondence: lumniczky.katalin@nnk.gov.hu or lumniczky.katalin@osski.hu; Tel.: +36-30-5549308
† These authors contributed equally to this work.

Abstract: Extracellular vesicles (EVs), through their cargo, are important mediators of bystander responses in the irradiated bone marrow (BM). MiRNAs carried by EVs can potentially alter cellular pathways in EV-recipient cells by regulating their protein content. Using the CBA/Ca mouse model, we characterised the miRNA content of BM-derived EVs from mice irradiated with 0.1 Gy or 3 Gy using an nCounter analysis system. We also analysed proteomic changes in BM cells either directly irradiated or treated with EVs derived from the BM of irradiated mice. Our aim was to identify key cellular processes in the EV-acceptor cells regulated by miRNAs. The irradiation of BM cells with 0.1 Gy led to protein alterations involved in oxidative stress and immune and inflammatory processes. Oxidative stress-related pathways were also present in BM cells treated with EVs isolated from 0.1 Gy-irradiated mice, indicating the propagation of oxidative stress in a bystander manner. The irradiation of BM cells with 3 Gy led to protein pathway alterations involved in the DNA damage response, metabolism, cell death and immune and inflammatory processes. The majority of these pathways were also altered in BM cells treated with EVs from mice irradiated with 3 Gy. Certain pathways (cell cycle, acute and chronic myeloid leukaemia) regulated by miRNAs differentially expressed in EVs isolated from mice irradiated with 3 Gy overlapped with protein pathway alterations in BM cells treated with 3 Gy EVs. Six miRNAs were involved in these common pathways interacting with 11 proteins, suggesting the involvement of miRNAs in the EV-mediated bystander processes. In conclusion, we characterised proteomic changes in directly irradiated and EV-treated BM cells, identified processes transmitted in a bystander manner and suggested miRNA and protein candidates potentially involved in the regulation of these bystander processes.

Keywords: bone marrow; ionising radiation; extracellular vesicles; miRNA content; proteome; pathway analysis; bystander effects

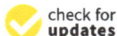

Citation: Csordás, I.B.; Rutten, E.A.; Szatmári, T.; Subedi, P.; Cruz-Garcia, L.; Kis, D.; Jezsó, B.; Toerne, C.v.; Forgács, M.; Sáfrány, G.; et al. The miRNA Content of Bone Marrow-Derived Extracellular Vesicles Contributes to Protein Pathway Alterations Involved in Ionising Radiation-Induced Bystander Responses. *Int. J. Mol. Sci.* **2023**, *24*, 8607. https://doi.org/10.3390/ijms24108607

Academic Editor: François Chevalier

Received: 19 April 2023
Revised: 4 May 2023
Accepted: 7 May 2023
Published: 11 May 2023

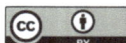

Copyright: © 2023 by the authors. Licensee MDPI, Basel, Switzerland. This article is an open access article distributed under the terms and conditions of the Creative Commons Attribution (CC BY) license (https://creativecommons.org/licenses/by/4.0/).

1. Introduction

Extracellular vesicles (EVs) are a heterogeneous class of nanoscale particles excreted by most cell types both under physiological and pathological conditions and under stress, and they serve primarily as intercellular communication vectors [1]. EVs include apoptotic bodies, microvesicles and exosomes, which are distinguished not primarily by size but by the method of biogenesis [2]. They shuttle several different kinds of cargo between cells, including lipids, proteins, DNA (DNA), mRNA, long non-coding RNA (lncRNA), and miRNA [3].

Apart from its cytotoxic and mutagenic effects, ionising radiation (IR) induces cellular stress and activates intercellular signalling mechanisms through which radiation damage can be transmitted in a bystander manner to cells not directly irradiated. This process is called the radiation-induced bystander effect, and it is a major mechanism through which tissue and systemic responses are elicited after local radiation damage [4–6]. Signals transmitted by chemokines, cytokines, small metabolites and various danger signal molecules released in the extracellular space play important roles in radiation-induced bystander responses. Given the complexity of bystander effects, it is less probable that single molecules mediate this response. EVs, with their complex cargo, are major candidates for mediating radiation-induced bystander responses, and several in vitro and in vivo studies actually proved the role of EVs in this process [7–10].

The role of bystander signalling is especially relevant in organs in which intercellular communication is a major element of proper organ functioning. Within the bone marrow (BM), interactions among the different stem and progenitor cells as well as the BM stroma are indispensable for normal haematopoiesis. In addition, BM is a particularly radiosensitive organ prone to the development of both IR-induced acute deterministic effects (acute BM damage) and late stochastic effects (radiation-induced leukaemia). EVs are known to play a major role in the communication with the BM microenvironment, being involved in the regulation of stem cell renewal, differentiation, proliferation and mobilisation [11,12].

Previously, we developed an in vivo model to study the role of EVs in mediating IR-induced bystander responses by injecting BM-derived EVs from irradiated into naïve, non-irradiated mice. We investigated local effects in the BM [9,10] and systemic effects in the blood and spleen [7,10,13]. In these studies, we showed that BM-derived EVs (1) induced changes in the pool of several of the BM haematopoietic and spleen immune cell subpopulations which mimicked direct irradiation effects; (2) induced DNA damage and apoptosis similarly to direct irradiation; (3) led to changes in several plasma protein levels involved in the inflammation and immune response, which were very similar to the effects observed after direct irradiation and (4) led to an increased oxidative stress. We also demonstrated that only EVs originating from the BM of acutely irradiated mice were able to initiate bystander responses, and these responses were long-lasting [9]. In the present study, we used a mouse model prone to radiation-induced leukaemia. We characterised IR-induced changes in the miRNA content of EVs and miRNA-regulated pathways as well as the proteome and related pathways of BM cells (BMC) treated with EVs from irradiated mice. By comparing pathways regulated by the differentially expressed miRNAs in the EVs with protein pathways altered in BMCs treated with EVs from irradiated mice, we identified miRNA candidates involved in bystander signalling in EV-recipient BMCs. The main steps of the workflow are presented in Figure 1.

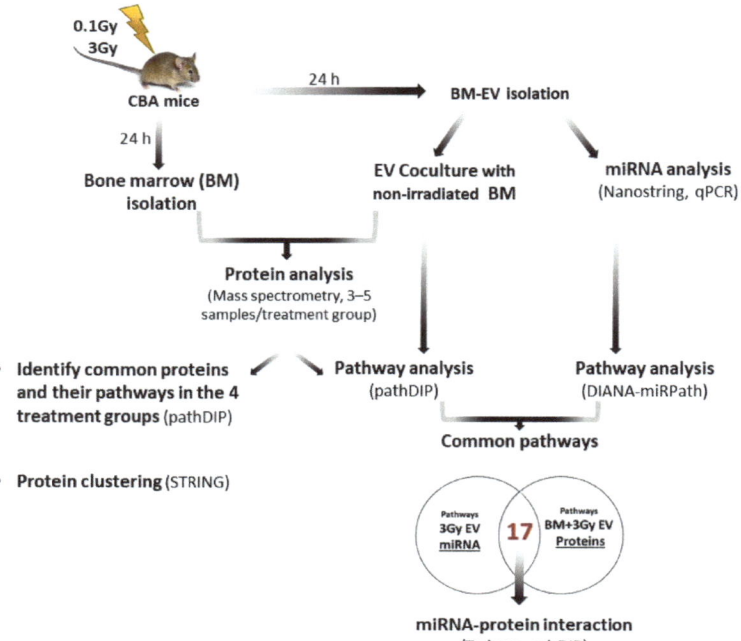

Figure 1. Schematic figure of the workflow. EV characterization is shown in Figure 2, EV uptake upon EV and BMC coculture is shown in Figure 5. Results of the miRNA expression analysis are shown in Figures 3 and 4 and Table 1. Summary of mass spectrometric results are presented in Figure 6. Results of miRNA and protein pathway analysis alongside with protein clustering results are shown in Figure 7. miRNA and protein interaction results are presented in Figures 8–10.

To simplify the terminology within the manuscript, we will use the following terms: EVs will refer to BM-derived EVs, since BM was the only source of EV isolation in the present study. Control EVs will refer to EVs isolated from the BM of control, sham-irradiated mice and, consecutively, 0.1 Gy and 3 Gy EVs will refer to EVs isolated from the BM of mice irradiated with either 0.1 Gy or 3 Gy.

2. Results

BM-derived EVs were isolated from the BM supernatant of total body-irradiated CBA/CA mice and characterised as described [14]. The electron microscopic characterisation of EV morphology and size indicated typical EV structures, while EV-specific proteins were identified by Western blotting (Figure 2A,B). The average particle size measured with TRPS was 150 nm, with no significant differences between EVs from control or irradiated mice (Figure 2C).

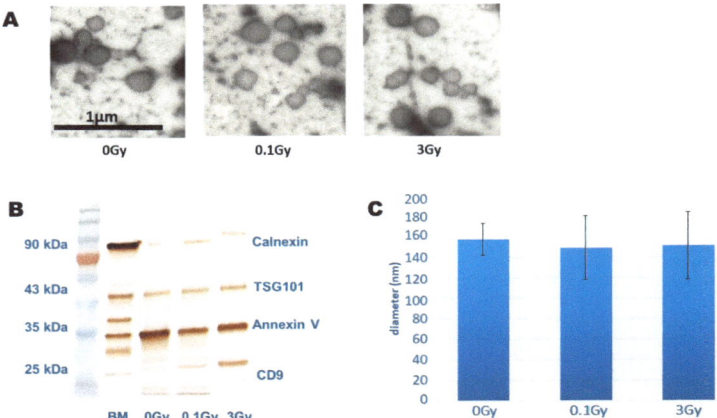

Figure 2. Characterisation of Bone Marrow-Derived Extracellular Vesicles. (**A**) Representative transmission electron microscopy images of extracellular vesicles isolated from the bone marrow of mice irradiated with the indicated doses of ionising radiation. (**B**) Representative Western blot analysis of whole cell lysates and extracellular vesicles isolated from the bone marrow of mice irradiated with the indicated doses of ionising radiation. Lane 1: protein ladder, lane 2: bone marrow whole cell lysate, lane 3–5: extracellular vesicle sample from control, nonirradiated, 0.1 Gy- and 3 Gy-irradiated mice. (**C**) Size of extracellular vesicle suspensions was examined by tunable resistance pulse sensing using an NP150 nanopore (measurement range: 70–420 nm). Mean values of extracellular vesicle size are shown, with bars representing standard deviations (SD). n = 3.

2.1. The miRNA Cargo of BM-Derived EVs Shows a Dose-Dependent Response to IR

The total RNA extracted from control, 0.1 Gy and 3 Gy EVs from three independent experiments was run in an nCounter panel which included probes to identify 800 different murine miRNAs. Analysis performed with the DIANA Tools, mirExTra2.0 software indicated that the level of two miRNAs (mmu-miR-761 and mmu-miR-129-5p) was increased in 0.1 Gy EVs compared to in EVs from controls (Supplementary Table S1). Pathway analysis based on the KEGG database using the Diana Tools miR path software identified two significantly altered pathways (TGF-beta signalling pathway and Signalling pathways regulating pluripotency of stem cells) relevant for the radiation response in the BM (Supplementary Table S2).

In the 3 Gy EVs, 17 miRNAs were differentially expressed; two of them (mmu-miR-709 and mmu-miR-706) had decreased levels, while the others had increased levels (Supplementary Table S1). The two miRNAs with increased levels in 0.1 Gy EVs were also increased in 3 Gy EVs. Both miRNAs were present at higher levels in 3 Gy EVs than in 0.1 Gy EVs, suggesting dose-dependent alteration. No EV-derived miRNAs unique for low doses were identified. Pathway analysis revealed 34 significantly altered pathways potentially regulated by the 17 differentially expressed miRNAs in 3 Gy EVs (Supplementary Table S2). The majority of the pathways were linked to cancer (29%), signal transduction (26%) and cellular processes (15%). Pathways relevant for BM functioning (signalling pathways regulating pluripotency of stem cells, acute myeloid leukaemia, chronic myeloid leukaemia) were among the significantly altered pathways.

Clustering analysis performed with the BRB array tool showed clear up- and down-regulated clusters of miRNAs, which also included the miRNAs identified using Diana tools software (Figure 3A,B). Dose correlation analysis identified 13 miRNAs that showed a strong dose-response (Table 1), with correlation coefficients between 0.95 and 0.84.

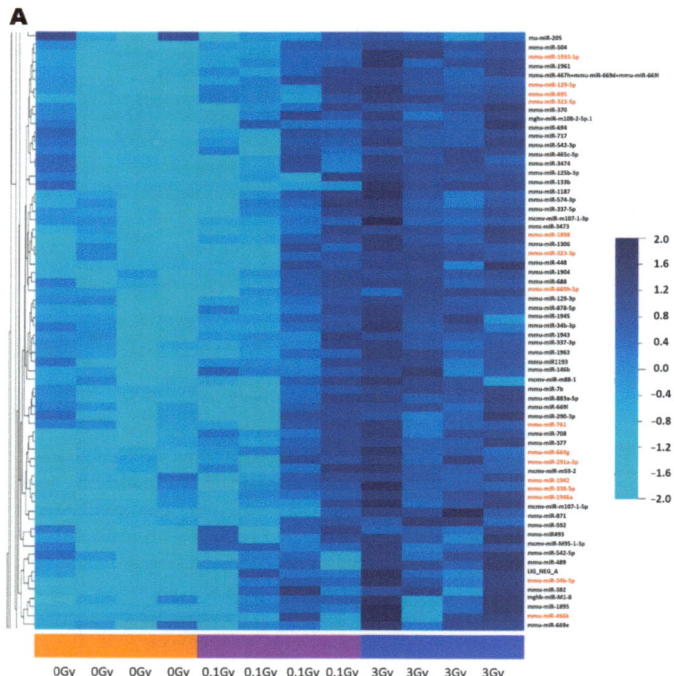

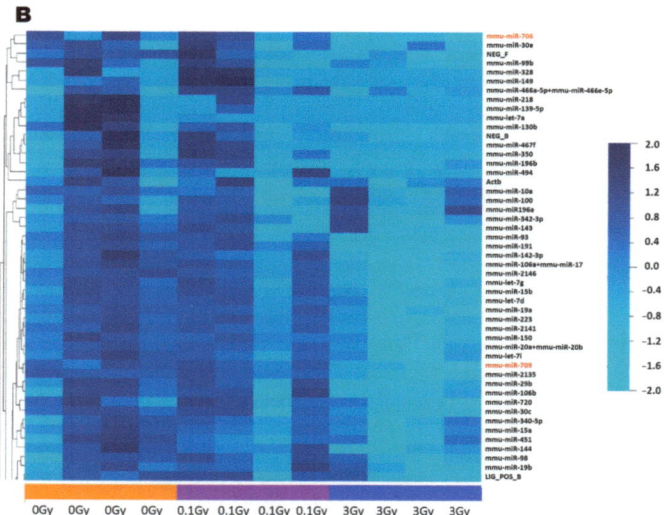

Figure 3. Based on clustering and dose correlation analysis, miRNAs from the bone marrow-derived extracellular vesicles of mice irradiated with 0.1 Gy and 3 Gy correlate with the dose. Heatmap and cluster dendrogram showing (**A**) a cluster of upregulated miRNAs and (**B**) a cluster of downregulated miRNAs from bone marrow extracellular vesicles of mice irradiated with 0.1 Gy and 3 Gy. MiRNAs highlighted in red are those miRNAs that were identified by Diana tools mirExTra 2.0. as significantly up- or downregulated. Clustering and dose correlation analysis was performed with the BRB array tools.

Table 1. MiRNAs correlating with the dose. Dose correlation analysis was performed with the BRB array tools. Correlations were considered at the nominal 0.001 level of the univariate test.

Correlation Coefficient	Parametric *p*-Value	FDR	miRNA Name
0.953	$<1 \times 10^{-7}$	$<1 \times 10^{-7}$	mmu-miR-323-5p
0.888	9.17×10^{-5}	0.00592	mmu-miR-1933-5p
0.888	9.17×10^{-5}	0.00592	mmu-miR-1961
0.888	9.17×10^{-5}	0.00592	mmu-miR-338-5p
0.888	9.17×10^{-5}	0.00592	mmu-miR-504
0.884	0.0001922	0.0103	mcmv-miR-m107-1-5p
0.875	0.0003089	0.0125	mmu-miR-290-5p
0.874	0.0003089	0.0125	mmu-miR-708
0.857	0.0005971	0.0161	mmu-miR-181c
−0.857	0.0005971	0.0161	mmu-miR-2146
0.859	0.0005971	0.0161	mmu-miR-467h + mmu-miR-669d + mmu-miR-669l
0.857	0.0005971	0.0161	mmu-miR-669j
−0.843	0.0009695	0.0222	mmu-miR-93

QRT-PCR measurements confirmed nCounter results for the downregulated miRNAs in the EVs identified by the DIANA Tools and mirExTra and also for most of the miRNAs correlating with the dose (based on BRB array analysis), though a dose–response relationship could not be identified for all miRNAs (Figure 4). Significant changes in miRNA levels were detected mostly after irradiation with 3 Gy (mmu-miR-669d-5p, mmu-miR-93-5p, mmu-miR-467h, mmu-miR-706, mmu-miR-1933-5p, mmu-miR-181c-5p, mmu-miR-338-5p), while 0.1 Gy induced significant changes only in two cases (mmu-miR-1933 and mmu-mi-34b-5p). Three miRNAs, which showed a positive dose correlation based on BRB array analysis, correlated negatively with the dose after qRT-PCR (mmu-miR-669d-5p, mmu-miR-504-5p and mmu-miR-467h). However, we have to point out that the nCounter system used the same ID for the identification of both mmu-miR-669d-5p and mmu-miR-467h, while individual miRNA-specific primers were used in the qRT-PCR reaction. Mmu-miR-34b-5p showed a positive dose correlation based on BRB array analysis, while qRT-PCR indicated an inverse dose relationship (decreased miRNA level after 0.1 Gy and enrichment after 3 Gy). For three miRNAs (miR-708-5p, mmu-miR-761 and miR-129-5p), we could not confirm any significant dose correlation with qRT-PCR (Figure 4).

2.2. Proteomic Changes in BMCs Treated with BM-Derived EVs from Irradiated Mice Indicate Partially Distinct Pathway Alterations to Directly Irradiated BMCs

Proteomic changes in BMCs treated with BM-derived EVs from irradiated mice have been compared to the proteome of directly irradiated BMCs. The ex vivo incubation of BMCs with fluorescently labelled EVs indicated that the rate of EV uptake was around 80%, with no significant difference in EV uptake if EVs originated from the BM of irradiated or control mice (Figure 5).

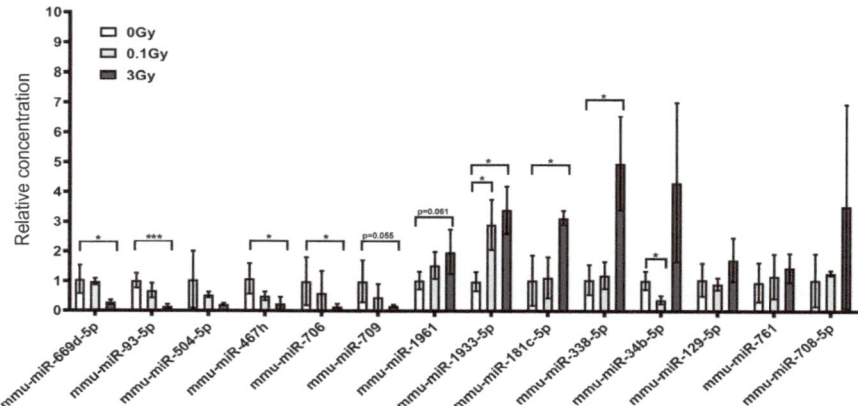

Figure 4. Ionising radiation influences the miRNA content of bone marrow-derived extracellular vesicles in irradiated mice. Extracellular vesicles were isolated from the bone marrow of control and irradiated mice, miRNAs were purified from the extracellular vesicles and the relative concentration of miRNAs was measured by qRT-PCR, as described in the Materials and Methods section. n = 3; Significant changes are indicated with * $p < 0.05$ and *** $p < 0.001$.

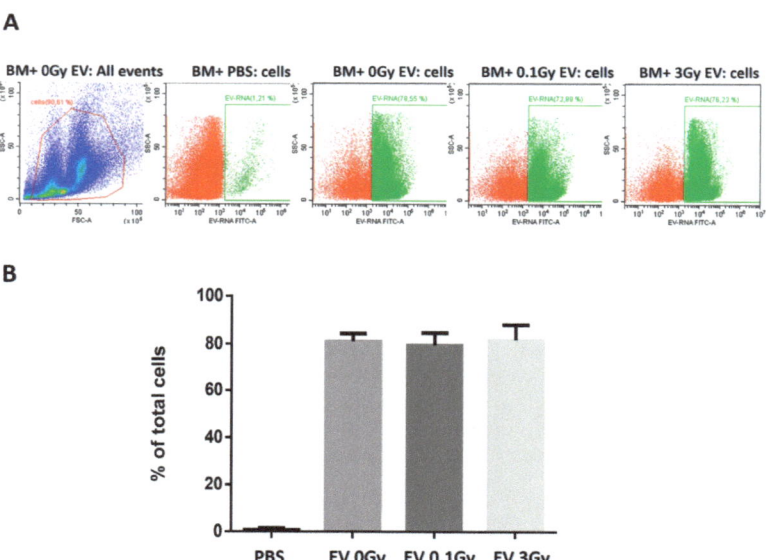

Figure 5. Irradiation does not influence the extracellular vesicle uptake by bone marrow cells. Bone marrow cells from control, non-irradiated mice were co-cultured in vitro with fluorescently labelled bone marrow-derived extracellular vesicles isolated from control, 0.1 Gy- and 3 Gy-irradiated mice, and the uptake rate was determined by flow cytometry, as described in Materials and Methods. (**A**) Flow cytometry blots showing the representative uptake rates of extracellular vesicles by bone marrow cells. Green colour indicates cells with EV uptake, red colour indicates cells without EV uptake. (**B**) The percentage of bone marrow cells taking up extracellular vesicles. n = 3. Error bars represent standard deviation (SD).

Proteomic changes were investigated in ex vivo cultured murine BMCs either non-irradiated (0 Gy or control), irradiated with 0.1 Gy or 3 Gy X-Rays or treated with BM-derived EVs isolated from mice irradiated with the same doses (0 Gy, 0.1 Gy or 3 Gy). A total of 3718 proteins were identified in the BMCs, among which 2707 proteins were qualified for further studies according to the selection criteria (FDR < 1% and identified with at least two unique peptides). Principal component analysis (PCA) and heat map clustering demonstrated that the 3 Gy group was the most different from all other experimental groups (Figure 6).

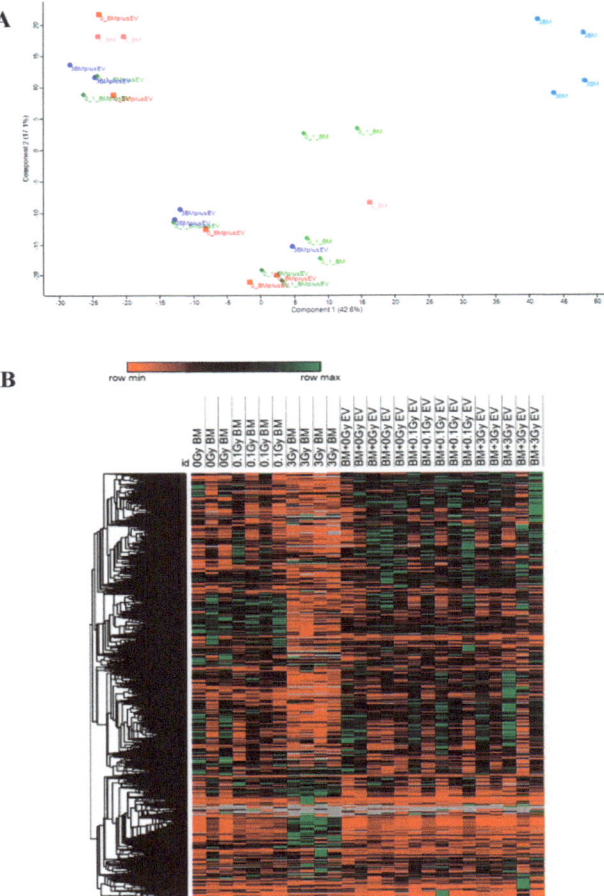

Figure 6. Irradiation of bone marrow cells with 3 Gy leads to a distinct proteomic pattern. (**A**) Principal component analysis was performed in Perseus software version 2.0.7.0. Proteome discoverer output with all proteins identified in all samples with more than two peptides was loaded. After log2 transformation, missing values were low-abundance-imputed according to program settings. Categorical annotations were added for experimental groups. Principal component analysis was performed using the standard settings of Perseus, displaying experimental groups. (**B**) Heatmap clustering. Proteins were characterised by hierarchical clustering (Euclidean distance algorithm and average distance method).

2.2.1. Proteomic Changes in Directly Irradiated BMCs

Irradiation with 0.1 Gy led to 142 deregulated (33 downregulated and 109 upregulated) proteins (Supplementary Table S3A, Figure 7A and Supplementary Figure S1A) compared to control samples. STRING clustering analysis indicated that the largest protein cluster included mitochondrial proteins involved in ATP synthesis and oxidative phosphorylation (Supplementary Table S7). Irradiation with 3 Gy led to 360 deregulated (236 downregulated and 124 upregulated) proteins in the BMCs (Supplementary Table S3B, Figure 7A and Supplementary Figure S1B) compared to control samples, which could be grouped into several clusters. One big cluster contained proteins involved in biological processes related to DNA repair, replication and DNA metabolism, stress response and metabolic pathways. A further cluster contained proteins involved in chromatin remodelling and histone proteins. Mitochondrial proteins involved in electron transport, oxidative phosphorylation and oxidation-reduction complexes constituted a third cluster (Supplementary Table S7). Seventy-two proteins were in common between BMCs irradiated with 0.1 Gy and 3 Gy. Changes in the expression of 35 proteins correlated with the dose, with 50% or higher difference in the protein abundance ratio between 0.1 Gy and 3 Gy samples (Figure 7A and Supplementary Table S3C; highlighted proteins indicate those correlating with the dose). Clustering analysis of the common proteins indicated that the largest protein clusters belonged to biological processes related to mitochondrial processes such as mitochondrial ATP synthesis and oxidative phosphorylation, as well as iron sulphur clusters (Figure 7B, Supplementary Table S7). The common proteins most significantly upregulated (highest abundance ratio and lowest p value) were putative transferase CAF17 homolog, mitochondrial (Iba57) and cysteine desulfurase mitochondrial (Nfs1) and also belonged to this cluster.

Based on pathway enrichment analysis using the PathDIP tool, deregulated proteins in BMCs irradiated with 0.1 Gy could be associated with 107 altered pathways (Supplementary Table S4A and Figure 7C). The vast majority of the deregulated pathways were associated with immune processes (15%), signal transduction (11%) as well as cancer (9%) and metabolism (9%, including oxidative phosphorylation and pyruvate metabolism); nevertheless, cell growth and death-related pathways were also deregulated (Figure 7D). In the BMCs irradiated with 3 Gy, the 360 altered proteins could be associated with 87 altered pathways (Supplementary Table S4B and Figure 7C). The highest number of altered pathways were related to metabolism (18%) and genetic information processing (17%). One-third of the pathways within genetic information processing were related to DNA damage and repair. Cancer-related pathways represented 10% of the total pathway alterations, including acute myeloid leukaemia. Immune-related and signal transduction pathways were also present but in lower percentages compared to BMCs irradiated with 0.1 Gy (Figure 7D).

Sixty-three pathways were in common between BMCs irradiated with 0.1 Gy and 3 Gy (Supplementary Table S4C and Figure 7C). Common pathways were related to metabolism (14%), cancer (11%), genetic information processing (11%), signal transduction (10%), the immune system (8%) and cell growth and death (Figure 7E).

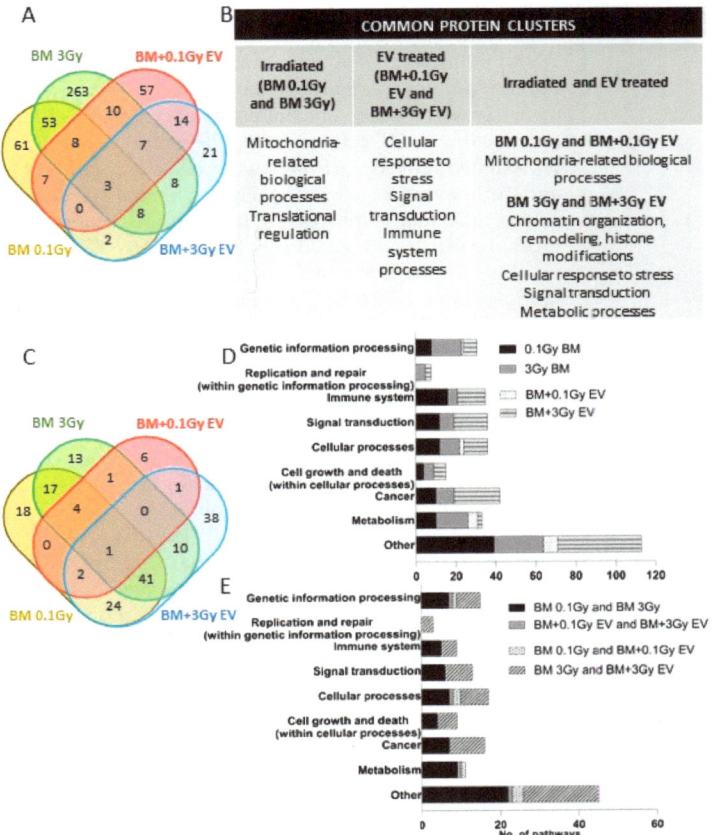

Figure 7. Significantly deregulated proteins and associated pathways in directly irradiated and extracellular vesicles-treated bone marrow cells. (**A**) Venn Diagram analysis of significantly deregulated proteins identified across all four treatment groups. (**B**) Common clusters formed by significantly deregulated proteins, as performed by STRING clustering analysis. (**C**) Venn diagram analysis of significant protein pathways. (**D**) Pathway distribution in the different treatment groups. (**E**) Pathway comparison between treatment groups. Pathway annotations and enrichment analysis were performed with the pathDIP database, integrating data from the KEGG database. BM: bone marrow; EV: extracellular vesicles.

2.2.2. Proteomic Changes in EV-Treated BMCs

The treatment of BMCs with 0.1 Gy EVs led to 106 deregulated (33 downregulated and 73 upregulated) proteins (Supplementary Table S5A, Figure 7A and Supplementary Figure S1C) compared to BMCs treated with control EVs, which could be clustered into several biological functions, out of which mitochondria-related biological processes (ATP synthesis, electron transport, oxidation-reduction), stress response, signal transduction and immune processes represented the largest clusters (Supplementary Table S7). Based on pathway enrichment analysis, the 106 proteins could be associated with 15 pathways (Supplementary Table S6A and Figure 7D), the majority of which were metabolism-related (Figure 7D). Treatment with 3 Gy EVs led to 63 deregulated (29 downregulated and 34 upregulated) proteins (Supplementary Table S5B, Figure 7A and Supplementary Figure S1D) compared to BMCs treated with control EVs. STRING clustering analysis indicated fewer protein clusters than in the other treatment groups, the largest clusters belonging to nuclear and nucleosomal proteins involved in chromatin organisation, the regulation of histone methylation and DNA binding as well as spliceosomal complex assembly, mRNA splicing and ribonucleoprotein complex assembly. Protein clusters involved in immune processes and metabolic processes were also present (Supplementary Table S7). The 63 deregulated proteins could be associated with 117 pathways (Supplementary Table S6B and Figure 7C). The most highly represented altered pathways were related to cancer (20%), signal transduction (16%) and the immune system (12%). Further altered pathways were endocrine system-related, genetic information processing including replication and repair and cellular processes including cell growth and death (Figure 7D).

Twenty-four proteins (Supplementary Table S5C and Figure 7A) and four pathways (Supplementary Table S6C and Figure 7C) were in common in BMCs treated with 0.1 Gy EVs and 3 Gy EVs, though common pathways could not be linked to either irradiation- or cancer- or BM damage-related processes (Figure 7E).

2.2.3. Comparison of Proteomic Changes between Directly Irradiated and EV-Treated BMCs

Next, we identified deregulated common proteins and pathways between directly irradiated and EV-treated BMCs. Eighteen proteins were common in BMCs irradiated with 0.1 Gy and treated with 0.1 Gy EVs, out of which eight (Carbonyl reductase NADPH1 (Cbr1), Cytochrome b-c1 complex subunit 6, mitochondrial (Uqcrh), RUN and FYVE domain-containing protein 1 (Rufy1), N-acetylglucosamine-1-phosphodiester alpha-N-acetylglucosaminidase (Nagpa), Mitochondrial 2-oxodicarboxylate carrier (Slc25a21), Thioredoxin domain-containing protein 5 (Txndc5), Enoyl-[acyl-carrier-protein] reductase, mitochondrial (Mecr) and Mitochondrial import inner membrane translocase subunit Tim8A (Timm8a1)) could be associated with redox and mitochondrial processes (Supplementary Table S8A and Figure 7A). Seven pathways were in common (Supplementary Table S8A and Figure 7C), out of which oxidative phosphorylation was the most significant and also the only relevant for IR-related processes.

Twenty-six common proteins and 52 common pathways could be identified between BMCs directly irradiated and treated with 3 Gy EVs (Supplementary Table S8B and Figure 7A). The 26 common proteins could not be grouped in big clusters; nevertheless, 3 common proteins (CD48 antigen (CD48), C-type lectin domain family 1 member B (Clec1b) and Integrin alpha-IIb (Itga2b)) were involved in platelet aggregation and activation, wound healing, cell adhesion and migration, 2 common proteins (p21-activated protein kinase-interacting protein 1 (Pak1ip1) and U4/U6 small nuclear ribonucleoprotein Prp31 (Prpf31)) were involved in spliceosomal complex assembly, mRNA splicing and ribonucleoprotein complex assembly, 2 proteins (Carbonyl reductase NADPH1 (Cbr1) and Carbonyl reductase NADPH2 (Cbr2)) were involved in NADPH activity and 2 other mitochondrial matrix proteins (Electron transfer flavoprotein-ubiquinone oxidoreductase, mitochondrial (Etfdh) and Propionyl-CoA carboxylase alpha chain, mitochondrial (Pcca)) were involved in propionyl-CoA carboxylase activity (Figure 7B). Pathway enrichment analysis indicated that out of the 52 common pathways, 17% were cancer-related, including acute myeloid leukaemia, 13% were signal transduction-related, 12% were related to genetic information processing, including replication and repair, 10% were linked to cell growth and death and 8% were linked to the immune system (Figure 7C,E).

2.3. Protein Pathways Regulated by EV-Containing miRNAs from Irradiated Mice Partially Overlap with Protein Pathways Altered in the EV-Treated BMCs

EV-derived miRNAs can potentially alter cellular pathways in EV-recipient cells by regulating their protein content. In order to identify those EV-derived miRNAs that are most probably involved in regulating cellular processes in the EV-recipient cells, we analysed overlaps in protein pathways predicted to be altered by EV-transmitted miRNAs and altered protein pathways based on proteomic data.

In 0.1 Gy EVs, two miRNAs had altered expression levels, which belonged to three pathways. BMCs treated with 0.1 Gy EVs led to 106 deregulated (up- or downregulated) proteins that could be linked to 15 pathways (Supplementary Tables S2 and S6A). The two pathway lists had no common elements; therefore, we assumed that EV-containing miRNAs after low-dose irradiation are not the major regulators of protein pathways in EV-acceptor BMCs.

The 17 miRNAs differentially expressed in 3 Gy EVs regulated 34 pathways. BMCs treated with 3 Gy EVs resulted in 63 (up- or downregulated) proteins which could be grouped in 117 pathways. Seventeen pathways were in common between miRNAs and proteins, and the vast majority of common pathways were cancer-related (59%) (Supplementary Table S9 and Figure 8). These findings suggested that miRNAs from 3 Gy EVs might have important roles in regulating protein pathways in EV-acceptor BMCs.

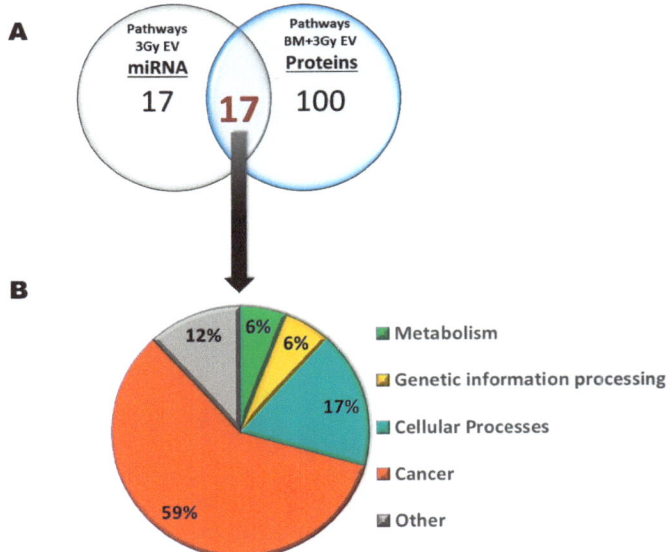

Figure 8. Common pathways between differentially expressed miRNAs from bone marrow-derived extracellular vesicles from mice irradiated with 3 Gy and deregulated proteins in bone marrow cells treated with bone marrow-derived extracellular vesicles of mice irradiated with 3 Gy. (**A**) Number of pathways; (**B**) Distribution of KEGG pathway classes.

In order to better characterise the interactions between EV-derived miRNAs and deregulated cellular proteins in the EV-acceptor BMCs, direct miRNA–protein interactions were analysed using the TARBASE database (for validated interactions) and the miRDB database (for predicted interactions). Out of the 17 miRNAs differentially expressed in the 3 Gy EVs, we identified those that could interact with at least one of the 63 deregulated proteins in the BMCs treated with 3 Gy EVs and found that 11 miRNAs could interact directly with 19 proteins. Nevertheless, only interactions between 6 miRNAs and 11 proteins were involved in the 17 altered pathways that were common between deregulated miRNAs in 3 Gy EVs and deregulated proteins in BMCs treated with 3 Gy EVs (Figure 9 and Supplementary Table S10). Alterations in the level of two highly significantly upregulated proteins ((Histone H2A.V (H2afv) and Cysteine protease ATG4B (Atg4b)) in the samples treated with 3 Gy EVs (for Atg4b $p = 4.51 \times 10^{-16}$ and for H2afv $p = 3.63 \times 10^{-5}$) and participating in validated interactions with miRNAs were investigated by Western blot analysis as well in order to confirm the proteomic data. The level of both proteins increased in the BMCs treated with 3 Gy EVs; nevertheless, changes were only significant for H2afv (Figure 10).

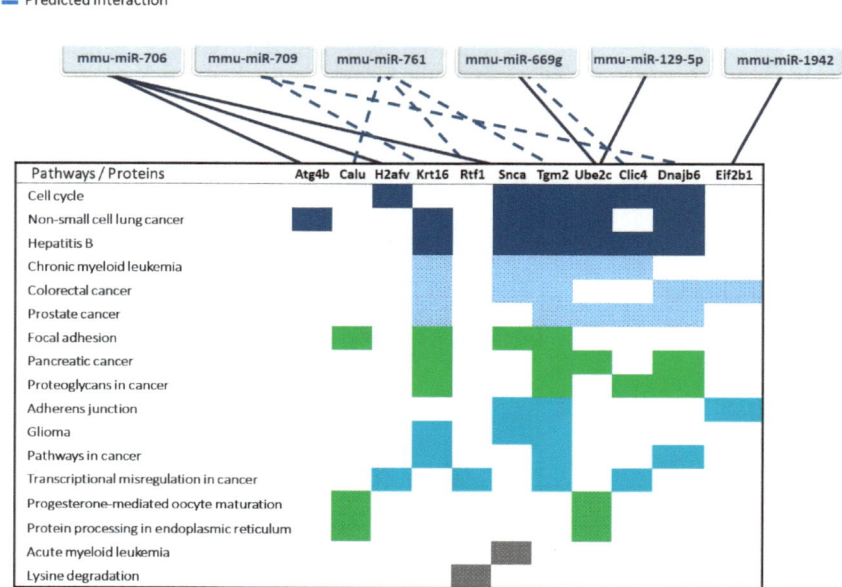

Figure 9. MiRNA–protein interactions involved in the common pathways between differentially expressed miRNAs from bone marrow-derived extracellular vesicles from mice irradiated with 3 Gy and deregulated proteins in bone marrow cells treated with bone marrow-derived extracellular vesicles of mice irradiated with 3 Gy. Only those miRNA and protein interactions are presented where both the miRNA and the protein could be linked to certain common pathways. MiRNA–protein interactions were searched for in the Tarbase (validated interactions) and miRDB databases (predicted interactions). Colour blocks indicate an identical number of proteins involved in a particular pathway.

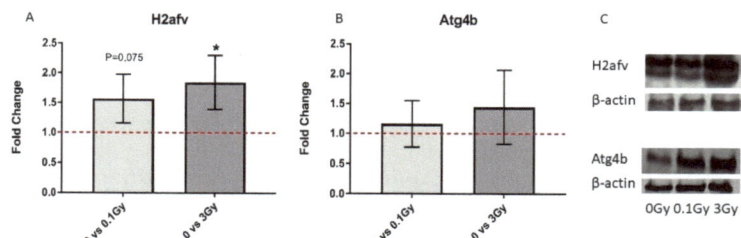

Figure 10. Western blot validation of deregulated proteins in bone marrow cells treated with bone marrow-derived extracellular vesicles from irradiated mice. A total of 40 µg of protein was loaded on the gel and hybridised to either anti-Atg4b or anti-H2afv or β-actin (loading control), as described in Materials and Methods. Quantification was performed with ImageJ software. Relative fold changes compared to bone marrow cells treated with extracellular vesicles from non-irradiated mice are shown in (**A**) for H2afv and (**B**) for Atg4b. (**C**) Representative blot image. n = 3. Error bars represent standard deviations (SD). Significant changes are indicated with * $p < 0.05$.

3. Discussion

In our previous studies, we reported that BM-derived EVs played an important role in transmitting IR-induced bystander effects in the BM [9,10,13]. Using the C57Bl/6 mouse model, we demonstrated that EVs isolated from the BM supernatant of irradiated mice, when injected systemically into naïve animals, induced changes in cell viability and cell subpopulation distribution in the BM and periphery that were similar to those for mice directly irradiated. We also highlighted the potential role of EV-derived miRNAs in mediating bystander effects. The aim of the present study was to identify those miRNAs in the BM-derived EVs of irradiated mice, which might interfere with cellular processes in the EV-acceptor cells. The CBA/CA mouse was used because this radiosensitive strain is prone to develop acute myeloid leukaemia exclusively upon irradiation [15].

Although blood is the most frequently used source of EVs for biological studies [16], blood-derived EVs are not optimal for characterising EV-mediated communication within a tissue microenvironment, since blood-derived EVs represent a mixture of EVs released from various parts of the body and, thus, they are not representative for a particular tissue microenvironment. Therefore, our study was performed using BM-derived EVs isolated from BM supernatant, in which EVs released by various BM cells are present in a concentrated form.

EVs carry a complex cargo comprising various proteins [17], different types of RNAs, various non-coding RNA types such as miRNAs [10,18], circular RNAs [19,20], long non-coding RNAs [21,22] as well as DNA of various sources such as genomic, mitochondrial [23], extrachromosomal [24], small metabolites [25] and possibly other biological structures present in the cells releasing the EVs. Out of these proteins and miRNAs are the best characterised molecules due to their role in regulating cellular processes in the EV-acceptor cells.

According to our results, the number of differentially expressed miRNAs in the EVs isolated from mice irradiated with low (0.1 Gy) or high (3 Gy) doses was low. In the EVs isolated from 0.1 Gy-irradiated mice, only two differentially expressed miRNAs were detected; nevertheless, they regulated important pathways involved in either signal transduction (TGF-β signalling pathway) or normal BM functioning (signalling pathways regulating the pluripotency of stem cells). Seventeen miRNAs were differentially expressed in EVs isolated from mice irradiated with 3 Gy, regulating mostly cancer-related pathways (including acute myeloid leukaemia) and multiple pathways relevant for either BM functioning (Wnt signalling pathway, signalling pathways regulating the pluripotency of stem cells) or for the cellular response to IR (Hippo signalling, cell cycle, TGF-β signalling, FoxO signalling, MAPK signalling, Erb signalling), suggesting the potential involvement of these miRNAs in mediating IR-induced bystander responses. The findings that all of the differentially expressed miRNAs of 0.1 Gy EVs were present in 3 Gy EVs and the expression level of several miRNAs in the EVs correlated with the applied dose suggest a dose-dependent regulation of miRNA packaging in EVs. Previous studies identified cellular and circulating miRNAs with various degrees of correlation with ionising radiation dose [26,27], but we are not aware of reports regarding the dose-dependent or dose-correlating expression of miRNAs in EVs.

Comparing our current results with the study of Szatmári et al., in which differentially expressed miRNAs in BM-derived EVs were investigated in C57Bl/6 mice irradiated with either 0.1 Gy or 2 Gy [10], only two miRNAs (miR709 and miR761) were in common in the EVs irradiated with high doses. Nevertheless, the number of common pathways regulated by the differentially expressed miRNAs in the two studies was largely overlapping. The two pathways regulated by miRNAs differentially expressed in the 0.1 Gy EVs (TGF-β signalling pathway and signalling pathways regulating the pluripotency of stem cells) and 80% of pathways regulated by the miRNAs from 3 Gy EVs were also present in the study by Szatmári et al.

We are not aware of any other publication investigating differentially expressed miRNAs in BM-derived EVs after IR. Comparing IR-induced differences in the miRNA content of EVs from different biological sources is difficult, since the miRNA content of the EVs largely reflects the miRNA panel of the EV-donor cells. Nevertheless, the majority of the EVs released by the BM should be present in the blood as well, although in a much lower yield. Therefore, we compared our current data with another study by Szatmári et al., in which they investigated differentially expressed miRNAs in EVs isolated from the blood of C57Bl/6 mice irradiated with either 0.1 Gy or 2 Gy [13]. Although identical miRNAs were not detected, several pathways relevant for cancer (such as acute myeloid leukaemia, chronic myeloid leukaemia, mTOR signalling) or signal transduction processes altered by IR (such as FoxO signalling, Hippo signalling, MAPK signalling, TGF-beta signalling) were in common. Moertl et al. investigated the effect of IR on the miRNA content of human peripheral blood mononuclear cell-derived EVs 72 h after irradiation with 2 Gy or 6 Gy. Similar to our data, they identified a limited number of differentially expressed miRNAs, and only the upregulated miRNA-338 was identical with the ones reported in our current study. MiRNA-regulated pathways related to the cell cycle, cell death and proliferation as well as DNA repair were also reported as altered [28]. The proteome of BMCs irradiated with 0.1 Gy revealed protein clusters involved in mitochondria-related processes, most notably ATP synthesis and oxidative phosphorylation, supporting that low-dose irradiation induces oxidative stress, as reported in other studies as well [29–31]. Pathway enrichment analysis indicated that immune system-related signalling pathways (such as NF-κB, T cell receptor, B cell receptor, Toll-like receptor, IL-17) and pathways related to immune cell differentiation and function were abundant, supporting the immune modulatory effect of low-dose irradiation, as reported [32–35].

The irradiation of the BMCs with 3 Gy led to a much higher number of deregulated proteins, clustered around biological processes relevant for cellular responses to high-dose radiation damage, such as DNA-related processes (repair, replication, DNA and nucleotide metabolism), stress response, chromatin remodelling, the regulation of transcription and mRNA maturation as well as several mitochondrial processes reflecting oxidative stress. Pathway enrichment analysis largely supported protein clustering, since the most significantly altered pathways were metabolism and genetic information processing, out of which one-third was related to DNA damage and repair (such as homologous recombination, DNA replication, mismatch repair, nucleotide excision repair). Metabolic pathways affected nucleotide metabolism, carbohydrate metabolism as well as oxidative phosphorylation. These data are in agreement with previous studies performed in various biological models indicating that high-dose irradiation leads to oxidative stress and the activation of DNA damage response pathways [36–39].

Approx. 50% of the common proteins between BMCs irradiated with 0.1 Gy and 3 Gy correlated with the dose, and these proteins clustered around the oxidative stress response, MAPK and NF-κB signalling and apoptosis, indicating that the severity of radiation-induced oxidative stress, inflammation and apoptosis is dose-dependent. Similar findings were reported by others as well [40–42]. Pathway enrichment analysis indicated 63 common pathways basically supporting protein clustering. Nevertheless, several important differences in pathway alterations between the two doses were also noted. Pathway alterations indicating radiation-induced DNA damage and pathways related to nucleotide metabolism were only present in BMCs irradiated with 3 Gy and were completely absent in low-dose-irradiated samples, indicating that low-dose irradiation does not activate DNA damage response pathways. These findings support previous reports with the same conclusion [43,44]. On the other hand, immune system-related and signal transduction pathways were less abundant in BMCs irradiated with high dose compared to low dose. While apoptosis was a common pathway for both doses, senescence-related pathways were only present after high-dose irradiation. Leukaemia-related pathway alterations were only present in BMCs irradiated with 3 Gy, which strongly supports previous data showing an increased incidence of myeloid leukaemia in the CBA/Ca mouse strain after irradiation with 3 Gy [15]. Altogether, commonalities and differences in the pathways between low- and high dose-irradiated BMCs highlight the major differences in the biological responses to the two doses. Systemic responses are markedly present after low-dose irradiation (increased number of immune system-related pathways), while mechanisms related to DNA damage repair (repair and replication-related pathways, metabolic pathways related to nucleotide metabolism) predominate in cellular responses to high-dose irradiation.

In order to study EV-induced changes in the protein profile of BMCs, first, we investigated whether the fact that EVs originate from irradiated mice influences their uptake rate by BMCs. Since we found no significant differences in the uptake rate, we concluded that changes in the protein pathways of BMCs treated with EVs were due to differences in the EV cargo and not due to differences in the number of internalised EV particles.

Proteomic changes in BMCs treated with 0.1 Gy EVs were clustered around mitochondrial processes involved in oxidative phosphorylation and were involved in 15 pathways, out of which 5 were metabolism-related such as oxidative phosphorylation and various components of lipid metabolism. The rest of the pathways were of less relevance for BM functioning and/or the response to IR. BMCs treated with 3 Gy EVs had 63 deregulated proteins that did not form big clusters except for a cluster of nuclear proteins involved in processes such as chromatin remodelling, histone methylation and DNA binding. Other smaller clusters were involved in immunological and metabolic processes. Pathway enrichment analysis indicated that, by far, the most highly represented group of pathways was cancer, followed by signal transduction and the immune response. Among cancer pathways, acute myeloid leukaemia- and chronic myeloid leukaemia-related pathways were significantly altered, indicating the potential role of EVs in leukemogenesis [45,46]. An additional important group of pathways was replication and repair, indicating that EVs could either transmit DNA damage into EV-recipient BMCs or signals leading to the activation of DNA damage response. This was also reflected in the alterations of certain signal transduction pathways interacting with the DNA damage response such as mTOR, PI3K-Akt, Wnt, cAMP, and NF-κB signalling pathways. Alterations in metabolism-related pathways were much less represented compared to either directly irradiated BMCs or BMCs treated with 0.1 Gy EVs. The comparison of common proteins and pathways between BMCs treated with 0.1 Gy EV and 3 Gy EV indicated that mostly proteins involved in energy metabolism and mitochondrial processes were in common; however, these were not reflected in identical pathway alterations.

Protein and pathway overlap between directly irradiated and EV-treated BMCs is a potential way to identify radiation-induced bystander signalling mechanisms transferred by EVs in the BM. As mentioned above, both direct irradiation with 0.1 Gy and the treatment of BMCs with 0.1 Gy EVs led to the deregulation of several mitochondrial proteins and protein pathways involved in energy metabolism. As such, 8 out of the 18 common deregulated proteins were involved in mitochondrial and redox-related processes, and the only common pathway that could be related to the IR response was oxidative phosphorylation. These data indicate that oxidative stress after the low-dose direct irradiation of BMCs can be transferred by EVs to non-irradiated BMCs in a bystander manner. EV-induced oxidative stress has been reported by other groups as well [47–49].

While we could not identify strong synergies between BMCs directly irradiated with 3 Gy or treated with 3 Gy EVs at the level of individual proteins, several altered pathways highly relevant for the IR response were identical between the two groups based on pathway enrichment analysis. Most importantly, all three pathways related to DNA replication and repair that were altered in BMCs treated with 3 Gy EVs were also altered in the directly irradiated cells, indicating that DNA damage response-related signals can be transmitted by EVs in a bystander manner. In addition, several of the signalling pathways related to DNA damage (PI3K-Akt, NF-κB) as well as cell death pathways characteristic of high-dose irradiation (apoptosis, senescence) were also in common between directly irradiated and EV-treated BMCs. The acute myeloid leukaemia pathway was present both in the directly irradiated and EV-treated BMCs. The number of cancer-related pathways was much higher in BMCs treated with 3 Gy EVs compared to their directly irradiated counterparts (23 vs. 9). Nevertheless, the majority of these pathways were related to cancer in specific organs other than BM, which might be due to signals originating from EVs present in the BM but released by cells from other organs, reaching the BM through the circulation.

Altogether, common protein and pathway alterations between directly irradiated and EV-treated BMCs indicated that cellular and molecular processes highly relevant for cellular responses to IR damage could be transmitted by EVs in a bystander manner. However, several important differences in the pathways could also be seen, as summarised in Supplementary Figure S2.

Next, we were curious to see to what extent differentially expressed miRNAs of EVs isolated from irradiated mice were responsible for the transmission of bystander responses. Since the number of differentially expressed miRNAs in 0.1 Gy EVs was very low (only two miRNAs involved in three pathways, out of which one was unrelated to either IR or BM), we assumed that miRNAs from 0.1 Gy EVs do not play a major role in IR-induced bystander effects. On the other hand, the 17 differentially expressed miRNAs from 3 Gy EVs regulated several pathways relevant for IR-induced damage in the BM which overlapped with protein pathways identified in BMCs treated with 3 Gy EVs. Such common pathways with relevance in IR-induced BM damage were the cell cycle, pathways in cancer, transcription misregulation in cancer and acute and chronic myeloid leukaemia. Based on direct miRNA–protein interaction studies, 6 miRNAs and 11 proteins were identified that could directly interact and were involved in the mentioned pathways (Figure 9). This raises the possibility that alterations in the abovementioned protein pathways in the BMCs treated with 3 Gy EVs could be attributed to the regulatory role of the six EV-derived miRNAs. Further studies are needed to confirm the direct miRNA–protein interactions and their impact on the cell cycle and BM malignancies.

While several other pathways relevant for IR response were altered in the BMCs treated with 3 Gy EVs, the majority of these pathways could not be linked to specific miRNAs transmitted by 3 Gy EVs. This suggests that proteomic changes in BMCs treated with 3 Gy EVs might be only in small part regulated by the EV-derived miRNAs, highlighting the role of other molecules within the EVs able to transmit IR-induced bystander effects.

4. Materials and Methods

4.1. Mouse Model and Irradiation

CBA/Ca mice were used in all experiments. Mice were kept and investigated in accordance with the guidelines and all applicable sections of the 2011 CLVIII Hungarian law about animal protection and welfare and the European 2010/63/EU directives and regulations. All animal studies were approved, and permission was issued by the Budapest and Pest County Administration Office Food Chain Safety and Animal Health Board (ethical permission: PE/EA/392-7/2017).

Nine- to twelve-week-old male mice randomly selected from at least five different litters were either sham-irradiated (0 Gy, controls) or total-body-irradiated with 0.1 Gy and 3 Gy X-rays using an X-RAD 225/XLi X-ray source (Precision X-ray, North Branford, CT, USA). The mice were sacrificed 24 h after irradiation by using a 100 mg/kg (0.25 mL/kg) intraperitoneal (i.p.) injection of sodium pentobarbital.

4.2. Isolation of BMCs and Co-Culture of BM-Derived EVs with BMCs

Twenty-four hours after irradiation, the BMs were isolated from the femur and tibia of mice by flushing out the tissue from the diaphyses of the bones and suspended in PBS. A BM single-cell suspension was made by the mechanical disaggregation of the tissue; then, the cells were filtered by a 40 μm mesh filter. The cells were pelleted by centrifugation at $500\times g$ and 4 °C for 10 min. The supernatant was removed and used for BM-derived EV isolation, as described below. Cell pellets were used for proteomic analysis, as described below.

BMCs from control (0 Gy or sham-irradiated) mice were prepared as described above and were incubated with EVs isolated from the BM supernatant of either control (0 Gy), 0.1 Gy- or 3 Gy-irradiated mice. Cell pellets were resuspended in RPMI1640 (Lonza

Bioscience, Verviers, Belgium) containing 10% foetal bovine serum (FBS) (Euroclone S.p.a., Pero(MI), Italy). Live BMCs were determined by trypan blue exclusion, and 20×10^6 BMCs per sample were incubated with EVs isolated from the supernatant of 100×10^6 BMCs for 3 h at 37 °C and 5% CO_2. BMCs from directly irradiated mice were processed in a similar manner, without adding EVs. After the three-hour incubation time, 20×10^6 cells per sample were pelleted at $500 \times g$ and 4 °C, and cell pellets were snap-frozen in liquid nitrogen and kept at −70 °C until proteomic analysis.

Part of the EVs and BMCs were used to trace the EV uptake. EVs were isolated from the BM supernatant of 0 Gy-, 0.1 Gy- or 3 Gy-irradiated mice, as described above. Isolated EVs were stained with a cell permeant nucleic acid stain that is selective for RNA (SYTO® RNASelect™ Green Fluorescent Cell Stain Invitrogen, Waltham, MA, USA), following the manufacturer's protocol. Briefly, EVs were incubated with the dye (1 µM final concentration) at 37 °C in the dark for 20 min, and the excess of nonincorporated dye was removed using a GE Healthcare PD SpinTrap G-25 desalting column (GE Healthcare Life Science, Chicago, IL, USA). Stained EVs were incubated with freshly isolated BMCs at a 1/5 ratio for 3 h at 37 °C; the non-internalised EVs were removed by centrifugation at $400 \times g$ for 10 min. As a control, PBS was stained and incubated with BMCs in the same way. The EV uptake was assessed by measuring the acquired fluorescence with a CytoFlex flow cytometer (Beckman Coulter, Brea, CA, USA). The results were analysed using the Cytexpert software version 2.3.0.84 (Beckman Coulter, Brea, CA, USA).

4.3. Isolation, Validation and Quantification of Mouse BM-Derived EVs

BM-derived EVs were isolated from the BMC supernatant of control and irradiated mice by pooling the supernatants of five mice/irradiation doses/experiments. EV isolation was conducted 24 h after irradiation using the ExoQuick-TC kit (System Biosciences, Palo Alto CA, USA), as described previously [10]. EVs were used for miRNA analysis and for co-culture with BMCs.

BM-derived EVs were investigated by transmission electron microscopy (TEM) as described [14]. The size distribution analysis of EVs was conducted by tunable resistance pulse sensing (TRPS) using an NP150 nanopore (measurement range: 70–420 nm) [9]. EV-specific protein markers were investigated by Western blot analysis, as detailed below.

4.4. RNA Extraction from BM-Derived EVs for miRNA Analysis

Total RNA extraction from BM-derived EVs was performed using the RNeasy mini extraction kit (Qiagen, Hilden, Germany), according to the manufacturer's instructions. The MiRNA concentration was measured on a BioAnalyzer 2100 (Agilent, Santa Clara, CA, USA) according to the manufacturer's instructions. Briefly, the concentrations of the samples to be measured were standardised according to the total RNA concentration, as measured by NanoDrop (ThermoFisher, Waltham, MA, USA), between 20 ng/µL and 50 ng/µL depending on the available sample amount. These were then loaded onto the BioAnalyzer small RNA chip (Agilent, part number 5067-1548) and read by the BioAnalyzer 2100. The resultant miRNA concentration was calculated by multiplying the measured miRNA concentration by the dilution factor of the sample, yielding the miRNA concentration in the undiluted sample.

4.5. nCounter Analysis of BM-Derived EV miRNAs and Their Quantitative Validation by Real-Time Polymerase Chain Reaction (RT-PCR)

An nCounter Mouse v1.5 miRNA Expression Panel including 800 miRNAs (NanoString Technologies, Seattle, WA, USA) was used to analyse the levels of miRNA expression in EVs, according to the manufacturer's instructions. MiRNA expression was analysed in four biological replicates in each experimental group (0 Gy, 0.1 Gy and 3 Gy EV, respectively). Briefly, the miRNA samples prepared as described above were hybridised to a miRNA-specific probe, which in turn hybridises to a barcoded fluorescent reporter specific to that probe; the barcode identifies which miRNA it is attached to. These were then fixed to a chip, which was read by the nCounter machine, giving counts based on recorded fluorescence intensities. This allows for a molecule-by-molecule resolution of the relative abundance of the miRNA in a sample.

The nCounter-reported raw counts were normalised according to the top 100 miRNAs using nSolver 4.0 software, and the normalised data were then analysed with BRBArray Tools, an open-source analysis extension used by the National Cancer Institute [50]. Dose correlation analysis and heat maps were also generated using BRBArray Tools. Statistical relevance was tested with DIANA Tools, mirExTra2.0. [51], using the LIMMA statistical method. The p-value threshold for relevance was set at 0.05.

cDNA synthesis and miRNA analysis by RT-qPCR were carried out by using the miRCURY™ LNA™ miRNA PCR System (Qiagen). cDNA was prepared from 2 μL RNA with a concentration of 40 ng/μL in a 10 μL reaction volume. The cDNA was diluted 20-fold and assayed in a 10 μL PCR reaction volume. The amplification was performed in a Rotor-Gene Q real-time PCR cycler (Qiagen). The following PCR primers (all purchased from Qiagen) were used: miR-669d-5p (YP00205051), miR-93-5p (YP00204715), miR-504-5p (YP00204396), miR-467h (YP00205922), miR-706 (YP00205976), miR-709 (YP00205463), miR-1961 (YP00205381), miR-1933-5p (YP00205351), miR-181c-5p (YP00204683), miR-338-5p (YP00204114), miR-34b-5p (YP00205075), miR-761 (YP00205475), miR-129-5p (YP00204534) and miR-708-5p (YP00204490). The amplification curves were analysed using the Rotor-Gene Q Series software (software version 2.1.0.9) both for the determination of quantification cycles and for the melting curve (T_m) analysis. In order for the data to be considered for further analysis, the following criteria had to be met: appropriate melting curves, T_m had to be within known specifications for the assay and the Cq value had to be ≤37. The relative concentration of each miRNA was calculated by the Rotor-Gene Q software, where sham-irradiated (0 Gy) samples were used as controls. To achieve optimal relative expression results, mmu-miR-423-3p was used as a normaliser, since mmu-miR-423-3p was present in a constant and well-detectable concentration in BM-derived EVs, which did not change due to 0.1 Gy or 3 Gy irradiation.

4.6. Western Blot Analysis of EV and BMC Proteins

BMCs and BM-derived EVs were isolated as described above. After the EV isolation protein content was measured by the Bradford protein assay kit (Thermo Fisher Scientific, Waltham, MA, USA) using a Synergy HT (Biotek, Winooski, VT, USA) plate reader, EVs with a 60 μg protein content and 2.6×10^6 BMCs were lysed with radioimmunoprecipiation assay (RIPA) lysis buffer containing 2% protease inhibitor (Protease Inhibitor Cocktail (P8340), Kenilworth, NJ, USA); then, the protein concentration was determined by the bichinchoninic acid (BCA) assay kit (Pierce™ BCA Protein Assay Kit, Thermo Fisher Scientific, Waltham, MA, USA). For further steps, 40 μg protein was precipitated by trichloroacetic acid (TCA) solution (one part of the TCA was added to three parts of the protein solution), incubated on ice for 5 min and pelleted at 3800× g and 4 °C for 5 min. The pellet was washed with ice-cold acetone twice, and the protein samples were diluted 1:2 in 2× Laemmli buffer (Bio-Rad Hercules, CA, USA) supplemented with β-mercaptoetanol, boiled at 95 °C for 5 min and cooled on ice for 5 min before loading on the gel. A total of 40 μg of the protein was loaded and electrophoresed on 4–20% sodium dodecyl sulphate-polyacrylamide (SDS-PAGE) gel (4–20% Mini-PROTEAN® TGX™ Precast Protein Gels, Bio-Rad Hercules, CA, USA) and transferred to a polyvinylidene fluoride (PVDF) membrane. After blotting, the PVDF membrane was blocked with blocking buffer (containing 3% bovine serum albumin (BSA) in Tris Buffered Saline, with Tween 20) at room temperature (RT) for 30 min. The blocked membrane was incubated with the primary antibodies: recombinant Anti-ATG4B (ab154843), H2AFV Polyclonal Antibody (PA5109802) and beta Actin Polyclonal Antibody (PA1-183) (Thermo Fisher Scientific, Waltham, MA, USA) at RT for 2 h, followed by 1 h of incubation with horseradish peroxidase-conjugated goat anti-rabbit secondary antibody (Goat Anti-Rabbit IgG H&L (HRP), (ab6721 Abcam). Antibodies were diluted in the blocking buffer according to the manufacturer's instructions. As a protein standard, the Spectra™ Multicolor Broad Range Protein Ladder was used (Thermo Fisher Scientific). The membrane was washed in Tris-buffered saline-tween buffer three times, and protein bands were visualised using 3,3′-diaminobenzidine substrate (Pierce™ DAB Substrate Kit, Thermo Fisher Scientific) by the chromogenic method. The density of each protein band was recorded and analysed by ImageJ software (Image Processing and Analysis in Java, National Institutes of Health, Bethesda, MD, USA). The measured density values were normalised to the density value of the loading control, β-actin.

4.7. Mass Spectrometry (MS) Sample Preparation and Measurement

BMCs from directly irradiated mice (n = 3 for 0 Gy BM, n = 4 for 0.1 Gy and 3 Gy BM) as well as BMCs co-cultured with BM-derived EVs from irradiated mice (n = 4 for 0 Gy BM + EV, n = 5 for 0.1 Gy BM + EV, 3 Gy BM + EV) were placed in 100 μL RIPA buffer (Thermo Fisher Scientific) that contained 25 mM Tris.HCl ph 7.6, 150 mM NaCl, 1% NP-40, 1% sodium deoxycholate and 0.1% SDS and incubated at 4 °C for 30 min [52]. They were then subjected to an ice-cold sonication bath for 30 s and another incubation (4 °C, 15 min). The protein concentration of the individual samples was determined using a BCA assay following the instruction manual (Thermo Fisher Scientific) on an Infinite M200 Spectrophotometer (Tecan GmbH, Crailsheim, Germany). BSA was used as an internal standard.

A total of 10 μg of the sample was enzymatically digested using a modified filter-aided sample preparation (FASP) protocol, as described in [53,54]. Peptides were stored at −20 °C until the MS measurement.

The MS measurement was performed in the data-dependent (DDA) mode. MS data were acquired on a Q Exactive (QE) high-field (HF) mass spectrometer (Thermo Fisher Scientific Inc.), as described in [55].

4.8. MS Data Processing and Protein Identification

Proteome Discoverer 2.4 software (Thermo Fisher Scientific; version 2.4.1.15) was used for peptide and protein identification via a database search (Sequest HT search engine) against the Swissprot mouse database (Release 2020_02, 17061 sequences), considering full tryptic specificity and allowing for up to one missed tryptic cleavage site, a precursor mass tolerance of 10 ppm and a fragment mass tolerance of 0.02 Da. Carbamidomethylation of cysteine was set as a static modification. Dynamic modifications included the deamidation of asparagine and glutamine, the oxidation of methionine and a combination of methionine loss with acetylation on protein N-terminus. The percolator was used for validating peptide spectrum matches and peptides, accepting only the top-scoring hit for each spectrum and satisfying the cut-off values for FDR < 1% and a posterior error probability < 0.01. The final list of proteins complied with the strict parsimony principle.

A schematic illustration of the workflow used for MS data processing and protein identification can be seen in Supplementary Figure S3.

4.9. Data Processing and Label-Free Quantification

The quantification of proteins was based on the area value of the abundance values for unique plus razor peptides. Abundance values were normalised in a retention time-dependent manner to account for sample loading errors. The protein abundances were calculated by summing up the abundance values for admissible peptides. The final protein ratio was calculated using the median abundance values of three replicate analyses each. The statistical significance of the ratio change was ascertained by employing the t-test approach described in [56], which is based on the presumption that we look for expression changes for proteins that are just a few in number in comparison to the number of total proteins being quantified. The quantification variability of the non-changing "background" proteins can be used to infer which proteins change their expression in a statistically significant manner.

The T-test was solely used for pairwise comparisons of two conditions. The following pairwise conditions were compared: (0.1 Gy BM)/(0 Gy BM); (3 Gy BM)/(0 Gy BM); (0.1 Gy BM + EV)/(0 Gy BM + EV); (3 Gy BM + EV)/(0 Gy BM + EV).

Proteins identified with an FDR <1% and a fold change above ±1.33 in treated samples, along with a Benjamini–Hochberg adjusted p-value < 0.05, were considered deregulated.

4.10. Pathway Analysis of Significantly Altered EV-Derived miRNAs and BMC Proteins

Statistically significant miRNAs differentially expressed in the EVs from irradiated mice were used in the miRNA functional KEGG pathway analysis, which was performed with DIANA mirPath v.3. Experimentally validated interactions from TarBase v.8 (http://www.microrna.gr/tarbase (accessed on 20 September 2022)) [57] were used primarily, and data generated by the microT-CDS algorithm [58] were used only if no experimentally validated interaction was found for the miRNA. The p-value threshold was set at <0.05.

For protein analysis, all four treatment groups (0.1 Gy or 3 Gy directly irradiated BMCs, and BMCs treated with 0.1 Gy- or 3 Gy-irradiated EVs) were considered separately, and the results were compared to their respective controls (either 0 Gy sham-irradiated or treated with BM-derived EVs from 0 Gy-irradiated mice) and to each other. Only significantly deregulated proteins based on MS analysis were included in the analysis, where the official gene symbol of the proteins was used in the query data. To calculate the number of protein–protein interactions (PPI) and form protein clusters, the STRING database version 11.0 (https://string-db.org/ (accessed on 12 September 2022)) was used. In the analysis, all interaction sources (text mining, experiments, databases, co-expression, neighbourhood, gene fusion, co-occurrence) were used, and the minimum required interaction score was 0.4 (medium confidence); protein clustering was performed using the MCL clustering algorithm within STRING. Pathway annotations and enrichment analysis were performed with the pathDIP database, version 4.0.7.0 (http://ophid.utoronto.ca/pathDIP/ (accessed on 19 September 2022)), which is an annotated database integrating data from several pathway databases. The advantage of using PathDIP was that it gave a greater protein coverage by using both literature-curated (core), orthologue and extended pathways. Extended pathways integrate core pathways with experimentally detected and orthologous PPIs. PPIs are either experimentally detected or high-confidence computationally predicted. Due to the pathway extension method, more than 36,000 pathway orphans (proteins with no annotations available in curated or orthologue pathways) could be annotated in sixteen non-human organisms, which led to a 9.56 times increase in the protein coverage in model organisms [59]. In our PathDIP analysis, we only considered data originating from the KEGG database in order to use similar conditions as in the microRNA pathway analysis. We used extended pathway associations, where core pathways were integrated with experimentally detected and orthologous PPIs with a minimum confidence level of protein–pathway association predictions of 0.95. Only significant pathways ($p < 0.05$) were considered.

To detect possible interactions between the significantly altered proteins and microRNAs, two databases were used: Tarbase for experimentally validated interactions and miRDB (http://mirdb.org/ (accessed on 20 September 2022)) [60] for predicted interactions.

4.11. Statistical Analysis

Data are presented as the mean ± standard deviation (SD). If no other method was indicated, than Students's t-test was applied to determine statistical significance using GraphPad Prism version 6.00 for Windows (GraphPad Software, La Jolla, CA, USA). Data were considered statistically significant if the p-value was lower than 0.05. For the dose correlation calculation, Pearson Correlation was used. To identify significantly altered miRNAs, the LIMMA method was used in DIANA mirExTra 2.0.

5. Conclusions

In this study, we identified differentially expressed miRNAs in the BM-derived EVs from mice irradiated with low- or high-dose IR. We showed that miRNAs regulated pathways related to the IR response and to normal and malignant BM functioning. The miRNA profile of the EVs was only moderately affected by low-dose irradiation, but the deregulated miRNAs were involved in pathways that are important for a healthy bone marrow, such as signalling pathways regulating the pluripotency of stem cells and mitochondria-related biological processes. These data indicate that oxidative stress after low-dose irradiation can be transferred by EV-derived miRNAs to non-irradiated bone marrow cells in a bystander manner.

We performed detailed proteomic analysis of either directly irradiated BMCs or those treated with EVs from irradiated mice. Several proteins, protein clusters and protein pathways were in common between directly irradiated and EV-treated BMCs, most probably representing biological processes transmitted via EVs in a bystander manner. One such important common process was the induction of oxidative stress after low-dose direct irradiation and treatment with EVs from low-dose irradiated mice. While pathways related to the DNA damage response were altered in both high-dose-irradiated BMCs and in BMCs treated with 3 Gy EVs, there was an important difference at the protein level. In directly irradiated cells, protein clusters indicated alterations in processes directly involved in DNA damage recognition, repair and processes linked to the epigenetic control of the IR response such as chromatin remodelling or histone methylation. In the EV-treated cells, only protein clusters involved in biological processes related to chromatin remodelling and histone modifications were present, which we think indicates that EVs can transmit factors influencing the DNA damage response pathway only via epigenetic mechanisms. We are not aware of other studies comparing direct and EV-induced changes in the proteomic profile of BMCs after irradiation. Since EV-derived miRNAs have important roles in regulating cellular processes in EV acceptor cells, pathways regulated by differentially expressed miRNAs in the EVs and altered protein pathways in BMCs treated with BM-derived EVs were compared. Certain important pathways altered in BMCs treated with 3 Gy EVs were identified as also regulated by miRNAs differentially expressed in 3 Gy EVs such as the cell cycle and myeloid leukaemia. Within these common pathways, direct interactions were shown between six miRNAs (mmu-miR-706, mmu-miR-709, mmu-miR-761, mmu-miR-669g, mmu-miR-129-5p and mmu-miR-1942) and eleven proteins (Atg4b, Calu, H2afv, Krt16, Rtf1, Snca, Tgm2, Ube2c, Clic4, Dnajb6 and Eif2b1), which might represent potential biomarkers indicative of EV-mediated effects. The existence of such common pathways indicates that miRNAs can induce functional changes in EV acceptor cells, strengthening the possible regulatory role of EV-derived miRNAs. Nevertheless, the majority of altered protein pathways could not be linked with miRNA-regulated pathways, indicating that miRNAs are involved in the regulation of certain but not all EV-mediated bystander effects, and other molecules comprising the EV cargo also have their role. In order to understand IR-induced bystander signals mediated by EVs, it is important to perform the complex characterisation of EV cargo changes after IR and to link them to biological processes in the EV acceptor cells. Since bystander responses are very important modulators of radiation damage, a better knowledge of these processes helps in an improved understanding of tissue responses to IR and in the estimation of long-term risks after radiation exposure.

Supplementary Materials: The supporting information can be downloaded at: https://www.mdpi.com/article/10.3390/ijms24108607/s1.

Author Contributions: Conceptualisation: K.L., C.B. and S.T.; methodology: K.L., S.T., C.B., I.B.C., E.A.R., P.S. and B.J.; software: I.B.C., E.A.R., P.S. and C.v.T.; validation: T.S., I.B.C., K.L. and G.S.; formal analysis: I.B.C.; investigation: I.B.C., E.A.R., P.S., L.C.-G., C.v.T., D.K. and M.F.; resources: K.L., S.T. and C.B.; data curation: P.S., E.A.R. and K.L.; writing—original draft preparation: K.L., I.B.C. and E.A.R.; writing—review and editing: I.B.C., C.v.T., K.L. and G.S.; visualisation: I.B.C. and E.A.R.;

supervision: K.L., C.B. and S.T.; project administration: K.L.; funding acquisition: K.L., C.B. and S.T. All authors have read and agreed to the published version of the manuscript.

Funding: This research was funded by the Euratom research and training programme 2014–2018 under the grant agreement No 662287.

Institutional Review Board Statement: The animal study protocol was approved by the Budapest and Pest County Administration Office Food Chain Safety and Animal Health Board (ethical permission: PE/EA/392-7/2017).

Informed Consent Statement: Not applicable.

Data Availability Statement: Raw proteomic and miRNA profiling data have been uploaded to the Store^{db} database (www.storedb.org, accessed on 30 January 2023). Study ID: https://www.storedb.org/?STOREDB:STUDY1176 (accessed on 30 January 2023), DOI: http://dx.doi.org/10.20348/STOREDB/1176 (accessed on 30 January 2023).

Acknowledgments: We wish to acknowledge the expert technical assistance of Károly Haller and Mariann Csabádi in the experimental animal care and handling.

Conflicts of Interest: The authors declare no conflict of interest.

References

1. van Niel, G.; D'Angelo, G.; Raposo, G. Shedding light on the cell biology of extracellular vesicles. *Nat. Rev. Mol. Cell Biol.* **2018**, *19*, 213–228. [CrossRef] [PubMed]
2. Doyle, L.M.; Wang, M.Z. Overview of Extracellular Vesicles, Their Origin, Composition, Purpose, and Methods for Exosome Isolation and Analysis. *Cells* **2019**, *8*, 727. [CrossRef] [PubMed]
3. Margolis, L.; Sadovsky, Y. The biology of extracellular vesicles: The known unknowns. *PLoS Biol.* **2019**, *17*, e3000363. [CrossRef] [PubMed]
4. Nikitaki, Z.; Mavragani, I.V.; Laskaratou, D.A.; Gika, V.; Moskvin, V.P.; Theofilatos, K.; Vougas, K.; Stewart, R.D.; Georgakilas, A.G. Systemic mechanisms and effects of ionizing radiation: A new 'old' paradigm of how the bystanders and distant can become the players. *Semin. Cancer Biol.* **2016**, *37–38*, 77–95. [CrossRef] [PubMed]
5. Hu, L.; Yin, X.; Zhang, Y.; Pang, A.; Xie, X.; Yang, S.; Zhu, C.; Li, Y.; Zhang, B.; Huang, Y.; et al. Radiation-induced bystander effects impair transplanted human hematopoietic stem cells via oxidative DNA damage. *Blood* **2021**, *137*, 3339–3350. [CrossRef]
6. Dawood, A.; Mothersill, C.; Seymour, C. Low dose ionizing radiation and the immune response: What is the role of non-targeted effects? *Int. J. Radiat. Biol.* **2021**, *97*, 1368–1382. [CrossRef]
7. Hargitai, R.; Kis, D.; Persa, E.; Szatmari, T.; Safrany, G.; Lumniczky, K. Oxidative Stress and Gene Expression Modifications Mediated by Extracellular Vesicles: An In Vivo Study of the Radiation-Induced Bystander Effect. *Antioxidants* **2021**, *10*, 156. [CrossRef]
8. Jabbari, N.; Karimipour, M.; Khaksar, M.; Akbariazar, E.; Heidarzadeh, M.; Mojarad, B.; Aftab, H.; Rahbarghazi, R.; Rezaie, J. Tumor-derived extracellular vesicles: Insights into bystander effects of exosomes after irradiation. *Lasers Med. Sci.* **2020**, *35*, 531–545. [CrossRef]
9. Kis, D.; Csordas, I.B.; Persa, E.; Jezso, B.; Hargitai, R.; Szatmari, T.; Sandor, N.; Kis, E.; Balazs, K.; Safrany, G.; et al. Extracellular Vesicles Derived from Bone Marrow in an Early Stage of Ionizing Radiation Damage Are Able to Induce Bystander Responses in the Bone Marrow. *Cells* **2022**, *11*, 155. [CrossRef]
10. Szatmari, T.; Kis, D.; Bogdandi, E.N.; Benedek, A.; Bright, S.; Bowler, D.; Persa, E.; Kis, E.; Balogh, A.; Naszalyi, L.N.; et al. Extracellular Vesicles Mediate Radiation-Induced Systemic Bystander Signals in the Bone Marrow and Spleen. *Front. Immunol.* **2017**, *8*, 347. [CrossRef]
11. Durand, C.; Charbord, P.; Jaffredo, T. The crosstalk between hematopoietic stem cells and their niches. *Curr. Opin. Hematol.* **2018**, *25*, 285–289. [CrossRef] [PubMed]
12. Sarvar, D.P.; Effatpanah, H.; Akbarzadehlaleh, P.; Shamsasenjan, K. Mesenchymal stromal cell-derived extracellular vesicles: Novel approach in hematopoietic stem cell transplantation. *Stem Cell Res. Ther.* **2022**, *13*, 202. [CrossRef] [PubMed]
13. Szatmari, T.; Persa, E.; Kis, E.; Benedek, A.; Hargitai, R.; Safrany, G.; Lumniczky, K. Extracellular vesicles mediate low dose ionizing radiation-induced immune and inflammatory responses in the blood. *Int. J. Radiat. Biol.* **2019**, *95*, 12–22. [CrossRef] [PubMed]
14. Kis, D.; Persa, E.; Szatmari, T.; Antal, L.; Bota, A.; Csordas, I.B.; Hargitai, R.; Jezso, B.; Kis, E.; Mihaly, J.; et al. The effect of ionising radiation on the phenotype of bone marrow-derived extracellular vesicles. *Br. J. Radiol.* **2020**, *93*, 20200319. [CrossRef]
15. Major, I.R.; Mole, R.H. Myeloid leukaemia in X-ray irradiated CBA mice. *Nature* **1978**, *272*, 455–456. [CrossRef]
16. Alberro, A.; Iparraguirre, L.; Fernandes, A.; Otaegui, D. Extracellular Vesicles in Blood: Sources, Effects, and Applications. *Int. J. Mol. Sci.* **2021**, *22*, 8163. [CrossRef]

17. Mutschelknaus, L.; Azimzadeh, O.; Heider, T.; Winkler, K.; Vetter, M.; Kell, R.; Tapio, S.; Merl-Pham, J.; Huber, S.M.; Edalat, L.; et al. Radiation alters the cargo of exosomes released from squamous head and neck cancer cells to promote migration of recipient cells. *Sci. Rep.* **2017**, *7*, 12423. [CrossRef]
18. Pazzaglia, S.; Tanno, B.; De Stefano, I.; Giardullo, P.; Leonardi, S.; Merla, C.; Babini, G.; Tuncay Cagatay, S.; Mayah, A.; Kadhim, M.; et al. Micro-RNA and Proteomic Profiles of Plasma-Derived Exosomes from Irradiated Mice Reveal Molecular Changes Preventing Apoptosis in Neonatal Cerebellum. *Int. J. Mol. Sci.* **2022**, *23*, 2169. [CrossRef]
19. Shi, X.; Wang, B.; Feng, X.; Xu, Y.; Lu, K.; Sun, M. circRNAs and Exosomes: A Mysterious Frontier for Human Cancer. *Mol. Ther. Nucleic Acids* **2020**, *19*, 384–392. [CrossRef]
20. Wang, D.; Ming, X.; Xu, J.; Xiao, Y. Circ_0009910 shuttled by exosomes regulates proliferation, cell cycle and apoptosis of acute myeloid leukemia cells by regulating miR-5195-3p/GRB10 axis. *Hematol. Oncol.* **2021**, *39*, 390–400. [CrossRef]
21. Hinger, S.A.; Cha, D.J.; Franklin, J.L.; Higginbotham, J.N.; Dou, Y.; Ping, J.; Shu, L.; Prasad, N.; Levy, S.; Zhang, B.; et al. Diverse Long RNAs Are Differentially Sorted into Extracellular Vesicles Secreted by Colorectal Cancer Cells. *Cell Rep.* **2018**, *25*, 715–725.e4. [CrossRef] [PubMed]
22. Li, Y.; Zhao, J.; Yu, S.; Wang, Z.; He, X.; Su, Y.; Guo, T.; Sheng, H.; Chen, J.; Zheng, Q.; et al. Extracellular Vesicles Long RNA Sequencing Reveals Abundant mRNA, circRNA, and lncRNA in Human Blood as Potential Biomarkers for Cancer Diagnosis. *Clin. Chem.* **2019**, *65*, 798–808. [CrossRef] [PubMed]
23. Ariyoshi, K.; Miura, T.; Kasai, K.; Fujishima, Y.; Nakata, A.; Yoshida, M. Radiation-Induced Bystander Effect is Mediated by Mitochondrial DNA in Exosome-Like Vesicles. *Sci. Rep.* **2019**, *9*, 9103. [CrossRef] [PubMed]
24. Baba, T.; Yoshida, T.; Tanabe, Y.; Nishimura, T.; Morishita, S.; Gotoh, N.; Hirao, A.; Hanayama, R.; Mukaida, N. Cytoplasmic DNA accumulation preferentially triggers cell death of myeloid leukemia cells by interacting with intracellular DNA sensing pathway. *Cell Death Dis.* **2021**, *12*, 322. [CrossRef]
25. Li, Z.; Jella, K.K.; Jaafar, L.; Moreno, C.S.; Dynan, W.S. Characterization of exosome release and extracellular vesicle-associated miRNAs for human bronchial epithelial cells irradiated with high charge and energy ions. *Life Sci. Space Res.* **2021**, *28*, 11–17. [CrossRef]
26. Song, M.; Xie, D.; Gao, S.; Bai, C.J.; Zhu, M.X.; Guan, H.; Zhou, P.K. A Biomarker Panel of Radiation-Upregulated miRNA as Signature for Ionizing Radiation Exposure. *Life* **2020**, *10*, 361. [CrossRef]
27. Małachowska, B.; Tomasik, B.; Stawiski, K.; Kulkarni, S.; Guha, C.; Chowdhury, D.; Fendler, W. Circulating microRNAs as Biomarkers of Radiation Exposure: A Systematic Review and Meta-Analysis. *Int. J. Radiat. Oncol. Biol. Phys.* **2020**, *106*, 390–402. [CrossRef]
28. Moertl, S.; Buschmann, D.; Azimzadeh, O.; Schneider, M.; Kell, R.; Winkler, K.; Tapio, S.; Hornhardt, S.; Merl-Pham, J.; Pfaffl, M.W.; et al. Radiation Exposure of Peripheral Mononuclear Blood Cells Alters the Composition and Function of Secreted Extracellular Vesicles. *Int. J. Mol. Sci.* **2020**, *21*, 2336. [CrossRef]
29. Tharmalingam, S.; Sreetharan, S.; Kulesza, A.V.; Boreham, D.R.; Tai, T.C. Low-Dose Ionizing Radiation Exposure, Oxidative Stress and Epigenetic Programing of Health and Disease. *Radiat. Res.* **2017**, *188*, 525–538. [CrossRef]
30. Veeraraghavan, J.; Natarajan, M.; Herman, T.S.; Aravindan, N. Low-dose γ-radiation-induced oxidative stress response in mouse brain and gut: Regulation by NFκB-MnSOD cross-signaling. *Mutat. Res.* **2011**, *718*, 44–55. [CrossRef]
31. Rodrigues-Moreira, S.; Moreno, S.G.; Ghinatti, G.; Lewandowski, D.; Hoffschir, F.; Ferri, F.; Gallouet, A.S.; Gay, D.; Motohashi, H.; Yamamoto, M.; et al. Low-Dose Irradiation Promotes Persistent Oxidative Stress and Decreases Self-Renewal in Hematopoietic Stem Cells. *Cell Rep.* **2017**, *20*, 3199–3211. [CrossRef] [PubMed]
32. Bogdandi, E.N.; Balogh, A.; Felgyinszki, N.; Szatmari, T.; Persa, E.; Hildebrandt, G.; Safrany, G.; Lumniczky, K. Effects of low-dose radiation on the immune system of mice after total-body irradiation. *Radiat. Res.* **2010**, *174*, 480–489. [CrossRef] [PubMed]
33. Lumniczky, K.; Impens, N.; Armengol, G.; Candeias, S.; Georgakilas, A.G.; Hornhardt, S.; Martin, O.A.; Rodel, F.; Schaue, D. Low dose ionizing radiation effects on the immune system. *Environ. Int.* **2021**, *149*, 106212. [CrossRef] [PubMed]
34. Hekim, N.; Cetin, Z.; Nikitaki, Z.; Cort, A.; Saygili, E.I. Radiation triggering immune response and inflammation. *Cancer Lett.* **2015**, *368*, 156–163. [CrossRef]
35. Shimura, N.; Kojima, S. Effects of low-dose-gamma rays on the immune system of different animal models of disease. *Dose-Response A Publ. Int. Hormesis Soc.* **2014**, *12*, 429–465. [CrossRef]
36. McBride, W.H.; Schaue, D. Radiation-induced tissue damage and response. *J. Pathol.* **2020**, *250*, 647–655. [CrossRef]
37. Ward, J.F. DNA damage produced by ionizing radiation in mammalian cells: Identities, mechanisms of formation, and reparability. *Prog. Nucleic Acid Res. Mol. Biol.* **1988**, *35*, 95–125. [CrossRef]
38. Hariharan, P.V.; Hutchinson, F. Neutral sucrose gradient sedimentation of very large DNA from Bacillus subtilis: II. Double-strand breaks formed by gamma ray irradiation of the cells. *J. Mol. Biol.* **1973**, *75*, 479–494. [CrossRef]
39. Morales, A.; Miranda, M.; Sánchez-Reyes, A.; Biete, A.; Fernández-Checa, J.C. Oxidative damage of mitochondrial and nuclear DNA induced by ionizing radiation in human hepatoblastoma cells. *Int. J. Radiat. Oncol. Biol. Phys.* **1998**, *42*, 191–203. [CrossRef]
40. Rainaldi, G.; Ferrante, A.; Indovina, P.L.; Santini, M.T. Induction of apoptosis or necrosis by ionizing radiation is dose-dependent in MG-63 osteosarcoma multicellular spheroids. *Anticancer. Res.* **2003**, *23*, 2505–2518.
41. Katsura, M.; Cyou-Nakamine, H.; Zen, Q.; Zen, Y.; Nansai, H.; Amagasa, S.; Kanki, Y.; Inoue, T.; Kaneki, K.; Taguchi, A.; et al. Effects of Chronic Low-Dose Radiation on Human Neural Progenitor Cells. *Sci. Rep.* **2016**, *6*, 20027. [CrossRef] [PubMed]

42. Karabulutoglu, M.; Finnon, R.; Cruz-Garcia, L.; Hill, M.A.; Badie, C. Oxidative Stress and X-ray Exposure Levels-Dependent Survival and Metabolic Changes in Murine HSPCs. *Antioxidants* **2021**, *11*, 11. [CrossRef] [PubMed]
43. Sampadi, B.; Vermeulen, S.; Mišovic, B.; Boei, J.J.; Batth, T.S.; Chang, J.G.; Paulsen, M.T.; Magnuson, B.; Schimmel, J.; Kool, H.; et al. Divergent Molecular and Cellular Responses to Low and High-Dose Ionizing Radiation. *Cells* **2022**, *11*, 3794. [CrossRef] [PubMed]
44. Henry, E.; Souissi-Sahraoui, I.; Deynoux, M.; Lefèvre, A.; Barroca, V.; Campalans, A.; Ménard, V.; Calvo, J.; Pflumio, F.; Arcangeli, M.L. Human hematopoietic stem/progenitor cells display reactive oxygen species-dependent long-term hematopoietic defects after exposure to low doses of ionizing radiations. *Haematologica* **2020**, *105*, 2044–2055. [CrossRef] [PubMed]
45. Kumar, B.; Garcia, M.; Weng, L.; Jung, X.; Murakami, J.L.; Hu, X.; McDonald, T.; Lin, A.; Kumar, A.R.; DiGiusto, D.L.; et al. Acute myeloid leukemia transforms the bone marrow niche into a leukemia-permissive microenvironment through exosome secretion. *Leukemia* **2018**, *32*, 575–587. [CrossRef]
46. Shahrokh, B.; Allahbakhshian, F.M.; Ahmad, G.; Fatemeh, F.; Hossein, M.M. AML-derived extracellular vesicles negatively regulate stem cell pool size: A step toward bone marrow failure. *Curr. Res. Transl. Med.* **2022**, *71*, 103375. [CrossRef]
47. Meziani, F.; Tesse, A.; David, E.; Martinez, M.C.; Wangesteen, R.; Schneider, F.; Andriantsitohaina, R. Shed membrane particles from preeclamptic women generate vascular wall inflammation and blunt vascular contractility. *Am. J. Pathol.* **2006**, *169*, 1473–1483. [CrossRef]
48. Dutta, S.; Warshall, C.; Bandyopadhyay, C.; Dutta, D.; Chandran, B. Interactions between exosomes from breast cancer cells and primary mammary epithelial cells leads to generation of reactive oxygen species which induce DNA damage response, stabilization of p53 and autophagy in epithelial cells. *PLoS ONE* **2014**, *9*, e97580. [CrossRef]
49. van Meteren, N.; Lagadic-Gossmann, D.; Podechard, N.; Gobart, D.; Gallais, I.; Chevanne, M.; Collin, A.; Burel, A.; Dupont, A.; Rault, L.; et al. Extracellular vesicles released by polycyclic aromatic hydrocarbons-treated hepatocytes trigger oxidative stress in recipient hepatocytes by delivering iron. *Free. Radic. Biol. Med.* **2020**, *160*, 246–262. [CrossRef]
50. Simon, R.; Lam, A.; Li, M.C.; Ngan, M.; Menenzes, S.; Zhao, Y. Analysis of gene expression data using BRB-ArrayTools. *Cancer Inform.* **2007**, *3*, 11–17. [CrossRef]
51. Vlachos, I.S.; Zagganas, K.; Paraskevopoulou, M.D.; Georgakilas, G.; Karagkouni, D.; Vergoulis, T.; Dalamagas, T.; Hatzigeorgiou, A.G. DIANA-miRPath v3.0: Deciphering microRNA function with experimental support. *Nucleic Acids Res.* **2015**, *43*, W460–W466. [CrossRef] [PubMed]
52. Subedi, P.; Schneider, M.; Philipp, J.; Azimzadeh, O.; Metzger, F.; Moertl, S.; Atkinson, M.J.; Tapio, S. Comparison of methods to isolate proteins from extracellular vesicles for mass spectrometry-based proteomic analyses. *Anal. Biochem.* **2019**, *584*, 113390. [CrossRef] [PubMed]
53. Grosche, A.; Hauser, A.; Lepper, M.F.; Mayo, R.; von Toerne, C.; Merl-Pham, J.; Hauck, S.M. The Proteome of Native Adult Müller Glial Cells From Murine Retina. *Mol. Cell. Proteom. MCP* **2016**, *15*, 462–480. [CrossRef] [PubMed]
54. Wiśniewski, J.R.; Zougman, A.; Nagaraj, N.; Mann, M. Universal sample preparation method for proteome analysis. *Nat. Methods* **2009**, *6*, 359–362. [CrossRef]
55. Hladik, D.; Dalke, C.; von Toerne, C.; Hauck, S.M.; Azimzadeh, O.; Philipp, J.; Ung, M.C.; Schlattl, H.; Rößler, U.; Graw, J.; et al. CREB Signaling Mediates Dose-Dependent Radiation Response in the Murine Hippocampus Two Years after Total Body Exposure. *J. Proteome Res.* **2020**, *19*, 337–345. [CrossRef]
56. Navarro, P.; Trevisan-Herraz, M.; Bonzon-Kulichenko, E.; Núñez, E.; Martínez-Acedo, P.; Pérez-Hernández, D.; Jorge, I.; Mesa, R.; Calvo, E.; Carrascal, M.; et al. General statistical framework for quantitative proteomics by stable isotope labeling. *J. Proteome Res.* **2014**, *13*, 1234–1247. [CrossRef]
57. Karagkouni, D.; Paraskevopoulou, M.D.; Chatzopoulos, S.; Vlachos, I.S.; Tastsoglou, S.; Kanellos, I.; Papadimitriou, D.; Kavakiotis, I.; Maniou, S.; Skoufos, G.; et al. DIANA-TarBase v8: A decade-long collection of experimentally supported miRNA-gene interactions. *Nucleic Acids Res.* **2018**, *46*, D239–D245. [CrossRef]
58. Paraskevopoulou, M.D.; Georgakilas, G.; Kostoulas, N.; Vlachos, I.S.; Vergoulis, T.; Reczko, M.; Filippidis, C.; Dalamagas, T.; Hatzigeorgiou, A.G. DIANA-microT web server v5.0: Service integration into miRNA functional analysis workflows. *Nucleic Acids Res.* **2013**, *41*, W169–W173. [CrossRef]
59. Rahmati, S.; Abovsky, M.; Pastrello, C.; Jurisica, I. pathDIP: An annotated resource for known and predicted human gene-pathway associations and pathway enrichment analysis. *Nucleic Acids Res.* **2017**, *45*, D419–D426. [CrossRef]
60. Chen, Y.; Wang, X. miRDB: An online database for prediction of functional microRNA targets. *Nucleic Acids Res.* **2020**, *48*, D127–D131. [CrossRef]

Disclaimer/Publisher's Note: The statements, opinions and data contained in all publications are solely those of the individual author(s) and contributor(s) and not of MDPI and/or the editor(s). MDPI and/or the editor(s) disclaim responsibility for any injury to people or property resulting from any ideas, methods, instructions or products referred to in the content.

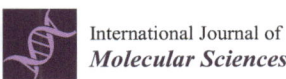

Article

Differential Expression of ATM, NF-KB, PINK1 and Foxo3a in Radiation-Induced Basal Cell Carcinoma

Rim Jenni [1], Asma Chikhaoui [1], Imen Nabouli [1], Anissa Zaouak [2], Fatma Khanchel [3], Houda Hammami-Ghorbel [2] and Houda Yacoub-Youssef [1,*]

[1] Laboratory of Biomedical Genomics and Oncogenetics (LR16IPT05), Institut Pasteur de Tunis, University Tunis El Manar, Tunis 1002, Tunisia
[2] Department of Dermatology, Habib Thameur Hospital (LR12SP03), Medicine Faculty, University Tunis El Manar, Tunis 1008, Tunisia
[3] Anatomopathology Department, Habib Thameur Hospital (LR12SP03), Medicine Faculty, University Tunis El Manar, Tunis 1008, Tunisia
* Correspondence: houda.yacoub@pasteur.utm.tn

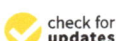

Citation: Jenni, R.; Chikhaoui, A.; Nabouli, I.; Zaouak, A.; Khanchel, F.; Hammami-Ghorbel, H.; Yacoub-Youssef, H. Differential Expression of ATM, NF-KB, PINK1 and Foxo3a in Radiation-Induced Basal Cell Carcinoma. *Int. J. Mol. Sci.* 2023, 24, 7181. https://doi.org/10.3390/ijms24087181

Academic Editor: François Chevalier

Received: 22 February 2023
Revised: 22 March 2023
Accepted: 27 March 2023
Published: 13 April 2023

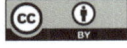

Copyright: © 2023 by the authors. Licensee MDPI, Basel, Switzerland. This article is an open access article distributed under the terms and conditions of the Creative Commons Attribution (CC BY) license (https://creativecommons.org/licenses/by/4.0/).

Abstract: Research in normal tissue radiobiology is in continuous progress to assess cellular response following ionizing radiation exposure especially linked to carcinogenesis risk. This was observed among patients with a history of radiotherapy of the scalp for ringworm who developed basal cell carcinoma (BCC). However, the involved mechanisms remain largely undefined. We performed a gene expression analysis of tumor biopsies and blood of radiation-induced BCC and sporadic patients using reverse transcription-quantitative PCR. Differences across groups were assessed by statistical analysis. Bioinformatic analyses were conducted using miRNet. We showed a significant overexpression of the *FOXO3a*, *ATM*, *P65*, *TNF-α* and *PINK1* genes among radiation-induced BCCs compared to BCCs in sporadic patients. *ATM* expression level was correlated with *FOXO3a*. Based on receiver-operating characteristic curves, the differentially expressed genes could significantly discriminate between the two groups. Nevertheless, *TNF-α* and *PINK1* blood expression showed no statistical differences between BCC groups. Bioinformatic analysis revealed that the candidate genes may represent putative targets for microRNAs in the skin. Our findings may yield clues as to the molecular mechanism involved in radiation-induced BCC, suggesting that deregulation of ATM-NF-kB signaling and *PINK1* gene expression may contribute to BCC radiation carcinogenesis and that the analyzed genes could represent candidate radiation biomarkers associated with radiation-induced BCC.

Keywords: radiotherapy; radiation-induced BCC; low-dose effects; DNA repair; ATM-NF-kb signaling; *PINK1* gene; microRNA; biomarkers

1. Introduction

Basal cell carcinoma (BCC) is the most frequent skin cancer, accounting for 90% of cutaneous cancer, and the most common human malignancy worldwide, characterized by an increasing incidence [1]. According to the Global Cancer Observatory (GLOBOCAN) database, 1,198,073 new cases of non-melanoma skin cancer, including BCC, were reported in 2020 [2]. While ultraviolet radiation (UV) is the most known carcinogen involved in skin malignancy, ionizing radiation (IR) exposure is an established etiological risk factor. In fact, radiotherapy is a standard treatment regimen for numerous solid tumors, and it was adopted for the treatment of some benign lesions of the skin, notably ringworm of the scalp (tinea capitis) [3]. Indeed, epidemiological studies have reported that previous depilatory radiotherapy is associated with a fourfold increased risk of cutaneous malignancy in irradiated skin, primarily BCC [4]. BCC occurs after a long period, up to decades after exposure, as a late effect of irradiation, with an inverse correlation between carcinogenesis risk and age at radiation exposure [5,6].

In addition, conflicting data exist concerning the clinical profile and the prognosis of radio-induced BCC compared to BCC in sporadic cases. Although some studies have reported a similar clinical course independently of radiotherapy history, other reports have described a more aggressive response associated with higher recurrence rates and difficult-to-treat radiation-induced BCC [7–9].

Aberrant activation of Hedgehog signaling is defined as a key common driver of BCC development. Moreover, high-throughput analyses have highlighted the potential contribution of other signaling pathways in BCC tumorigenesis, notably the WNT, Hippo, NOTCH, and mTOR pathways [10,11]. Nevertheless, little attention has been paid to the underlying molecular mechanisms involved in radiation-induced BCC, and studies that were conducted to identify molecular signatures unique to these tumors are controversial [12,13]. It was suggested that identifying the molecular link between the DDR pathway and Hedgehog signaling could unveil the pathogenesis of BCC developed post-radiotherapy [14].

Furthermore, studies based on genomic and transcriptomic profiling are ongoing to decipher the molecular mechanisms of radiogenic cancer and to identify molecular signatures that are discriminatory between radio-induced cancer and its sporadic counterpart. These were explored notably in radiation-induced hematological malignancies [15], sarcoma [16] and thyroid cancer [17]. While some reports have revealed molecular patterns unique to radiation-induced cancer with a lack of consistency, others have failed to identify these signatures, and the mechanisms underlying radiation-induced carcinogenesis are still largely misunderstood [18–20]. In fact, IR induces double-strand DNA breaks (DSBs) which activate ATM protein, a master regulator of the DNA damage response (DDR) pathway, leading subsequently to a cascade of cellular responses that may ultimately contribute to different cell fates [21]. It was reported that different signaling pathways are activated in response to IR in normal and tumor cells, including cellular senescence [22], mitochondrial signaling [23], inflammation [24], oxidative stress response [25], autophagy [26] and microRNA signaling [27–29]. Indeed, it was suggested that tumor recurrence following radiotherapy may be explained by radiation-induced cellular senescence of adjacent normal cells surrounding the tumor [22,30,31].

In this study, we aimed to decipher the molecular mechanism(s) of radiation-induced BCC tumorigenesis by investigating the expression patterns of genes of interest in radio-induced BCC and exploring their potential usefulness as candidate biomarkers specific to this tumoral entity. Moreover, we aimed to study the microRNA-mRNA regulatory network to understand the potential contribution of microRNA regulators in this pathogenesis. Our results identified differential gene expression between radiation-induced and non-radiation-induced BCC, suggesting that the deregulation of ATM-NF-kB signaling and *PINK1* expression could be involved in the pathogenesis of radiation-induced BCC.

2. Results
2.1. Clinical Features of BCC Patients

Patients were separated into two groups depending on history of radiotherapy of the scalp for tinea capitis during their childhood: radiation-induced (radio-induced) BCC and non-radiation-induced (non-radio-induced) BCC developed in sporadic patients.

According to the experience of the referral center, the "Dermatology department of Habib Thameur Hospital", the majority of patients treated with radiotherapy for tinea capitis develop nodular BCC on the scalp.

To avoid any bias due to patient selection that may have affected gene expression levels, the patients enrolled in both groups were selected to match different parameters (age at BCC diagnosis, UV exposure, etc.) as closely as possible. All collected tumors were localized on the face (six cases) and on the scalp (two cases). All tumors were primary BCCs. Mean age at diagnosis was 66.25 and 65.5 for the radio-induced and non-radio-induced groups, respectively. The tumors were of nodular or adenoid histology independently of radiation etiology. The majority of patients, especially radio-BCC patients, showed multiples lesions. Adenoid tumors coexisted with basosquamous carcinoma at the same anatomical site or with morphea form BCC ata nearby site in the cases of BCC2 and BCC5, respectively. Basosquamous carcinoma and morphea form BCC are aggressive BCC subtypes. Within our cohort, BCC patients presented different clinical phenotypes (according to the numbers and sites of lesions and histopathological subtypes) independently of IR exposure. Clinical and anatomopathological parameters were obtained from medical records and are summarized in Table 1. Different clinical and histopathological BCC subtypes are presented in Figures 1 and 2 respectively.

Table 1. Patients' characteristics.

Patient	Gender	Ethnicity	Age	History of Radiotherapy	Histology	Tumor Size	Multifocality	Tumor Location
BCC2	M	Tunisia	60	Yes	Adenoid	3 cm	Yes (n = 7)	Temporal region of the face
BCC4	M	Tunisia	60	Yes	Adenoid	3 cm	Yes (n = 2)	Temporal region of the face
BCC5	M	Tunisia	79	No	Adenoid	1 cm	Yes (n = 3)	Temporal region of the face
BCC8	M	Tunisia	85	Yes	Nodular	2.5 cm	No	Scalp
BCC12	F	Tunisia	63	No	Nodular	3 cm	Yes (n = 2)	Ala of nose
BCC16	M	Tunisia	40	No	Nodular	3 cm	No	Ala of nose
BCC19	M	Tunisia	80	No	Nodular	3 cm	No	Cheek
BCC22	M	Tunisia	60	Yes	Nodular	2 cm	Yes (n = 2)	Scalp

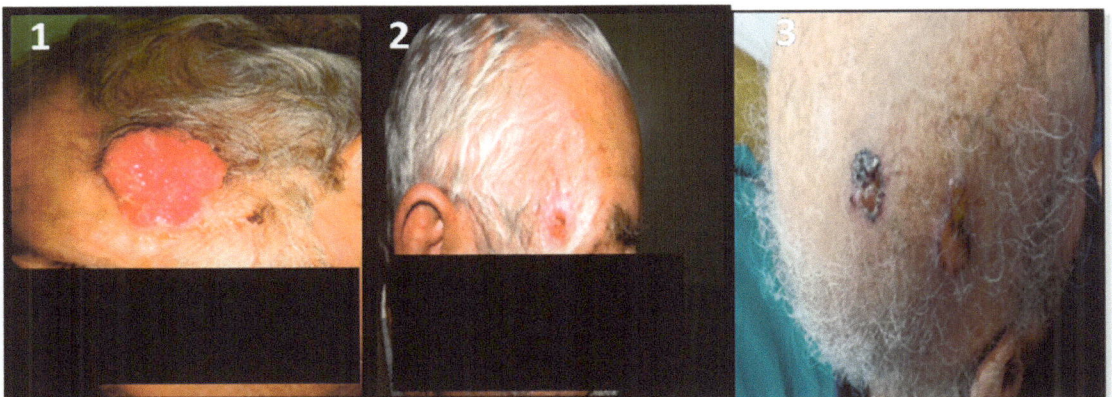

Figure 1. Radio-induced and non-radio-induced BCC patients. 1-corresponds to a non-radio-induced BCC patient. 2,3-correspond to two radio-induced patients: 2-presents one small malignant lesion; 3-presents multiple lesions on the scalp. The aggressive form of BCC is independent of radiation etiology in this cohort.

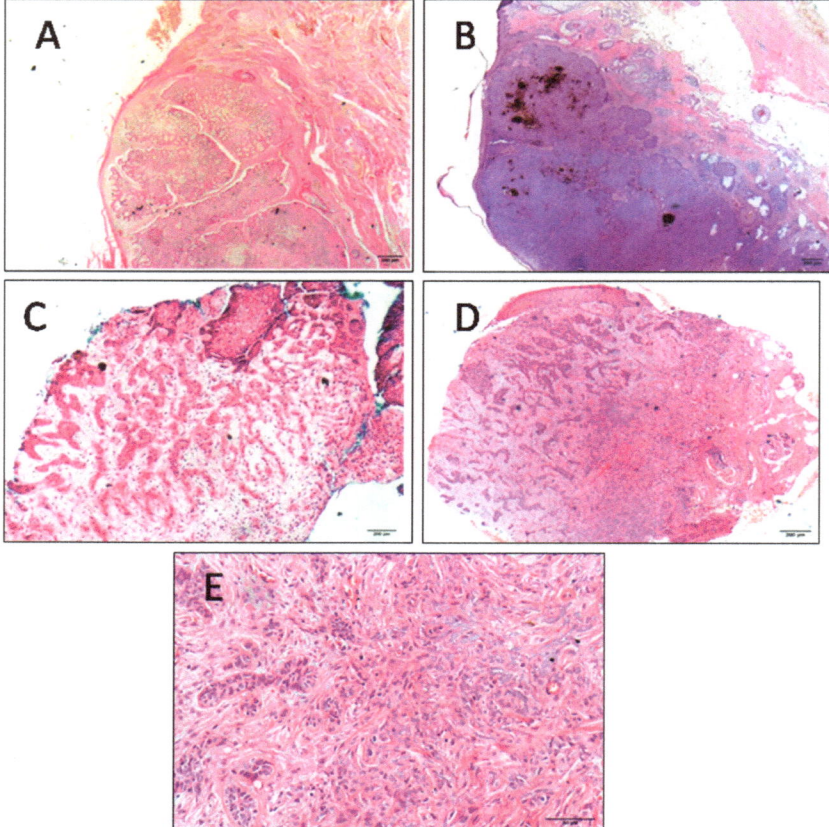

Figure 2. Hematoxylin-and-eosin-stained section of BCC tumor tissues representative of different histopathological subtypes of BCC. (**A**) Adenoid basal cell carcinoma with pseudo-glandular appearance. The stroma is fibrous (×100). (**B**) Nodular subtype of basal cell carcinoma with melanin deposit (×100). (**C**) Morphea form basal cell carcinoma with narrow cords of basaloid cells which are compressed by abundant sclerotic collagenous stroma (×100). (**D**) Basosquamous basal cell carcinoma (×100). (**E**) A focal squamous differentiation (×200). Scale bars = 200 μm for (**A**–**D**) and 50 μm for (**E**).

2.2. Molecular Analysis

All tumors located on the head was selected as an inclusion criterion. This decision was made in order to exclude any differential gene expression associated with molecular signatures linked to UV exposure. First, we investigated *FOXO3a*, *ATM*, *P65*, *PINK1* and *TNF-α* expression in radio-induced BCC and non-radio-induced BCC and in age-matched healthy controls using the rt-qPCR technique. Our data revealed significant upregulation of *FOXO3a*, *ATM*, *P65*, *PINK1* and *TNF-α* genes among the radio-induced BCC patients compared to the non-radio-induced BCC group ($p = 0.021$ for each of the *ATM*, *P65*, *PINK1* and *TNF-α* genes; $p = 0.043$ for *FOXO3a*) (Figure 3).

Furthermore, a significant strong positive correlation was observed between *ATM* and *FOXO3a*' expression among BCC patients using the Pearson correlation test ($r = 0.951$, $p = 0.000289$) (Figure 4). A positive correlation was also observed between *ATM* and *P65* ($r = 0.984$, $p = 0.000009$) and between *ATM* and *TNF-α* ($r = 0.976$, $p = 0.000036$).

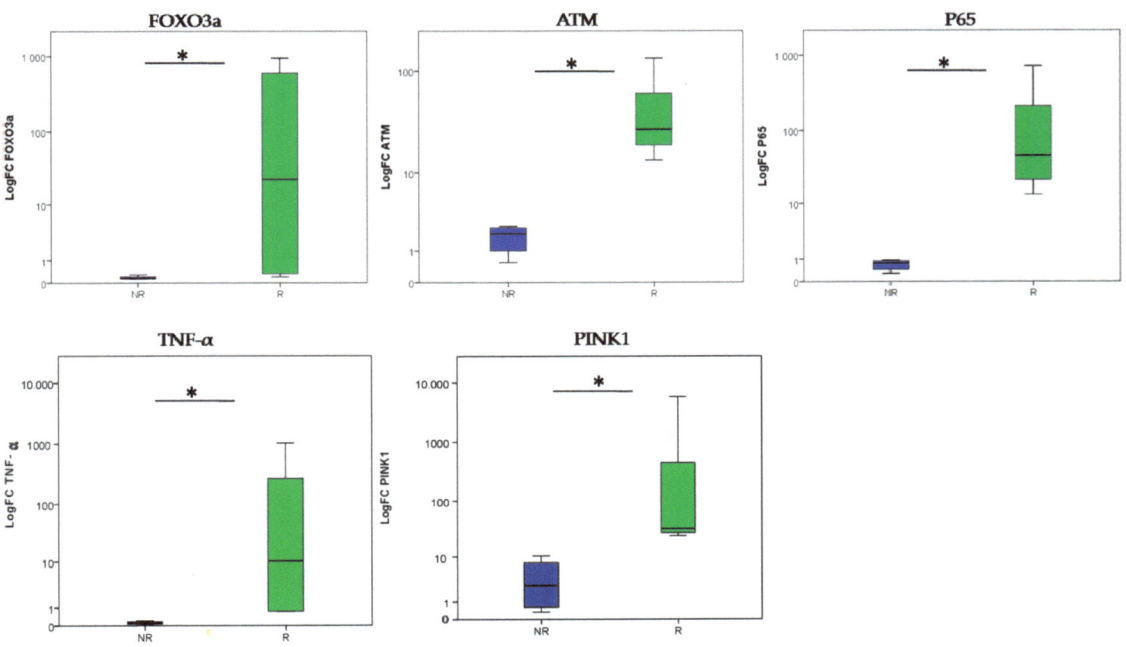

Figure 3. Differential gene expression profiles for radio-induced and non-radio-induced BCC biopsies. Blue box plot: non-radio-induced BCC (NR); green box plot: radio-induced BCC (R). (* = $p < 0.05$).

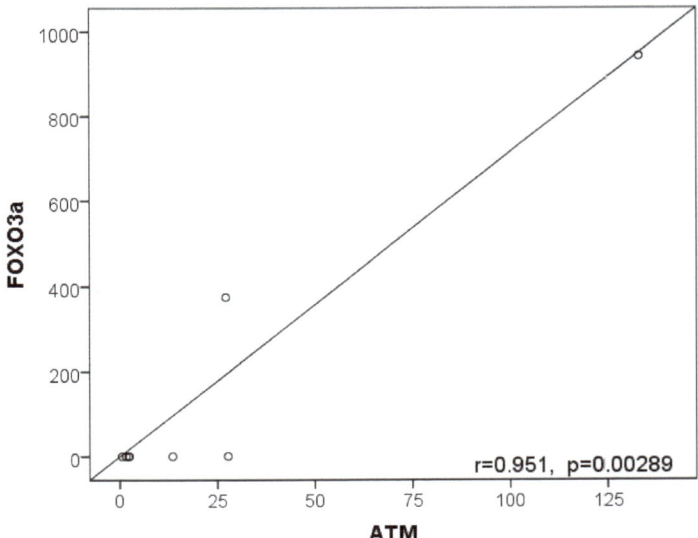

Figure 4. Correlation between *FOXO3a* and *ATM* expression in BCC patients' biopsies. Pearson correlation of *FOXO3a* and *ATM* gene expression fold changes among BCC patients revealed a strong positive correlation of these genes with a Pearson correlation coefficient (r) = 0.951 (p = 0.00289). Each circle represents the expression levels of both genes for each patient.

We further examined the potential of *FOXO3a*, *ATM*, *P65*, *PINK1* and *TNF-α* genes to discriminate between radio-induced and non-radio-induced BCC using ROC curve analysis. We defined cut-off values of 0.179, 7.956, 7.09, 16.78 and 0.46 for *FOXO3a*, *ATM*, *P65*, *PINK1* and *TNF-α*, respectively, based on the Youden index method. Our results revealed that the gene expression levels could significantly differentiate between BCC groups (area under the curve (AUC) = 1, $p = 0.021$, for the *ATM*, *P65*, *PINK1* and *TNF-α* genes, with 100% specificity and 100% sensitivity, and AUC = 0.938, $p = 0.043$, with 100% sensitivity and 75% specificity, for *FOXO3a*) (Figure 5). In fact, these genes showed an excellent diagnostic performance, which suggests their usefulness as potential diagnostic biomarkers for radio-induced BCC.

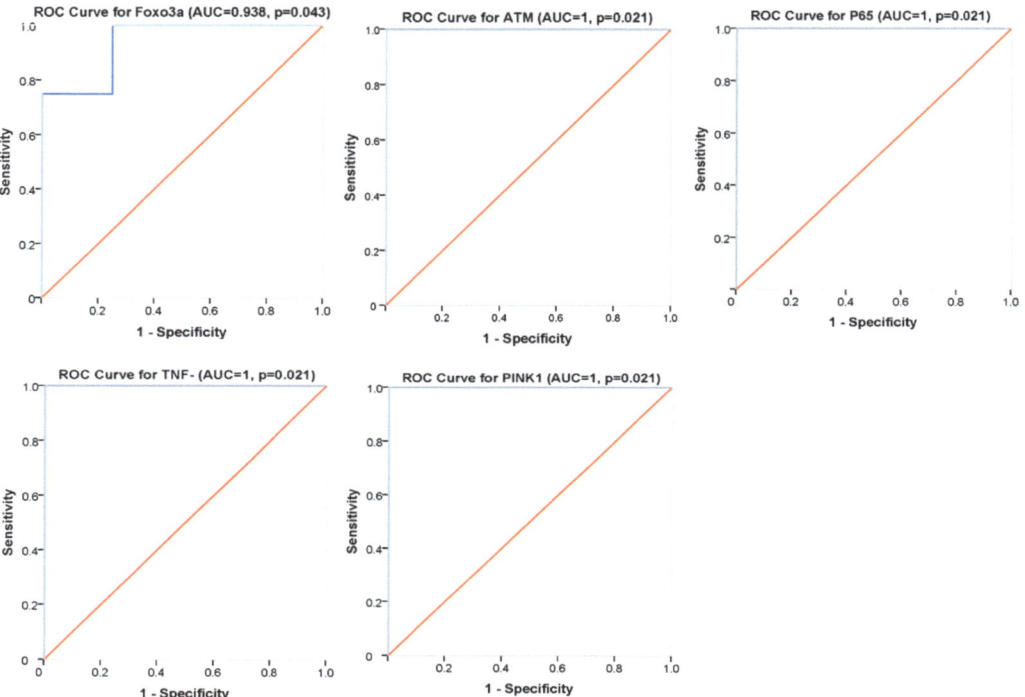

Figure 5. ROC curve analysis of differentially expressed genes between radio-induced and non-radio-induced BCC. ROC analysis for the *FOXO3a*, *ATM*, *P65*, *PINK1* and *TNF-α* genes in different plots. The *p*-value is the probability that the observed sample AUC-ROC is found when the true AUC-ROC is 0.5 (null hypothesis: the variable cannot distinguish between the two groups; area = 0.5 if the ROC coincides with the reference line). We found that the area under the curve is significantly different from 0.5. *ATM*, *P65*, *PINK1* and *TNF-α* have excellent discrimination performance, with AUCs = 1 (100%specificity and 100% sensitivity). The ROC curve foreach of them passes through the upper left corner of the plot, while *FOXO3a* has an ROC curve close to the upper left corner, with an AUC = 0.938 that represents an excellent diagnostic value.

Subsequently, the expression levels of the *TNF-α* and *PINK1* genes were analyzed in the blood of patients with BCC to assess their potential as non-invasive biomarkers for radio-induced BCC. Our data showed a similar expression profile for *TNF-α* among BCC patients in both groups ($p > 0.05$). Inaddition, *PINK1* analysis revealed upregulation among radio-induced BCC compared to non-radio-induced BCC, which was in accordance with the *PINK1* expressionin patients' biopsies. However, this differential expression failed to reach statistical significance ($p > 0.05$) (Figure 6).

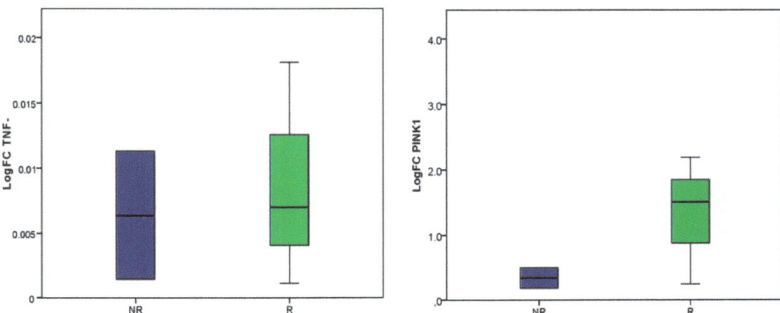

Figure 6. Differential gene expression profiles between radio-induced and non-radio-induced BCC in patients' blood. Blue box plot: non-radio-induced BCC NR; green box plot: radio-induced BCC R.

2.3. Bioinformatic Analysis

We examined putative interactions between the differentially expressed genes and microRNAs (miRNAs) in the skin using the miRNet database. An miRNA-target interaction network was created that included several upstream miRNAs that interact directly with FOXO3a, ATM, P65, TNF-α and PINK1 mRNAs, representing a complex landscape of functional associations. Each node represents an mRNA or miRNA (Figure 7). In fact, miRNAs are intricately involved in the DDR pathway by targeting ATM in the skin. FOXO3a and ATM had the highest interaction (highest connectivity degree) and hence were the most important hubs in this network analysis. miR-24-3p was the most important miRNA regulating the network based on its having the highest node degree (Table 2). According to the Reactome database, cellular senescence was the most enriched pathway ($p = 0.0026$, adj. $p < 0.05$).

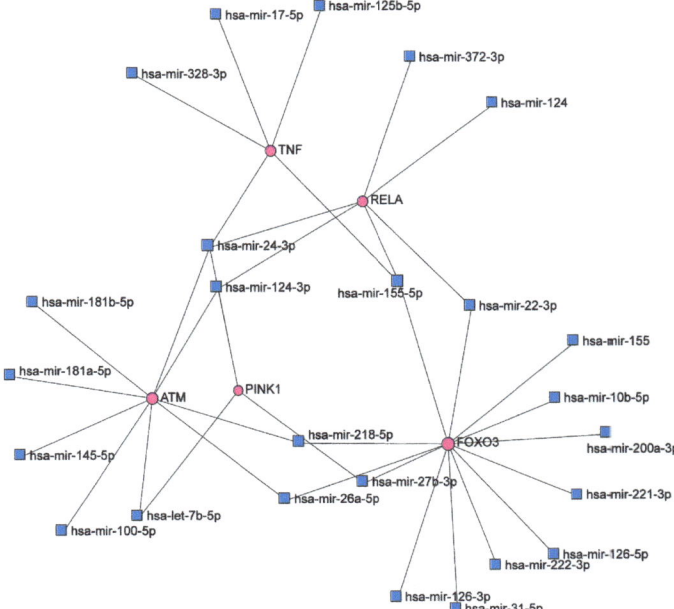

Figure 7. miRNA-mRNA interaction network with differentially expressed genes in the skin, constructed using miRNet database data.

Table 2. Top miRNAs and targeted mRNAs in the network interactions determined via miRNet.

Node	Degree
FOXO3a	13
ATM	9
RELA	6
TNF	5
hsa-mir-24-3p	4
PINK1	4
hsa-mir-124-3p	3
hsa-mir-155-5p	3
hsa-mir-26a-5p	2
hsa-mir218-5p	2
hsa-mir-27b-3p	2
hsa-mir-22b-3p	2
hsa-mir-22b	2
hsa-mir-let-7b-5p	3

The majority of these miRNAs are described in the literature as IR-responsive and are primarily involved in cellular senescence (this will be discussed below). Hence, we suggest that deregulation of these miRNAs in response to IR may affect skin cells' response to irradiation, notably linked to the analyzed pathways, which may be associated with the carcinogenesis process.

3. Discussion

In our study, we aimed to identify differentially expressed genes between radio-induced and non-radio-induced BCC which may provide insights into the molecular contributors to or the under pinning sofradio-induced carcinogenesis. To the best of our knowledge, our study was the first to explore the ATM-NF-kB pathway and *PINK1* expression in radio-induced BCC. In addition, we suggest that miRNA regulation of these pathways may shed light on radio-induced BCC.

BCC represents a significant health and socio-economic burden given its high frequency and incidence [32]. BCC is rarely invasive or metastatic an dis usually associated with a good prognosis. However, it may lead to significant morbidity due to its locally destructive potential and its relatively high recurrence rate [33]. In addition, different BCC entities exist, though the genetic basis of the carcinogenic process and clinical differences are not fully elucidated [34]. Moreover, it is unclear whether mechanisms of BCC carcinogenesis differ according to etiological factors.

IR is a well-known risk factor for skin malignancies. Clinical and epidemiological studies have reported a high rate of BCC cancer following IR exposure, which has primarily been described in the context of treatment for tinea capitis during childhood [4]. It was suggested that cancer risk may persist throughout the life of exposed individuals [35]. Conflicting data exist concerning the prognosis of radio-induced BCC.

- Clinical features of radio-induced BCC and non-radio-induced BCC

In the present study, patients were characterized by different clinical profiles independently of radiation etiology, presenting adenoid or nodular subtypes. Although nodular BCC is the most frequent subtype, adenoid tumors are very rare histopathological variants that are considered low-grade BCCs [36]. Adenoid tumors were isolated or associated with other subtypes, notably basosquamous and morphea form BCC, for BCC2 and 5, respectively, which are aggressive BCC subtypes [37,38]. Nodular BCC was classified as a low-risk tumor according to the WHO classification. According to BCC risk stratification, BCC8 and BCC19 are associated with an intermediate prognosis, as they are characterized as nodular subtypes, with sizes> 2 cm, and are located in low-risk areas [39]. Based on the new BCC classification, tumors may be classified as "easy-to-treat" or "difficult-to-treat", which classifications are associated with different clinical outcomes [40,41]. Although some tumors included in our study were "easy-to-treat" BCCs, some of them presented specific features that may pose treatment difficulties, which may be linked to tumor location, as with BCC12 and BCC16 sporadic cases (located in patients' noses).These tumors have a high risk of recurrence. In fact, our data are consistent with a study which reported that IR exposure does not affect clinical and histopathological features or even patient prognosis [42]. However, other studies have reported a more aggressive phenotype among radio-induced BCC [9]. Herein, prognosis was assessed based on clinical prognostic factors.

- Gene expression analysis to decipher radio-induced BCC carcinogenesis mechanisms

Despite radiation exposure being a known carcinogenic factor for BCC, the underlying molecular mechanisms are not yet fully understood. Although those studies have reported the absence of molecular signatures that could discriminate between radio-induced and non-radio-induced BCC, particularly linked to the *PTCH* and *TP53* genes [13,43], it was suggested that the Hh signaling pathway could be linked to susceptibility to BCC radiation carcinogenesis and that *PTCH* could contribute to this process [43]. In fact, it was reported that the genetic background of Ptch-mutated mice may affect susceptibility to BCC development after IR exposure [44,45]. Furthermore, it was suggested that genomic instability could explain genetic susceptibility to radio-induced BCC carcinogenesis [46], which may predispose to mitochondrial DNA mutations [47]. Recently, a genomic characterization of radio-induced BCC versus sporadic cases has revealed specific chromosomal rearrangements that could discriminate between both groups [12].

- ATM-NF-kB signaling and PINK1-mediated mitophagy in response to irradiation

In our study, we report differentially expressed genes between BCC groups that are radiation-responsive and mainly involved in IR-driven BCC carcinogenesis. *ATM* and *FOXO3a* expression were significantly increased in BCC biopsies from irradiated patients compared to sporadic cases. In fact, IR induces DSBs which trigger the DDR pathway. *ATM* is a master regulator involved in the coordination of cellular response to radiation-induced DNA damage and a key determinant of radio-sensitivity [48]. In addition, *ATM* expression was significantly correlated with *FOXO3a* expression level in BCC patients. This suggests a potential regulation, at least in part, of *ATM* by *FOXO3a* transcription factors. Indeed, it was reported that in the DDR pathway, FOXO3a interacts directly with ATM, which is required for ATM autophosphorylation, promoting the ATM response network [49]. However, our findings were in agreement with the fact that FOXO3a regulates *ATM* gene expression, which has been reported in hematopoietic stem cells [50]. Nonetheless, it was described that, in response to DNA damage, *FOXO3a* upregulation maintains genomic stability and is mediated by H2AX, a downstream target of ATM [51,52]. However, *FOXO3a* and *ATM* expression levels were not correlated among three radio-induced patients, which may suggest that other factors are involved in *ATM* regulation in BCC radiation carcinogenesis. Moreover, we revealed upregulation of *P65*, which coded for an NF-kB subunit, and of *TNF-α*, which coded for a pro-inflammatory cytokine and a senescence-associated secretory phenotype (SASP) factor, among irradiated patients. A positive correlation was observed between ATM and P65 and between ATM and TNF-α, which could suggest a molecular link between ATM and NF-kB. In fact, IR triggers cellular senescence in normal and cancer cells. ATM is a key driver of NF-kB-induced cellular senescence following DNA damage through the secretion of SASP factors, which enhance NF-kB signaling in an autocrine manner via cytokine receptors [22]. Our data suggest an aberrant activation/over-presentation of the ATM-NF-kB signaling pathway in response to IR. Despite this, we did not directly analyze NF-kb signaling activation. The high expression levels of *TNF-α* and *P65* are indicative markers of NF-kB activation. A few studies have been performed to assess the biological effect of IR on human skin cells which revealed the activation of the DDR pathway, an inflammatory response [53–55], and the expression of cellular senescence markers [56]. Moreover, in the context of cancer radiotherapy, IR induced cellular senescence of normal cells adjacent to tumors, leading to either tissue fibrosis and organ dysfunction or to tumorigenesis [22,30,31]. Indeed, it was suggested that transient senescent cells are associated with an anti-tumoral effect, while their accumulation is linked to a detrimental effect leading to increased cancer susceptibility [57].

Furthermore, ATM plays an important role in mitochondrial responses to irradiation, following recognition of nuclear DNA damage and subsequent damage signal transduction to mitochondria, playing an important role in the crosstalk between these two organelles in irradiated fibroblast cells, which enhance mitochondrial biogenesis and ROS generation [58]. Although nuclear DNA was primarily considered as a main target of IR, the involvement of mitochondria as key targets of IR and as contributors to radio-induced cell impairment is becoming increasingly evident [23,59] and could explain the high risk of carcinogenesis [60]. Despite the role of mitochondrial dysfunction in response to irradiation being well understood, the involvement of mitochondrial integrity and dynamics has been less explored. In fact, ATM can promote selective elimination of defective mitochondria, termed mitophagy, via activation of the PINK1/Parkin pathway; however, the mechanism involved is not fully elucidated. It was described that ATM impacts this pathway via kinase-dependent [61] or -independent mechanisms through the regulation of *PINK1* (PTEN-induced putative kinase1) expression or interaction with Parkin [62,63]. In addition, ATM-deficient cells revealed that mitophagy induction following irradiation is ATM-dependent [64]. We analyzed *PINK1* gene expression, a key contributor to mitophagy, and observed over expression in radio-induced BCC compared to non-radio-induced cases. In addition, FOXO3a enhances *PINK1* gene expression, leading to a pro-survival signal in response to oxidative stress [65]. This was in accordance with another study which suggested that under extensive mitochondrial alterations, mitophagy activation enhances cell survival following irradiation [66]. However, it was suggested that post-irradiation mitophagy induction could maintain cellular redox control and that disruption of this pathway leads to tumorigenesis [60]. Another report has described that mitophagy effect depends on irradiation dose [67].

In summary, our results suggest that the ATM-NF-kB signaling pathway and the *PINK1* gene, related to cellular senescence and mitophagy, are involved in radio-induced BCC carcinogenesis.

- Biomarkers of radio-induced BCC

ROC curve analysis revealed that the differentially expressed genes could significantly discriminate between radio-induced BCC and non-radio-induced BCC and may consequently represent candidate radio-induced BCC biomarkers. This could guide further validation studies aiming to investigate the relevance of these candidate biomarkers with larger cohorts based on independent sets of samples. Such studies could provide straightforward evidence of potential radiation biomarkers and be a step toward understanding radio-susceptibility to BCC. Indeed, accumulating studies are seeking to identify molecular peculiarities unique to radiation-induced cancer compared to sporadic counterparts, as they are often clinically indistinguishable, which may lead to the decipherment of key events involved in radiation carcinogenesis [15]. Conflicting data have been generated, while some reports have identified specific signatures associated with molecular fingerprints of radiation-induced cancer. Others have often described similar molecular patterns independently of radiation etiology, and no accurate molecular signature/biomarker has yet been settled [16,18,68]. Further studies are warranted to untangle the underlying mechanisms. Therefore, we examined whether these biomarkers in particular, *TNF-α* and *PINK1* could serve as non-invasive tools by analyzing their expression profiles in patients' blood. *TNF-α* was under-expressed in BCC patients, with a similar pattern independent of radiation etiology. These data may support that *TNF-α* alteration was tumor-specific. This finding was supported by a loop between radio-induced inflammation, mobilization of immune cells and sustained tissular damage, mediated by DNA damage and SASP factors following irradiation [69]. However, our results were in discordance with previous studies that reported persistent systemic inflammation in individuals with a history of IR exposure [70]. This was explained by possible confounding factors or by the combinatorial effect of patient age and irradiation [71–73]. In fact, the BCC patients included in our study were age-matched; accordingly, the differences in gene expression probably reflect cellular response to irradiation. In addition, inflammatory systemic response may be explained by blood cell response to irradiation, since these individuals were exposed to whole-body rather than localized irradiation. On the other hand, PINK1 was differentially expressed between the two BCC groups, with overexpression in irradiated cases; however, this differential expression failed to reach statistical significance. In fact, an increase in PINK1 expression in rat thyroids was reported following irradiation [74]. Our results point out, at least, that the analyzed genes could not represent non-invasive radio-BCC biomarkers.

- miRNA regulators in BCC radiation carcinogenesis

Our current understanding of cellular response to irradiation has evolved to a more complex network that involves different molecular determinants, such as epigenetic regulators, mainly miRNAs [75]. miRNAs mediate cellular radio-response via regulating components of key signaling pathways involved in this process, specifically DDR signaling [76]. Indeed, it was suggested that gene expression profile alterations following irradiation are largely explained by miRNAs, which play a crucial role in defining cell fates, controlling subsequent radiosensitivity [77]. Moreover, it was described that miRNAs participate in radiation carcinogenesis [78–80]. In this study, miRNAs represented in the network analysis created by miRNet are mostly described as radio-responsive. miR-24-3p represents the most important miRNA in the generated network, targeting the ATM, RELA (P65) and PINK1 genes. In fact, it was reported that miR-24-3p plays a crucial role in carcinogenesis and therapeutic response associated with radiosensitivity [81]. miR-24 was described as a regulator of cellular response to DNA damage, and its downregulation enhances tumor cell radio-resistance [82]. Furthermore, miR-24 expression decreases with cellular senescence [83], and it was defined as a mitochondrial miR (mitomiR) [84]. It was described that miR-24-3p and miR-124 attenuate the expression of pro-inflammatory mediators via NF-kB signaling [85,86]. miR-124 also increases in senescent skin, while it decreases during tumorigenesis, particularly in squamous cell carcinoma [87]. In addition, it was reported that Let-7 family expression patterns are altered upon irradiation, characterized by ATM-dependent downregulation in skin fibroblasts [88]. miR-26a and miR-100a were described as enhancing tumor cell radio-sensitivity via targeting DNA repair proteins [89,90]. miR-145 is described as a regulator of the DDR pathway and cellular senescence in different cell types [91,92]. Downregulation of miR-145-5p was also reported in basal cell carcinoma [93]. Indeed, it was revealed that senescence-associated miRNAs (SA-miRs) are implicated in radiation-induced premature cellular senescence and that the knockdown of miR-155 stimulates this process [94]. miR-181a/b are involved in keratinocyte replicative senescence and are dysregulated in cancers [95]. According to miRNA transcriptome profiling, miR-222 was repressed in irradiated cells [96]. Moreover, miR-24 is a radiation-responsive miRNA that may represent a potential biomarker of radiation-induced gastric cancer [97]. We suggest that this network may give insights into the regulatory role of microRNAs in radio-induced BCC; some of these miRNAs may contribute to the pathogenesis of BCC through the regulation of ATM-NF-kB signaling and PINK1 expression level in response to irradiation. Experimental studies are warranted to validate these interactions in radio-induced BCC.

Further research in the field of normal tissue radiobiology is of paramount importance to decipher the mechanisms involved in cellular radio-response. In fact, even though depilatory radiotherapy is no longer used, IR is still used as a clinical diagnostic tool and a therapeutic modality, besides being used for occupationally/accidentally exposed individuals, and the incidence of BCC is continuously increasing. Moreover, patients with cancers, including some BCCs amenable to radiotherapy, may develop a second malignancy due to the radiosensitivity of healthy tissues surrounding the tumor, which affects treatment efficiency. The identification of promising biomarkers is an unmet need to improve long-term risk assessment following IR exposure, which may aid clinicians in monitoring exposed individuals. These biomarkers may represent novel targets to prevent or at least minimize cellular radiotoxicity linked to carcinogenesis risk.

To our knowledge, our study represents the first investigation of ATM-NF-kB signaling and *PINK1* gene expression, implicated in cellular senescence and mitophagy in BCC pathogenesis following radiotherapy. Further studies are needed to deeply characterize and explore these processes in a larger cohort of radio-induced BCC patients. Moreover, proteins encoded by the studied genes should be analyzed to further confirm the activation of these pathways. In addition, further studies are mandatory to shed light on the complexity of the interactions between genes of interest and microRNAs in response to irradiation.

4. Materials and Methods

4.1. Human Specimens and Sample Collection

We conducted a comparative study using patients' fresh frozen skin biospecimens and blood. According to histological evaluation, confirmed by an atomopathologist, a total of eight patients diagnosed with basal cell carcinoma were enrolled in this study. Four of the BCC samples were obtained from sporadic patients and four were obtained from patients with a history of radiotherapy of the scalp for tinea capitis during their childhood and were considered as radio-induced BCC. All tumors being located on the face and scalp area was an inclusion criterion. One healthy skin biopsy from a UV-exposed area from the head of a healthy age- and geographically matched control was included after screening for the absence of any signs of malignancy. Systemic investigation was performed for five of the patients, including three radio-induced BCCs and two BCCs from sporadic cases (or non-radiation-induced BCC), and the sample from the healthy control. BCC and healthy control biopsies were collected from the Dermatology department of "Habib Thameur" Hospital.

All participants included in this study provided written informed consent, and the study was carried out in accordance with the Helsinki principles and approved by the Institute Pasteur Ethics Committee in Tunisia under the ethical accord number (reference PCI/22/2012/v2).

4.2. Gene Expression Analysis

4.2.1. RNA Extraction and cDNA Synthesis

Total RNA from the tissue and blood samples of patients with BCC and the healthy control were extracted using trizol and the miRNeasy Mini Kit (QIAGEN), following the manufacturer's instructions. The concentration and purity of isolated RNA was assessed using the Nanodrop spectrophotometer DeNovix DS-11 (Thermo Fisher Scientific, Wilmington, DE, USA).

Prior to total isolated RNA reverse transcription (RT), a Dnase treatment was carried out in a Qsp of 10 µL, using 1 µg of RNA, 10X DNase Buffer and 1 U/µL of DNase I enzyme. After RNA sample incubation at ambient temperature for 15 min, 25 mM of EDTA was added, and RNA was then placed at 65 °C for 10 min. The cDNA synthesis was performed using the Superscript II RT Kit (Cat. No:18064014 Invitrogen, Carlsbad, CA, USA), starting with 1µg of purified RNA in a total reaction volume of 20 µL, according to the manufacturer's protocol.

4.2.2. Quantitative Real-Time PCR

The *ATM*, *FOXO3a*, *P65* (*RELA*), *TNF-α* and *PINK1* genes were investigated by quantitative real-time PCR (qPCR) using the Syber Green kit, according to the manufacturer's protocol. Among genes involved in cellular senescence and mitophagy, this set of genes was selected after exploring gene expression data generated by the GTEx (Genotype-Tissue Expression) database. These genes are expressed in human skin cells and showed no differences between sun-exposed and non-sun-exposed skin areas. Specific primers were used. The qPCR reaction was carried out in a 96-well plate using the Light Cycler L480 (Roche Applied System) with a reaction volume containing Sybr Green Mix (Invitrogen), Quantities of 10 µM of each forward and reverse primer for 17 µL of Mix and 100 ng/µL of cDNA were used. cDNA amplification was performed in a cycling protocol with 35 cycles (at 95 °C for 15 s and for 60 °C for 1 min) preceded by a pre-amplification step at 95 °C for 10 min. Relative gene expression levels were normalized to the expression of the housekeeping gene *RPLP0*. Experiments were performed in duplicate for each candidate target gene and for each reference gene. Relative fold changes were calculated using the comparative cycle threshold (ct) method ($2^{-\Delta\Delta Ct}$). The sequences of the primers are listed in Table 3.

Table 3. Primer sequences used for qPCR.

Gene	Sequence (5'-3')	Length	Tm (°C)
FOXO3a	F: CGGACAAACGGCTCACTCT	19	61.9
	R: GGACCCGCATGAATCGACTAT	21	61.7
ATM	F: GCACGAAGTGCCTCCAATTC	21	61.1
	R: ACATTCTGGCACGCTTTGG	19	61.4
TNF-α	F: CCTCTCTCTAATCAGCCCTCTG	22	62.1
	R: GAGGACCTGGGAGTAGATGAG	21	62.8
PINK1	F: CCCAAGCAACTAGCCCCTC	19	64.5
	R: GGCAGCACATCAGGGTAGTC	20	63.1
P65	F: ATGTGGAGATCATTGAGCAGC	21	60
	R: CCTGGTCCTGTGTAGCCATT	20	60.2

4.3. Statistical Analysis

IBM SPSS version 21.0 was used for statistical analysis. Differences across specimen groups and gene expression correlations were inspected using the Mann–Whitney U and Pearson exact tests, respectively. Area under the curve–receiver operating characteristic (AUC-ROC) analysis was performed to evaluate the potential of candidate genes to discriminate between radio-induced BCC and non-radio-induced BCC groups. An excellent model for a good separation performance was considered when the AUC value was near to 1. Cut-off values were determined according to the Youden index method. Maximizing the Youden index enabled the identification of the cut-off point of the curve with the highest value for the sum of sensitivity and specificity. For all tests, a p-value < 0.05 was considered statistically significant.

4.4. Bioinformatic Analysis

We explored the miRNet 2.0 database to identify putative upstream microRNAs that target the candidate genes and generate an miRNA-target gene interaction network-based visual analysis of the skin. In fact, node degrees (the numbers of connections with other nodes) indicate important hubs in the generated network. In addition, miRNet offers a functional enrichment analysis, which was performed with the Reactome pathway tool (adjusted $p < 0.05$).

5. Conclusions

We suggest that aberrant regulation of ATM-NF-kB signaling and *PINK1* gene expression could be related to BCC radiation carcinogenesis and that biomarkers involved in these pathways may discriminate between BCCs according to their radiation etiologies. Furthermore, we suggest that microRNAs may play an important role as well, highlighting their potential implication in the pathogenesis of radio-induced BCC. Our study highlights the importance of the exploration of radio-induced carcinogenesis and extends our understanding to a more complex network involving different interconnected cellular and molecular components.

Author Contributions: R.J. performed the experiments, analyzed the data and drafted the manuscript. A.C. collected the biospecimens, helped with the experiments and reviewed the manuscript draft. I.N. helped with the biospecimen collections. A.Z. performed the skin biopsies. F.K. performed the anatomopathological analysis for tumor biopsies. H.H.-G. undertook the patient recruitment and clinical follow-up of patients. H.Y.-Y. was responsible for the study conception, supervised the study and revised the manuscript. All authors have read and agreed to the published version of the manuscript.

Funding: The study was supported by the Tunisian Ministry of Public Health, the Ministry of Higher Education and Scientific Research (LR16IPT05) and the "Project Collaborative Interne" (PCI_Melanoma, IPT).

Institutional Review Board Statement: This study was carried out in accordance with the Helsinki principles and approved by the Institute Pasteur Ethics Committee in Tunisia under the ethical accord number (reference PCI/22/2012/v2).

Informed Consent Statement: Written informed consent was obtained from all subjects involved in the study for the molecular investigation and publication of the article.

Data Availability Statement: All data have been provided in the manuscript. The data generated in this study can be provided by the corresponding author upon reasonable request.

Acknowledgments: We would like to thank the patients for their collaboration and trust.

Conflicts of Interest: The authors declare no conflict of interest.

References

1. Fania, L.; Didona, D.; Morese, R.; Campana, I.; Coco, V.; Di Pietro, F.R.; Ricci, F.; Pallotta, S.; Candi, E.; Abeni, D.; et al. Basal Cell Carcinoma: From Pathophysiology to Novel Therapeutic Approaches. *Biomedicines* **2020**, *8*, 449. [CrossRef] [PubMed]
2. Global Cancer Observatory. Estimated Number of New Cases in 2020, World, Both Sexes, All Ages. Available online: https://gco.iarc.fr/today/online-analysis-table (accessed on 13 November 2022).
3. McKeown, S.R.; Hatfield, P.; Prestwich, R.J.; Shaffer, R.E.; Taylor, R.E. Radiotherapy for benign disease; assessing the risk of radiation-induced cancer following exposure to intermediate dose radiation. *Br. J. Radiol.* **2015**, *88*, 20150405. [CrossRef]
4. Ron, E.; Modan, B.; Preston, D.; Alfandary, E.; Stovall, M.; Boice, J.D., Jr. Radiation-induced skin carcinomas of the head and neck. *Radiat. Res.* **1991**, *125*, 318–325. [CrossRef] [PubMed]
5. Lichter, M.D.; Karagas, M.R.; Mott, L.A.; Spencer, S.K.; Stukel, T.A.; Greenberg, E.R. Therapeutic ionizing radiation and the incidence of basal cell carcinoma and squamous cell carcinoma. The New Hampshire Skin Cancer Study Group. *Arch. Dermatol.* **2000**, *136*, 1007–1011. [CrossRef]
6. Ekmekçi, P.; Bostanci, S.; Anadolu, R.; Erdem, C.; Gürgey, E. Multiple basal cell carcinomas developed after radiation therapy for tinea capitis: A case report. *Dermatol. Surg. Off. Publ. Am. Soc. Dermatol. Surg.* **2001**, *27*, 667–669. [CrossRef]
7. Hassanpour, S.E.; Kalantar-Hormozi, A.; Motamed, S.; Moosavizadeh, S.M.; Shahverdiani, R. Basal cell carcinoma of scalp in patients with history of childhood therapeutic radiation: A retrospective study and comparison to nonirradiated patients. *Ann. Plast. Surg.* **2006**, *57*, 509–512. [CrossRef]
8. Thorsness, S.L.; Freites-Martinez, A.; Marchetti, M.A.; Navarrete-Dechent, C.; Lacouture, M.E.; Tonorezos, E.S. Nonmelanoma Skin Cancer in Childhood and Young Adult Cancer Survivors Previously Treated With Radiotherapy. *J. Natl. Compr. Cancer Netw. JNCCN* **2019**, *17*, 237–243. [CrossRef] [PubMed]
9. Oshinsky, S.; Baum, S.; Huszar, M.; Debby, A.; Barzilai, A. Basal cell carcinoma induced by therapeutic radiation for tinea capitis-clinicopathological study. *Histopathology* **2018**, *73*, 59–67. [CrossRef] [PubMed]
10. Bonilla, X.; Parmentier, L.; King, B.; Bezrukov, F.; Kaya, G.; Zoete, V.; Seplyarskiy, V.B.; Sharpe, H.J.; McKee, T.; Letourneau, A.; et al. Genomic analysis identifies new drivers and progression pathways in skin basal cell carcinoma. *Nat. Genet.* **2016**, *48*, 398–406. [CrossRef]
11. Bakshi, A.; Chaudhary, S.C.; Rana, M.; Elmets, C.A.; Athar, M. Basal cell carcinoma pathogenesis and therapy involving hedgehog signaling and beyond. *Mol. Carcinog.* **2017**, *56*, 2543–2557. [CrossRef]
12. Cardoso, J.C.; Ribeiro, I.P.; Caramelo, F.; Tellechea, O.; Barbosa de Melo, J.; Marques Carreira, I. Basal cell carcinomas of the scalp after radiotherapy for tinea capitis in childhood: A genetic and epigenetic study with comparison with basal cell carcinomas evolving in chronically sun-exposed areas. *Exp. Dermatol.* **2021**, *30*, 1126–1134. [CrossRef] [PubMed]
13. Tessone, A.; Amariglio, N.; Weissman, O.; Jacob-Hirsch, J.; Liran, A.; Stavrou, D.; Haik, J.; Orenstein, A.; Winkler, E. Radiotherapy-induced basal cell carcinomas of the scalp: Are they genetically different? *Aesthetic Plast. Surg.* **2012**, *36*, 1387–1392. [CrossRef] [PubMed]
14. Li, C.; Athar, M. Ionizing Radiation Exposure and Basal Cell Carcinoma Pathogenesis. *Radiat. Res.* **2016**, *185*, 217–228. [CrossRef] [PubMed]

15. Fleenor, C.J.; Higa, K.; Weil, M.M.; DeGregori, J. Evolved Cellular Mechanisms to Respond to Genotoxic Insults: Implications for Radiation-Induced Hematologic Malignancies. *Radiat. Res.* **2015**, *184*, 341–351. [CrossRef] [PubMed]
16. Lesluyes, T.; Baud, J.; Perot, G.; Charon-Barra, C.; You, A.; Valo, I.; Bazille, C.; Mishellany, F.; Leroux, A.; Renard-Oldrini, S. Genomic and transcriptomic comparison of post-radiation versus sporadic sarcomas. *Mod. Pathol.* **2019**, *32*, 1786–1794. [CrossRef] [PubMed]
17. Maenhaut, C.; Detours, V.; Dom, G.; Handkiewicz-Junak, D.; Oczko-Wojciechowska, M.; Jarzab, B. Gene expression profiles for radiation-induced thyroid cancer. *Clin. Oncol. R Coll. Radiol.* **2011**, *23*, 282–288. [CrossRef]
18. Suzuki, K.; Saenko, V.; Yamashita, S.; Mitsutake, N. Radiation-Induced Thyroid Cancers: Overview of Molecular Signatures. *Cancers* **2019**, *11*, 1290. [CrossRef]
19. Thiagarajan, A.; Iyer, N. Radiation-induced sarcomas of the head and neck. *World J. Clin. Oncol.* **2014**, *5*, 973–981. [CrossRef]
20. Detours, V.; Wattel, S.; Venet, D.; Hutsebaut, N.; Bogdanova, T.; Tronko, M.D.; Dumont, J.E.; Franc, B.; Thomas, G.; Maenhaut, C. Absence of a specific radiation signature in post-Chernobyl thyroid cancers. *Br. J. Cancer* **2005**, *92*, 1545–1552. [CrossRef]
21. Li, L.; Story, M.; Legerski, R. Cellular responses to ionizing radiation damage. *Int. J. Radiat. Oncol. Biol. Phys.* **2001**, *49*, 1157–1162. [CrossRef]
22. Li, M.; You, L.; Xue, J.; Lu, Y. Ionizing Radiation-Induced Cellular Senescence in Normal, Non-transformed Cells and the Involved DNA Damage Response: A Mini Review. *Front. Pharmacol.* **2018**, *9*, 522. [CrossRef] [PubMed]
23. Averbeck, D.; Rodriguez-Lafrasse, C. Role of Mitochondria in Radiation Responses: Epigenetic, Metabolic, and Signaling Impacts. *Int. J. Mol. Sci.* **2021**, *22*, 11047. [CrossRef] [PubMed]
24. Najafi, M.; Motevaseli, E.; Shirazi, A.; Geraily, G.; Rezaeyan, A.; Norouzi, F.; Rezapoor, S.; Abdollahi, H. Mechanisms of inflammatory responses to radiation and normal tissues toxicity: Clinical implications. *Int. J. Radiat. Biol.* **2018**, *94*, 335–356. [CrossRef] [PubMed]
25. Azzam, E.I.; Jay-Gerin, J.; Pain, D. Ionizing radiation-induced metabolic oxidative stress and prolonged cell injury. *Cancer Lett.* **2012**, *327*, 48–60. [CrossRef] [PubMed]
26. Classen, F.; Kranz, P.; Riffkin, H.; Pompsch, M.; Wolf, A.; Göpelt, K.; Baumann, M.; Baumann, J.; Brockmeier, U.; Metzen, E. Autophagy induced by ionizing radiation promotes cell death over survival in human colorectal cancer cells. *Exp. Cell Res.* **2019**, *374*, 29–37. [CrossRef]
27. Mao, A.; Liu, Y.; Zhang, H.; Di, C.; Sun, C. microRNA expression and biogenesis in cellular response to ionizing radiation. *DNA Cell Biol.* **2014**, *33*, 667–679. [CrossRef]
28. Chen, Y.; Cui, J.; Gong, Y.; Wei, S.; Wei, Y.; Yi, L. MicroRNA: A novel implication for damage and protection against ionizing radiation. *Environ. Sci. Pollut. Res. Int.* **2021**, *28*, 15584–15596. [CrossRef]
29. Jia, M.; Wang, Z. MicroRNAs as Biomarkers for Ionizing Radiation Injury. *Front Cell Dev. Biol.* **2022**, *10*, 861451. [CrossRef]
30. Nguyen, H.Q.; To, N.H.; Zadigue, P.; Kerbrat, S.; De La Taille, A.; Le Gouvello, S.; Belkacemi, Y. Ionizing radiation-induced cellular senescence promotes tissue fibrosis after radiotherapy. A review. *Crit. Rev. Oncol. Hematol.* **2018**, *129*, 13–26. [CrossRef]
31. Chen, Z.; Cao, K.; Xia, Y.; Li, Y.; Hou, Y.; Wang, L.; Li, L.; Chang, L.; Li, W. Cellular senescence in ionizing radiation (Review). *Oncol. Rep.* **2019**, *42*, 883–894. [CrossRef]
32. Verkouteren, J.A.C.; Ramdas, K.H.R.; Wakkee, M.; Nijsten, T. Epidemiology of basal cell carcinoma: Scholarly review. *Br. J. Dermatol.* **2017**, *177*, 359–372. [CrossRef] [PubMed]
33. Basset-Seguin, N.; Herms, F. Update in the Management of Basal Cell Carcinoma. *Acta Derm. Venereol.* **2020**, *100*, adv00140. [CrossRef]
34. Pellegrini, C.; Maturo, M.G.; Di Nardo, L.; Ciciarelli, V.; Gutiérrez García-Rodrigo, C.; Fargnoli, M.C. Understanding the Molecular Genetics of Basal Cell Carcinoma. *Int. J. Mol. Sci.* **2017**, *18*, 2485. [CrossRef] [PubMed]
35. Shore, R.E.; Moseson, M.; Xue, X.; Tse, Y.; Harley, N.; Pasternack, B.S. Skin cancer after X-ray treatment for scalp ringworm. *Radiat. Res.* **2002**, *157*, 410–418. [CrossRef]
36. Sethi, N.; Sharma, A.; Singh, C.; Pandia, K.; Gupta, A. Adenoid basal cell carcinoma: A rare variant and a diagnostic dilemma. *Clin. Dermatol. Rev.* **2021**, *5*, 114. [CrossRef]
37. Tarallo, M.; Cigna, E.; Frati, R.; Delfino, S.; Innocenzi, D.; Fama, U.; Corbianco, A.; Scuderi, N. Metatypical basal cell carcinoma: A clinical review. *J. Exp. Clin. Cancer Res.* **2008**, *27*, 65. [CrossRef]
38. Conforti, C.; Pizzichetta, M.A.; Vichi, S.; Toffolutti, F.; Serraino, D.; Di Meo, N.; Giuffrida, R.; Deinlein, T.; Giacomel, J.; Rosendahl, C.; et al. Sclerodermiform basal cell carcinomas vs. other histotypes: Analysis of specific demographic, clinical and dermatoscopic features. *J. Eur. Acad Dermatol. Venereol.* **2021**, *35*, 79–87. [CrossRef]
39. McDaniel, B.; Badri, T.; Steele, R.B. *Basal Cell Carcinoma*; StatPearls Publishing: Treasure Island, FL, USA, 2022.
40. Peris, K.; Fargnoli, M.C.; Garbe, C.; Kaufmann, R.; Bastholt, L.; Seguin, N.B.; Bataille, V.; Marmol, V.D.; Dummer, R.; Harwood, C.A.; et al. Diagnosis and treatment of basal cell carcinoma: European consensus-based interdisciplinary guidelines. *Eur. J. Cancer* **2019**, *118*, 10–34. [CrossRef]
41. Grob, J.J.; Gaudy-Marqueste, C.; Guminski, A.; Malvehy, J.; Basset-Seguin, N.; Bertrand, B.; Fernandez-Penas, P.; Kaufmann, R.; Zalaudek, I.; Fargnoli, M.C.; et al. Position statement on classification of basal cell carcinomas. Part 2: EADO proposal for new operational staging system adapted to basal cell carcinomas. *J. Eur. Acad. Dermatol. Venereol.* **2021**, *35*, 2149–2153. [CrossRef]
42. Zaraa, I.; Ben Taazayet, S.; Zribi, H.; Chelly, I.; El Euch, D.; Trojjet, S.; Mokni, M.; Haouet, S.; Ben Osman, A. Cutaneous carcinoma induced by radiotherapy: A report of 31 cases. *Tunis. Med.* **2013**, *91*, 191–195.

43. Mizuno, T.; Tokuoka, S.; Kishikawa, M.; Nakashima, E.; Mabuchi, K.; Iwamoto, K.S. Molecular basis of basal cell carcinogenesis in the atomic-bomb survivor population: p53 and PTCH gene alterations. *Carcinogenesis* **2006**, *27*, 2286–2294. [CrossRef] [PubMed]
44. Pazzaglia, S.; Mancuso, M.; Tanori, M.; Atkinson, M.J.; Merola, P.; Rebessi, S.; Di Majo, V.; Covelli, V.; Hahn, H.; Saran, A. Modulation of patched-associated susceptibility to radiation induced tumorigenesis by genetic background. *Cancer Res.* **2004**, *64*, 3798–3806. [CrossRef] [PubMed]
45. Chaudhary, S.C.; Tang, X.; Arumugam, A.; Li, C.; Srivastava, R.K.; Weng, Z.; Xu, J.; Zhang, X.; Kim, A.L.; McKay, K.; et al. Shh and p50/Bcl3 signaling crosstalk drives pathogenesis of BCCs in Gorlin syndrome. *Oncotarget* **2015**, *6*, 36789–36814. [CrossRef] [PubMed]
46. Naruke, Y.; Nakashima, M.; Suzuki, K.; Kondo, H.; Hayashi, T.; Soda, M.; Sekine, I. Genomic instability in the epidermis induced by atomic bomb (A-bomb) radiation: A long-lasting health effect in A-bomb survivors. *Cancer* **2009**, *115*, 3782–3790. [CrossRef] [PubMed]
47. Boaventura, P.; Pereira, D.; Mendes, A.; Batista, R.; da Silva, A.F.; Guimarães, I.; Honavar, M.; Teixeira-Gomes, J.; Lopes, J.M.; Máximo, V.; et al. Mitochondrial D310 D-Loop instability and histological subtypes in radiation-induced cutaneous basal cell carcinomas. *J. Dermatol. Sci.* **2014**, *73*, 31–39. [CrossRef] [PubMed]
48. Ghosh, S.; Ghosh, A. Activation of DNA damage response signaling in mammalian cells by ionizing radiation. *Free Radic. Res.* **2021**, *55*, 581–594. [CrossRef]
49. Tsai, W.B.; Chung, Y.M.; Takahashi, Y.; Xu, Z.; Hu, M.C. Functional interaction between FOXO3a and ATM regulates DNA damage response. *Nat. Cell Biol.* **2008**, *10*, 460–467. [CrossRef]
50. Yalcin, S.; Zhang, X.; Luciano, J.P.; Mungamuri, S.K.; Marinkovic, D.; Vercherat, C.; Sarkar, A.; Grisotto, M.; Taneja, R.; Ghaffari, S. Foxo3 is essential for the regulation of ataxia telangiectasia mutated and oxidative stress-mediated homeostasis of hematopoietic stem cells. *J. Biol. Chem.* **2008**, *283*, 25692–25705. [CrossRef]
51. White, R.R.; Maslov, A.Y.; Lee, M.; Wilner, S.E.; Levy, M.; Vijg, J. FOXO3a acts to suppress DNA double-strand break-induced mutations. *Aging Cell* **2020**, *19*, e13184. [CrossRef]
52. Tarrade, S.; Bhardwaj, T.; Flegal, M.; Bertrand, L.; Velegzhaninov, I.; Moskalev, A.; Klokov, D. Histone H2AX is involved in FoxO3a-mediated transcriptional responses to ionizing radiation to maintain genome stability. *Int. J. Mol. Sci.* **2015**, *16*, 29996–30014. [CrossRef]
53. Trémezaygues, L.; Seifert, M.; Vogt, T.; Tilgen, W.; Reichrath, J. 1,25-dihydroxyvitamin D3 modulates effects of ionizing radiation (IR) on human keratinocytes: In vitro analysis of cell viability/proliferation, DNA-damage and -repair. *J. Steroid Biochem. Mol. Biol.* **2010**, *121*, 324–327. [CrossRef] [PubMed]
54. Warters, R.L.; Packard, A.T.; Kramer, G.F.; Gaffney, D.K.; Moos, P.J. Differential gene expression in primary human skin keratinocytes and fibroblasts in response to ionizing radiation. *Radiat. Res.* **2009**, *172*, 82–95. [CrossRef]
55. Zhang, Q.; Zhu, L.; Wang, G.; Zhao, Y.; Xiong, N.; Bao, H.; Jin, W. Ionizing radiation promotes CCL27 secretion from keratinocytes through the cross talk between TNF-α and ROS. *J. Biochem. Mol. Toxicol.* **2016**, *31*, e21868. [CrossRef] [PubMed]
56. Miyake, T.; Shimada, M.; Matsumoto, Y.; Okino, A. DNA Damage Response After Ionizing Radiation Exposure in Skin Keratinocytes Derived from Human-Induced Pluripotent Stem Cells. *Int. J. Radiat. Oncol. Biol. Phys.* **2019**, *105*, 193–205. [CrossRef]
57. Yang, J.; Liu, M.; Hong, D.; Zeng, M.; Zhang, X. The Paradoxical Role of Cellular Senescence in Cancer. *Front Cell Dev. Biol.* **2021**, *9*, 722205. [CrossRef]
58. Shimura, T. ATM-Mediated Mitochondrial Radiation Responses of Human Fibroblasts. *Genes* **2021**, *12*, 1015. [CrossRef]
59. Kam, W.W.-Y.; Banati, R. Effects of ionizing radiation on mitochondria. *Free. Radic. Biol. Med.* **2013**, *65*, 607–619. [CrossRef] [PubMed]
60. Kawamura, K.; Qi, F.; Kobayashi, J. Potential relationship between the biological effects of low-dose irradiation and mitochondrial ROS production. *J. Radiat. Res.* **2018**, *59* (Suppl. S2), ii91–ii97. [CrossRef]
61. Kawamura, K.; Qi, F.; Kobayashi, J. Lead (Pb) induced ATM-dependent mitophagy via PINK1/Parkin pathway. *Toxicol. Lett.* **2018**, *291*, 92–100.
62. Sarkar, A.; Stellrecht, C.M.; Vangapandu, H.V.; Ayres, M.; Kaipparettu, B.A.; Park, J.H.; Balakrishnan, K.; Burks, J.K.; Pandita, T.K.; Hittelman, W.N. Ataxia-telangiectasia mutated interacts with Parkin and induces mitophagy independent of kinase activity. Evidence from mantle cell lymphoma. *Haematologica* **2021**, *106*, 495. [CrossRef]
63. Qi, Y.; Qiu, Q.; Gu, X.; Tian, Y.; Zhang, Y. ATM mediates spermidine-induced mitophagy via PINK1 and Parkin regulation in human fibroblasts. *Sci. Rep.* **2016**, *6*, 1–11. [CrossRef] [PubMed]
64. Shimura, T.; Kobayashi, J.; Komatsu, K.; Kunugita, N. Severe mitochondrial damage associated with low-dose radiation sensitivity in ATM- and NBS1-deficient cells. *Cell Cycle* **2016**, *15*, 1099–1107. [CrossRef] [PubMed]
65. Mei, Y.; Zhang, Y.; Yamamoto, K.; Xie, W.; Mak, T.W.; You, H. FOXO3a-dependent regulation of Pink1 (Park6) mediates survival signaling in response to cytokine deprivation. *Proc. Natl. Acad. Sci. USA* **2009**, *106*, 5153–5158. [CrossRef]
66. Chaurasia, M.; Bhatt, A.N.; Das, A.; Dwarakanath, B.S.; Sharma, K. Radiation-induced autophagy: Mechanisms and consequences. *Free Radic. Res.* **2016**, *50*, 273–290. [CrossRef]
67. Meng, Q.; Zaharieva, E.K.; Sasatani, M.; Kobayashi, J. Possible relationship between mitochondrial changes and oxidative stress under low dose-rate irradiation. *Redox Rep.* **2021**, *26*, 160–169. [CrossRef] [PubMed]
68. Mito, J.K.; Qian, X.; Jo, V.Y.; Doyle, L.A. MYC expression has limited utility in the distinction of undifferentiated radiation-associated sarcomas from sporadic sarcomas and sarcomatoid carcinoma. *Histopathology* **2020**, *77*, 667–672. [CrossRef] [PubMed]

69. Boerma, M.; Davis, C.M.; Jackson, I.L.; Schaue, D.; Williams, J.P. All for one, though not one for all: Team players in normal tissue radiobiology. *Int. J. Radiat. Biol.* **2022**, *98*, 346–366. [CrossRef]
70. Hayashi, T.; Kusunoki, Y.; Hakoda, M.; Morishita, Y.; Kubo, Y.; Maki, M.; Kasagi, F.; Kodama, K.; Macphee, D.G.; Kyoizumi, S. Radiation dose-dependent increases in inflammatory response markers in A-bomb survivors. *Int. J. Radiat. Biol.* **2003**, *79*, 129–136. [CrossRef]
71. Hayashi, T.; Morishita, Y.; Khattree, R.; Misumi, M.; Sasaki, K.; Hayashi, I.; Yoshida, K.; Kajimura, J.; Kyoizumi, S.; Imai, K.; et al. Evaluation of systemic markers of inflammation in atomic-bomb survivors with special reference to radiation and age effects. *FASEB J.* **2012**, *26*, 4765–4773. [CrossRef]
72. Mukherjee, S.; Laiakis, E.C.; Fornace, A.J., Jr.; Amundson, S.A. Impact of inflammatory signaling on radiation biodosimetry: Mouse model of inflammatory bowel disease. *BMC Genom.* **2019**, *20*, 329. [CrossRef]
73. Hayashi, T.; Furukawa, K.; Morishita, Y.; Hayashi, I.; Kato, N.; Yoshida, K.; Kusunoki, Y.; Kyoizumi, S.; Ohishi, W. Intracellular reactive oxygen species level in blood cells of atomic bomb survivors is increased due to aging and radiation exposure. *Free. Radic. Biol. Med.* **2021**, *171*, 126–134. [CrossRef]
74. Matsuu-Matsuyama, M.; Shichijo, K.; Okaichi, K.; Kurashige, T.; Kondo, H.; Miura, S.; Nakashima, M. Effect of age on the sensitivity of the rat thyroid gland to ionizing radiation. *J. Radiat. Res.* **2015**, *56*, 493–501. [CrossRef] [PubMed]
75. Kraemer, A.; Anastasov, N.; Angermeier, M.; Winkler, K.; Atkinson, M.J.; Moertl, S. MicroRNA-mediated processes are essential for the cellular radiation response. *Radiat. Res.* **2011**, *176*, 575–586. [CrossRef]
76. Szatkowska, M.; Krupa, R. Regulation of DNA Damage Response and Homologous Recombination Repair by microRNA in Human Cells Exposed to Ionizing Radiation. *Cancers* **2020**, *12*, 1838. [CrossRef] [PubMed]
77. Rzeszowska-Wolny, J.; Hudy, D.; Biernacki, K.; Ciesielska, S.; Jaksik, R. Involvement of miRNAs in cellular responses to radiation. *Int. J. Radiat. Biol.* **2022**, *98*, 479–488. [CrossRef] [PubMed]
78. Iizuka, D.; Imaoka, T.; Nishimura, M.; Kawai, H.; Suzuki, F.; Shimada, Y. Aberrant microRNA expression in radiation-induced rat mammary cancer: The potential role of miR-194 overexpression in cancer cell proliferation. *Radiat. Res.* **2013**, *179*, 151–159. [CrossRef] [PubMed]
79. Kim, E.S.; Choi, Y.E.; Hwang, S.J.; Han, Y.H.; Park, M.J.; Bae, I.H. IL-4, a direct target of miR-340/429, is involved in radiation-induced aggressive tumor behavior in human carcinoma cells. *Oncotarget* **2016**, *7*, 86836–86856. [CrossRef]
80. Cui, J.; Cheng, Y.; Zhang, P.; Sun, M.; Gao, F.; Liu, C.; Cai, J. Down regulation of miR200c promotes radiation-induced thymic lymphoma by targeting BMI1. *J. Cell Biochem.* **2014**, *115*, 1033–1042. [CrossRef]
81. Wang, S.; Liu, N.; Tang, Q.; Sheng, H.; Long, S.; Wu, W. MicroRNA-24 in Cancer: A Double Side Medal With Opposite Properties. *Front. Oncol.* **2020**, *10*, 553714. [CrossRef] [PubMed]
82. Wang, S.; Pan, Y.; Zhang, R.; Xu, T.; Wu, W.; Zhang, R.; Wang, C.; Huang, H.; Calin, C.A.; Yang, H.; et al. Hsa-miR-24-3p increases nasopharyngeal carcinoma radiosensitivity by targeting both the 3′UTR and 5′UTR of Jab1/CSN5. *Oncogene* **2016**, *35*, 6096–6108. [CrossRef]
83. Lal, A.; Kim, H.H.; Abdelmohsen, K.; Kuwano, Y.; Pullmann, R., Jr.; Srikantan, S.; Subrahmanyam, R.; Martindale, J.L.; Yang, X.; Ahmed, F.; et al. p16(INK4a) translation suppressed by miR-24. *PLoS ONE* **2008**, *3*, e1864. [CrossRef] [PubMed]
84. Khorsandi, S.E.; Salehi, S.; Cortes, M.; Vilca-Melendez, H.; Menon, K.; Srinivasan, P.; Prachalias, A.; Jassem, W.; Heaton, N. An in silico argument for mitochondrial microRNA as a determinant of primary non function in liver transplantation. *Sci. Rep.* **2018**, *8*, 3105. [CrossRef] [PubMed]
85. Oladejo, A.O.; Li, Y.; Imam, B.H.; Ma, X.; Shen, W.; Wu, X.; Jiang, W.; Yang, J.; Lv, Y.; Ding, X.; et al. MicroRNA miR-24-3p Mediates the Negative Regulation of Lipopolysaccharide-Induced Endometrial Inflammatory Response by Targeting TNF Receptor-Associated Factor 6 (TRAF6). *J. Inflamm. Res.* **2022**, *15*, 807–825. [CrossRef] [PubMed]
86. Cao, Y.; Tang, S.; Nie, X.; Zhou, Z.; Ruan, G.; Han, W.; Zhu, Z.; Ding, C. Decreased miR-214-3p activates NF-κB pathway and aggravates osteoarthritis progression. *EBioMedicine* **2021**, *65*, 103283. [CrossRef] [PubMed]
87. Harada, M.; Jinnin, M.; Wang, Z.; Hirano, A.; Tomizawa, Y.; Kira, T.; Igata, T.; Masuguchi, S.; Fukushima, S.; Ihn, H. The expression of miR-124 increases in aged skin to cause cell senescence and it decreases in squamous cell carcinoma. *Biosci. Trends* **2017**, *10*, 454–459. [CrossRef] [PubMed]
88. Saleh, A.D.; Savage, J.E.; Cao, L.; Soule, B.P.; Ly, D.; DeGraff, W.; Harris, C.C.; Mitchell, J.B.; Simone, N.L. Cellular stress induced alterations in microRNA let-7a and let-7b expression are dependent on p53. *PLoS ONE* **2011**, *6*, e24429. [CrossRef] [PubMed]
89. Guo, P.; Lan, J.; Ge, J.; Nie, Q.; Guo, L.; Qiu, Y.; Mao, Q. MiR-26a enhances the radiosensitivity of glioblastoma multiforme cells through targeting of ataxia-telangiectasia mutated. *Exp. Cell Res.* **2014**, *320*, 200–208. [CrossRef]
90. Yan, D.; Ng, W.L.; Zhang, X.; Wang, P.; Zhang, Z.; Mo, Y.Y.; Mao, H.; Hao, C.; Olson, J.J.; Curran, W.J.; et al. Targeting DNA-PKcs and ATM with miR-101 sensitizes tumors to radiation. *PLoS ONE* **2010**, *5*, e11397. [CrossRef]
91. Hemmings, K.E.; Riches-Suman, K.; Bailey, M.A.; O'Regan, D.J.; Turner, N.A.; Porter, K.E. Role of MicroRNA-145 in DNA Damage Signalling and Senescence in Vascular Smooth Muscle Cells of Type 2 Diabetic Patients. *Cells* **2021**, *10*, 919. [CrossRef]
92. Xia, C.; Jiang, T.; Wang, Y.; Chen, X.; Hu, Y.; Gao, Y. The p53/miR-145a Axis Promotes Cellular Senescence and Inhibits Osteogenic Differentiation by Targeting Cbfb in Mesenchymal Stem Cells. *Front Endocrinol.* **2020**, *11*, 609186. [CrossRef]
93. Sand, M.; Hessam, S.; Amur, S.; Skrygan, M.; Bromba, M.; Stockfleth, E.; Gambichler, T.; Bechara, F.G. Expression of oncogenic miR-17-92 and tumor suppressive miR-143-145 clusters in basal cell carcinoma and cutaneous squamous cell carcinoma. *J. Dermatol. Sci.* **2017**, *86*, 142–148. [CrossRef] [PubMed]

94. Wang, Y.; Scheiber, M.N.; Neumann, C.; Calin, G.A.; Zhou, D. MicroRNA regulation of ionizing radiation-induced premature senescence. *Int. J. Radiat. Oncol. Biol. Phys.* **2011**, *81*, 839–848. [CrossRef] [PubMed]
95. Rivetti di Val Cervo, P.; Lena, A.M.; Nicoloso, M.; Rossi, S.; Mancini, M.; Zhou, H.; Saintigny, G.; Dellambra, E.; Odorisio, T.; Mahé, C.; et al. p63-microRNA feedback in keratinocyte senescence. *Proc. Natl. Acad. Sci. USA* **2012**, *109*, 1133–1138. [CrossRef] [PubMed]
96. Chaudhry, M.A.; Omaruddin, R.A.; Brumbaugh, C.D.; Tariq, M.A.; Pourmand, N. Identification of radiation-induced microRNA transcriptome by next-generation massively parallel sequencing. *J. Radiat. Res.* **2013**, *54*, 808–822. [CrossRef]
97. Naito, Y.; Oue, N.; Pham, T.T.; Yamamoto, M.; Fujihara, M.; Ishida, T.; Mukai, S.; Sentani, K.; Sakamoto, N.; Hida, E.; et al. Characteristic miR-24 Expression in Gastric Cancers among Atomic Bomb Survivors. *Pathobiology* **2015**, *82*, 68–75. [CrossRef] [PubMed]

Disclaimer/Publisher's Note: The statements, opinions and data contained in all publications are solely those of the individual author(s) and contributor(s) and not of MDPI and/or the editor(s). MDPI and/or the editor(s) disclaim responsibility for any injury to people or property resulting from any ideas, methods, instructions or products referred to in the content.

Review

High Resolution and Automatable Cytogenetic Biodosimetry Using In Situ Telomere and Centromere Hybridization for the Accurate Detection of DNA Damage: An Overview

Radhia M'Kacher [1,*], Bruno Colicchio [2], Steffen Junker [3], Elie El Maalouf [1], Leonhard Heidingsfelder [4], Andreas Plesch [4], Alain Dieterlen [2], Eric Jeandidier [5], Patrice Carde [6] and Philippe Voisin [1]

1. Cell Environment DNA Damage R&D, Genopole, 91000 Evry-Courcouronnes, France
2. IRIMAS, Institut de Recherche en Informatique, Mathématiques, Automatique et Signal, Université de Haute-Alsace, 69093 Mulhouse, France
3. Institute of Biomedicine, University of Aarhus, DK-8000 Aarhus, Denmark
4. MetaSystems GmbH, Robert-Bosch-Str. 6, D-68804 Altlussheim, Germany
5. Laboratoire de Génétique, Groupe Hospitalier de la Région de Mulhouse Sud-Alsace, 69093 Mulhouse, France
6. Department of Hematology, Institut Gustave Roussy, 94804 Villejuif, France
* Correspondence: radhia.mkacher@cell-environment.com; Tel.: +33-160878918

Abstract: In the event of a radiological or nuclear accident, or when physical dosimetry is not available, the scoring of radiation-induced chromosomal aberrations in lymphocytes constitutes an essential tool for the estimation of the absorbed dose of the exposed individual and for effective triage. Cytogenetic biodosimetry employs different cytogenetic assays including the scoring of dicentrics, micronuclei, and translocations as well as analyses of induced premature chromosome condensation to define the frequency of chromosome aberrations. However, inherent challenges using these techniques include the considerable time span from sampling to result, the sensitivity and specificity of the various techniques, and the requirement of highly skilled personnel. Thus, techniques that obviate these challenges are needed. The introduction of telomere and centromere (TC) staining have successfully met these challenges and, in addition, greatly improved the efficiency of cytogenetic biodosimetry through the development of automated approaches, thus reducing the need for specialized personnel. Here, we review the role of the various cytogenetic dosimeters and their recent improvements in the management of populations exposed to genotoxic agents such as ionizing radiation. Finally, we discuss the emerging potentials to exploit these techniques in a wider spectrum of medical and biological applications, e.g., in cancer biology to identify prognostic biomarkers for the optimal triage and treatment of patients.

Keywords: cytogenetic biodosimetry; radioprotection; telomere; centromere; chromosomal instability

1. Introduction

Biological dosimetry refers to the quantitative estimation of an absorbed dose of radiation in individuals exposed to ionizing radiation [1]. Radiation exposure may occur due to the geological environment, medical diagnostics and therapy, occupation in radiation facilities or the nuclear industry, or large-scale incidents such as accidents in nuclear industries, nuclear tests, fallouts, nuclear terrorism, or dirty bombs [2–4]. Individuals involved in large-scale incidents often do not have personal dosimeters. In cases of exposures requiring dose reconstruction, regardless of the circumstances, biological dosimetry becomes a valuable tool in the accurate assessment of the absorbed radiation dose in the shortest possible time for successful and effective triage and medical management.

The DNA-damaging effects of genotoxic stress such as ionizing radiation may result in chromosome aberrations that can be used as a biomarker, i.e., a biological endpoint to indicate an earlier event as a result of exposure [5]. Biological dosimetry based on cytogenetic assays, termed cytogenetic biodosimetry, has, for decades, been the most extensively studied system. The assays are usually performed on peripheral blood lymphocytes (PBL) because they are easily accessible. The assays are based on the quantification of radiation-induced chromosomal aberrations such as chromosome dicentrics (DC), cytokinesis-block micronuclei (CBMN), premature chromosome condensation (PCC), fragments/rings, or fluorescence in situ hybridization (FISH) for chromosome painting to monitor, e.g., translocations. Three of the techniques, i.e., DC assay (DCA), CBMN, and FISH have now been standardized for monitoring and quantifying the resulting chromosome aberrations in PBL. One of the assays, the DCA, is considered the "gold standard" for biological dosimetry in radiation emergency medicine by IAEA and other international agencies due to the radio-specificity of DCs. Of note, DCA has proven its utility in past large-scale nuclear accidents or accidents such as the Chernobyl accident in 1986 [6].

The assessment of individual doses of exposure in a population should be carried out within the shortest possible time for effective triage and medical intervention, especially in the event of a large-scale radiation incident involving a sizable population group. However, cytogenetic assays for scoring chromosome aberrations suffer from methodological limitations because most of them require a cell culture step, followed by cytological preparations of the cells, and finally scoring under microscopes. Therefore, the time required for performing such biodosimetric measurements and obtaining a result becomes longer than desirable (i.e., >50 h) [1,7–9]. The situation is even more challenging when a large number of samples need to be processed, e.g., in a large-scale nuclear incident. Further efforts are thus required to improve methods for scoring radiation-induced chromosome aberrations.

The introduction of peptide nucleic acid (PNA) probes to the scoring of radiation-induced DNA damage has opened new horizons for cytogenetic biodosimetry. Such probes have the advantage of short hybridization times, high specificity, and signal intensity, in addition to low cost [10]. By employing telomere and centromere-specific PNA probes (TC staining), we have obtained significant advances in the scoring of dicentric and ring chromosomes—the best biomarkers of radiation-induced DNA damage—on metaphases from mitosis-induced lymphocytes [10,11] and also on premature chromosome condensation (PCC) in nonstimulated lymphocytes [12,13]. Furthermore, the application of TC staining to the CBMN assay has vastly improved the identification of micronucleus formation, thus increasing the applicability of this assay [14]. Thus, not only have these improvements enhanced the precision of the cytogenetic assays but also obviated the need for personnel with high expertise [15,16].

More recently, as a result of the improvements in these techniques, their applicability has been explored in other fields of biology and their use by other biological non-DNA ionizing radiation assessors have been proposed. Thus, with the advance of cytogenetic techniques, they are not restricted to radiation biology and are not only applicable for the assessment of the effects of any genotoxic agent but also intrinsic defects in maintaining DNA integrity due to pathological gene variants. For instance, chromosomal instability is a prerequisite of ongoing cellular transformation and cancer development. These significantly improved cytogenetic techniques should constitute a valuable tool for the improved characterization of karyotypes in cancer patients, and hence, focused individual treatment and follow-up [17,18].

Here, we present an overview of the advantages of employing TC staining in current techniques used for cytogenetic biodosimetry, i.e., the shorter processing time, higher resolution, accuracy, and automatable recording, and we discuss the clinical utility of these approaches and their great potential in biological dosimetry.

2. Cytogenetic Markers of Irradiation

Cytogenetic biodosimetric assays are based on several biological endpoints essentially related to chromosomal aberrations that are consequences of DNA damage in peripheral blood lymphocytes (Figure 1). The markers of irradiation can be classified into three groups:

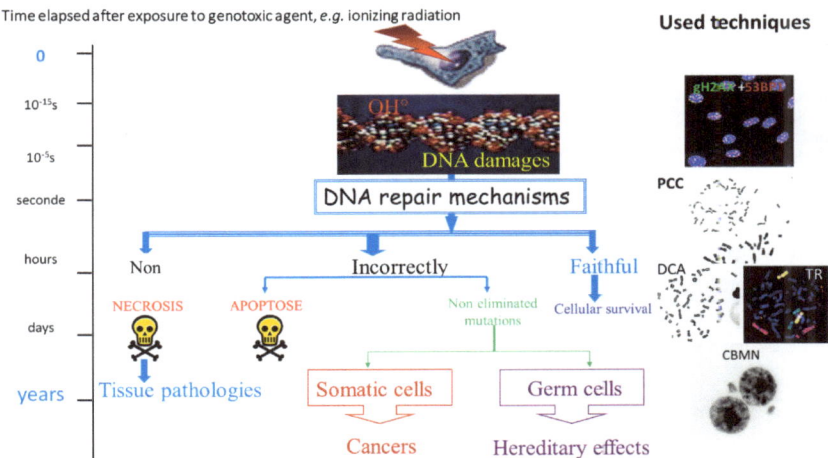

Figure 1. Schematic overview of the consequences of DNA repair mechanisms of varying efficiencies, induced after exposure to genotoxic agents. To the right are depicted examples of cytogenetic preparations using assays employed in cytogenetic biodosimetry. PCC: premature chromosome condensation; DCA: dicentric chromosome assay; TR: scoring of translocations; and MN: micronucleus assay.

(1) Direct molecular consequences such as single and double-strand breaks in the DNA molecule detected by fluorochrome-labeled antibodies specific for, e.g., γH2AX, MR11 proteins, or p53-binding protein (53BP1) that are markers of double-strand breaks (DSB) [19,20]. The preparation and analysis of the immunostainings can be automated [4,21]. The proteins are useful markers of DSB (Table 1) in analyses of putative biological effects of low doses of irradiation [22] and for the triage of exposed populations [23,24]. In addition, immunostaining can be used to assess interindividual sensitivity to radiation [25]. However, the specificity of the abovementioned markers to irradiation, the lack of stability of the fluorescent signals over time, the standardization of the technique, and the interindividual variation constitute the main drawbacks for their use in biological dosimetry [26,27].

(2) The kinetics of DNA break repair is monitored in prematurely condensed chromosomes (PCCs) in the form of single-stranded filaments. PCCs can be observed by ordinary light microscopy or by fluorescence microscopy after staining with appropriate DNA dyes [28,29]; however, the techniques are subject to significant constraints and low stability of the acentric breaks over time, which limit their use in particular investigations.

(3) The consequences of DNA misrepair on the integrity of chromosomes at the time of the first postirradiation cell division or during the second interphase. Such failures resulting in more or less stable dicentrics, translocations, acentric fragments, or micronuclei can be visualized microscopically by the employment of relevant cytogenetic techniques of high sensitivity, specificity, and accuracy. Moreover, the techniques are automatable and easy to implement.

The long-term consequences of irradiation on DNA integrity have been investigated in populations exposed to irradiation following nuclear accidents or medical treatments, and also in their offspring [30–36] (Figure 1). Based on the collected data, multiple models of radiation-induced carcinogenesis and the transmission of chromosome aberrations to offspring have been proposed [37].

Table 1. Different categories of commonly used cytogenetic biological dosimeters/indicators explored for radiation dose reconstruction and possible accidental exposure situations. The question marks indicate that the validity of the test is not yet recognized.

Techniques	Types of Exposure to Ionizing Radiation				Sensitivity
	Recent and Homogeneous Events	Recent and Heterogeneous Events	Past Event	Large-Scale Event	Sensitivity
Dicentric and centric rings	YES	YES	NO	YES	0.1 Gy
Micronuclei	YES	YES	NO	YES	0.3 Gy
Translocations	YES	YES	YES	NO	0.25–0.3 Gy
PCC—CHO	YES	YES	NO	YES	0.1 Gy
PCC—ring	YES	?	NO	?	?

3. TC Staining Allows Insight into Mechanisms of Formation of Chromosome Aberrations

TC staining represents a major advance in not only the sensitivity of detection and classification of complex chromosome aberrations but also in elucidating mechanisms of their formation based on their structural alterations. The staining of telomeres, i.e., the ends of each chromosome, allows a very precise determination of the chromosomal landscape. Centromere staining makes it possible to define the nature of the chromosome aberrations and ultimately predict how sustainable they will be during subsequent cell divisions.

Thus, using TC staining, the accurate nomenclature of chromosomal aberrations can be established: (1) Dicentric chromosome: two centromere signals with four telomere signals; (2) centric ring chromosome: one centromere signal without any telomere signal; (3) acentric ring without telomere and centromere signal; (4) acentric chromosomes with four telomere signals or acentric fusion accompanied by dicentric or ring or translocation formation; (5) acentric chromosome with two telomere signals related to terminal deletion; and (6) acentric chromosome without telomere and centromere signals are related to interstitial deletion (Figure 2).

Moreover, TC staining makes it possible to distinguish between metaphases in the first and second mitotic cell division without any supplementary step related to the cross-hybridization of the centromere signal [11].

Furthermore, the scoring of TC-stained chromosome preparations is fully automatable [11,12,17]. Therefore, we believe that the implementation of TC staining will open new fields of research and diagnosis offering the vastly improved visualization of chromosomes and the identification and definition of their associated aberrations.

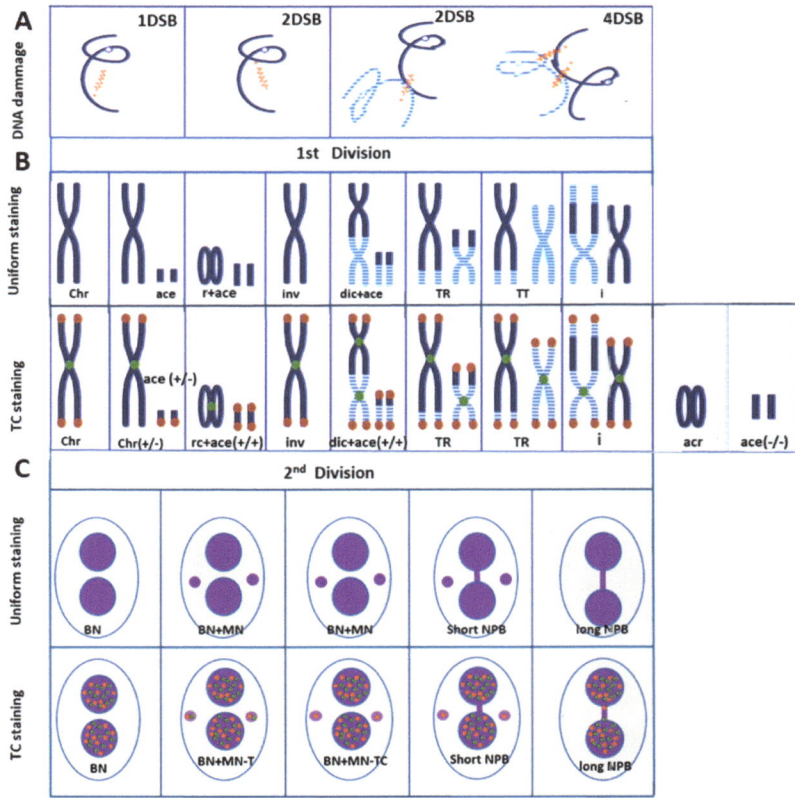

Figure 2. DNA damage and chromosomal aberrations after exposure to ionizing irradiation: (**A**) DNA damage after one, two, or four DSB. (**B**) Chromosomal aberrations in the first mitosis are visualized by uniform staining or TC staining. The latter permits the precise identification of chromosomal aberrations. Ace: acentric fragment; Rc: ring chromosome; Dic: dicentric chromosome; inv: inversion; TR: translocation; I: insertion; Gray: centromere; and red: telomere. (**C**) CBMN assay followed by TC staining for assessing DNA damage permits a distinction between aneugenic and clastogenic exposures. CBMN assay followed by TC staining allows the detection of the mechanisms of the formation of an anaphase bridge: a short anaphase bridge without TC staining related to the presence of a dicentric chromosome with centromere breakpoints and a long anaphase bridge with TC staining related to the presence of dicentric chromosomes with telomere fusions.

4. Employment of TC Staining Adds Distinctive Value to Commonly Used Cytogenetic Techniques

Table 1 summarizes the sensitivity of commonly used cytogenetic biological dosimetry techniques and the possible detection of recent or past irradiation as well as the homogeneous and heterogenous exposure (Table 1).

4.1. The "Gold Standard" Technique

Among the various assays employed in cytogenetic biodosimetry, the dicentric chromosome assay (DCA) is considered the "gold standard" in radiation emergency medicine.

It is medically and legally recognized [1,7–9] and is approved by the International Atomic Energy Agency (IAEA) because of its proven utility in past large-scale nuclear incidents and accidents [30,38].

A dicentric chromosome is an abnormal chromosome with two centromeres. It is formed through two double-strand breaks (DSB) and followed by the fusion of two chromosome fragments, each with a centromere, resulting in the formation of a dicentric chromosome together with acentric fragments (Figure 2B) [8].

Dicentric chromosomes, together with centric rings, the latter formed by the fusion of sticky chromosome ends (Figure 2B), occur in peripheral lymphocytes of individuals as a consequence of recent exposure to an external source of ionizing radiation. Their frequency is dose-dependent. However, they are unstable aberrations, and hence their frequencies decrease during subsequent cell divisions. The acentric fragments can also provide an aid in dose estimation, e.g., to substantiate the presence of other aberrations or, especially in cases of partial body exposure, to verify information about the incident.

Dicentrics and centric rings are relatively simple to score and enumerate. Moreover, their frequency is dose-dependent. For those reasons their enumeration in peripheral blood lymphocytes, termed the "dicentric chromosome assay" (DCA), constitutes the basis of the "Gold Standard" technique for estimating biological dosimetry.

The abovementioned chromosomal aberrations can be observed after uniform staining (Giemsa or DAPI) of metaphases of lymphocytes from a blood sample after their cultivation for 48 h in the presence of phytohemagglutinin (PHA), a stimulator of mitosis, followed by a 2–4 h colcemid-induced block of metaphase (Figure 3A).

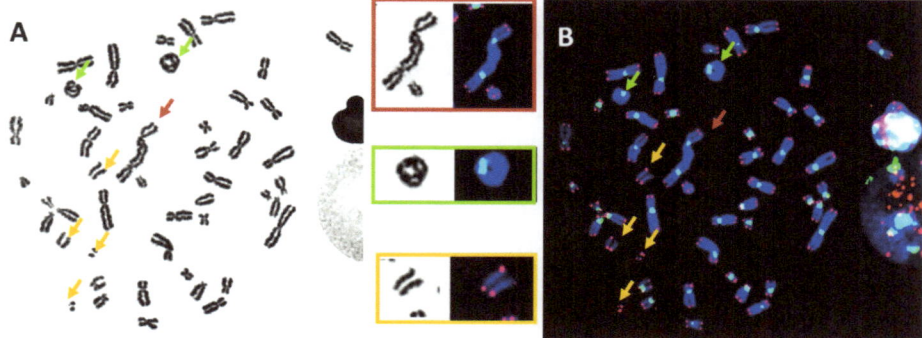

Figure 3. The identification of unstable chromosomal aberrations after the in vitro irradiation of blood lymphocytes (63× magnification) using (**A**) uniform chromosome staining (Giemsa staining) permits the detection of unstable chromosomal aberrations according to their morphologies; (**B**) telomere (red) and centromere (green) staining allow the accurate detection of all unstable chromosome aberrations: (*i*) dicentric chromosome with two green signals and four red signals (top insert), (*ii*) ring chromosomes with one green signal, but no red signals (2nd insert from the top), and (*iii*) acentric fragments with four red signals only (bottom insert).

Several studies have shown that frequencies of chromosome aberrations are similar in in vitro and in vivo irradiated blood lymphocytes, respectively. Hence, a calibration curve of the dose-effect relationship obtained after the in vitro irradiation of blood is used to estimate the dose of exposure from an irradiation event in vivo [39,40].

The operating conditions are described in numerous publications such as the IAEA technical guides [1,7–9]. Key points of the technique to validate its quality and reproducibility are defined in several ISO standards [41–43].

By incorporating TC staining into the "gold standard" technique, the identification of normal chromosomes as well as their aberrations has been vastly improved. The visualization of telomere sequences permits the identification of chromosome ends, and visualization of the centromere sequences, the nature of a chromosome, i.e., (*i*) dicentric: chromosome with two centromere signals (Figure 2B); (*ii*) centric ring: circular chromosome without telomere signal and with only centromere signal (Figure 2B); (*iii*) acentric: chromosome without centromere signal and with or without telomere signal (Figures 2 and 3) [10,11]. Thus, TC staining allows the accurate and reliable detection of all unstable chromosomal aberrations in a single analysis. Importantly, the analysis can be made operator independent [11,44]. Last, but not least, software has been developed that allows the satisfactory automation of chromosomal aberrations scoring [11,12,45–49]. Thus, the technique has significantly reduced the labor-intensive and time-consuming burden of enumerating chromosome aberrations in the classical "gold standard" assay. Moreover, this improved technique should also be applied to studies on the effects of any external genotoxic agent and intrinsic cellular factors affecting chromosome stability.

4.2. Detection of Translocations

Chromosomal anomalies that are the result of exchanges of genetic material between non-homologous chromosomes are termed translocations (Figure 2B) [50–56]. The frequency of radiation-induced translocations in a cell population depends on the dose of irradiation [57]. Some of the translocations may persist for decades because they remain compatible with cell division, as documented in biodosimetric studies on A-bomb survivors performed decades after exposure, and on patients observed for decades after their treatment with radiotherapy for ankylosing spondylitis [58]. Thus, in contrast to dicentrics, rings, and fragments that are lost progressively in subsequent mitotic divisions, a translocation is a better biomarker for retrospective dose evaluation when there has been a long delay between exposure and blood sampling.

In the past, the identification and analysis of translocations based on banding techniques required highly skilled staff to assess karyotypes. However, the introduction of the FISH technique has revolutionized this analysis by using one or several different chromosome-specific colors to "paint" each pair of chromosomes. Each chromosome-specific DNA probe is labeled with fluorescent molecules allowing each chromosome pair or group to be visualized individually or collectively. Any exchange of non-homologous chromosomal material can therefore be easily identified. The fastest method at present is to 'paint' three pairs of chromosomes, each pair being the same or different in color from another pair [54,55]. However, some imprecision in the detection of the nature of aberrations cannot be completely avoided, such as an incomplete translocation or terminal translocation, and the distinction between translocation and a specific configuration of a dicentric chromosome with both centromeres in close proximity [17,18]. However, by combining telomere and centromere staining with chromosome painting, the scoring of chromosomal aberrations becomes considerably simpler and more reliable. A further advantage of combining these techniques is that the nature of more complex aberrations can be established with high accuracy, as demonstrated in Figure 4.

4.3. The Cytokinesis-Blocked Micronucleus Assay (CBMN)

The scoring of micronuclei has been proposed as an alternative to the conventional quantification of chromosomal aberrations because the assay is faster and also easier. Micronuclei are biomarkers not only of DNA damage but also of genomic instability [59]. However, the high baseline frequency of micronuclei in healthy populations has limited the sensitivity and application of the CBMN assay for the follow-up of exposed populations [60].

Micronuclei containing acentric chromosome fragments or chromatid fragments arise due to non- or misrepaired DNA double-strand breaks as a result of exposure to clastogenic agents, e.g., ionizing radiation [61,62]. Micronuclei can also contain whole chromosomes that lag behind and do not attach to the mitotic spindle during the segregation process in anaphase. Such micronuclei arise as a result of exposure to aneugenic agents (e.g., intracellular oxidants and polycyclic aromatic hydrocarbons) [62], and they represent the main fraction (>70%) of spontaneously occurring micronuclei [14,63]. Irrespective of the cause of their origin, these chromosomes or chromosome fragments are subsequently enveloped by a nuclear membrane and appear in the cytoplasm as small nuclei, i.e., micronuclei, separated from the main nucleus (Figure 2C). The assay is based on peripheral lymphocytes stimulated to undergo mitosis by in vitro stimulation with phytohemagglutinin (PHA). Micronuclei can subsequently be observed in interphase cells.

Ionizing radiation is a strong clastogenic agent and thus a potent inducer of micronuclei, most of which lack centromeres. The CBMN assay has now been established as a reliable technique in radiobiology for the assessment of the radiation exposure of medical, occupational, or accidentally exposed individuals.

The enhanced resolution of the CBMN assay has been obtained by including TC staining or only centromere staining [14,63–65]. The achievements using that approach are significant: (1) The visualization of both the telomere and the centromere sequences enhances the sensitivity and detection of MN. (2) The determination of the nature of the genotoxic exposure: clastogenic effect (i.e., MN–T with only telomere sequences) and aneugenic (i.e., MN–TC with telomere and centromere staining) (cf. Figures 2C and 5). In addition, the introduction of TC staining into the CBMN assay may advance our insight into molecular mechanisms giving rise to dicentric chromosomes due to the improved scoring of long anaphase bridges with TC sequences and short anaphase bridges without any staining (Figure 2C).

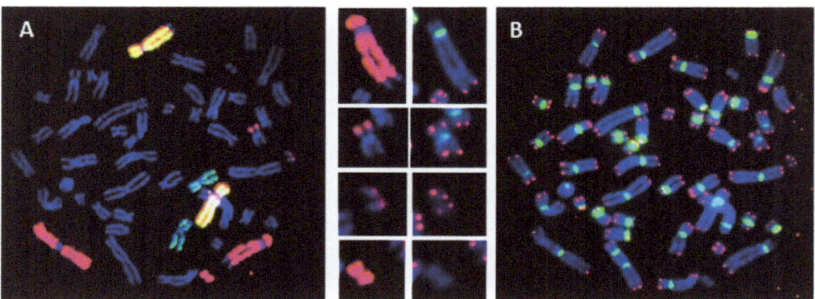

Figure 4. The detection of stable chromosomal aberrations after the in vitro irradiation of blood lymphocytes (63× magnification) using (**A**) chromosome 1 (red), 4 (yellow), and 11 (green) painting and the identification of a complex rearrangement involving chromosome 1 with a reciprocal translocation and of two other undefined aberrations. (**B**) By combining telomere and centromere staining with chromosome painting, the two other aberrations can be defined: telomere deletion (1st insert from the top) was detected in chromosome 1 implicated in this reciprocal translocation (2nd insert from the top); the precise detection of an acentric fragment accompanied the formation of this reciprocal aberration (3rd insert from the top); detection of an acentric ring lacking telomere and centromere staining (bottom insert).

4.4. Premature Chromosome Condensation (PCC) Assay

Occasionally, it is difficult to obtain sufficient numbers of metaphases in lymphocytes grown in a culture with PHA. An alternative useful method to the gold standard technique is the premature chromosome condensation (PCC) assay that facilitates the visualization of interphase chromatin as a condensed form of chromosomes. Usually, chromosomes condense during mitosis, following a strict order that is under strict cellular controls. However, it is possible to artificially uncouple chromosome condensation from the mitotic sequence, which makes it possible to visualize chromosomes in, e.g., resting PBL. Two different approaches are usually employed to induce PCC: (1) The PCC fusion approach (PCC–CHO), and (2) the chemical induction approach. In the fusion approach, Chinese hamster ovary (CHO) cells in the M-phase of their cell cycle are fused with the target interphase cells using a fusogen-like polyethylene glycol or inactivated Sendai virus. Prior to fusion, mitotic CHO cells have been synchronized and stocks are frozen and stored until used [28,66].

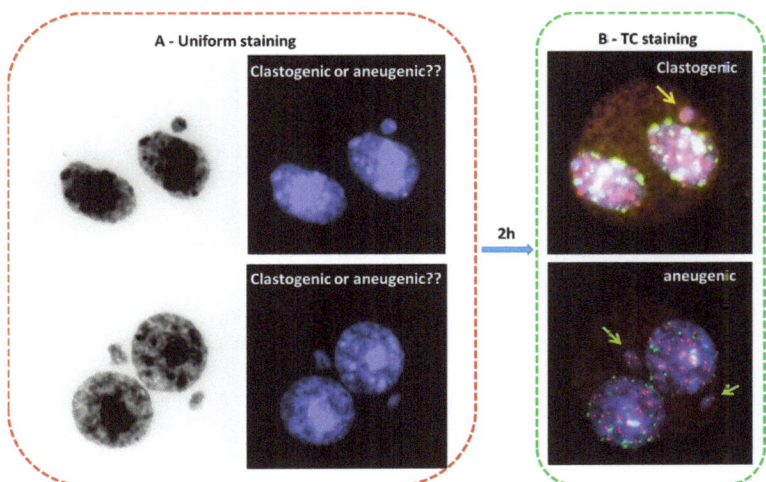

Figure 5. A combination of telomere (red) and centromere (green) staining in the CBMN assay allows the easy identification of the nature of a genotoxic exposure. (**A**) The detection of micronuclei after uniform DNA staining. The staining does not allow the identification of their chromosomal contents. (**B**) Micronuclei with only telomere staining (yellow arrow) as a consequence of exposure to the clastogenic agent, and micronuclei with telomere and centromere staining (green arrow) due to exposure to the aneugenic agent (63× magnification).

Alternatively, PCC can be induced chemically in PBL at any stage of the cell cycle by treatment with okadaic acid or calyculin, which are specific inhibitors of serine/threonine protein phosphatase [13,67,68]. The technique is very easy to practice, simply by substituting colcemid with either of the two chemicals. Incubation times of only 30 min, sometimes only 5–10 min (in contrast to the 2–4 h colcemid block) induce a sufficient number of chromosomes. The PCC index is usually much higher (>10%) than the mitotic index (1–2% at best), which makes chromosome analysis much easier. In addition, the drug-induced PCC has outstanding merit that allows the metaphase chromatin, i.e., G_1-, S-, and G_2-phase chromatin to be visualized as condensed forms of chromosome structure.

The induction of PCC allows the observation of chromosomes with a light microscope not only during mitosis but also in interphase and hence the analysis of (*i*) chromosome breakage and repair after exposure to ionizing radiation or chemical mutagens; (*ii*) DNA duplication; (*iii*) conformational changes during the cell cycle. Thus, PCCs constitute a useful alternative in cases where metaphase analysis may fail [69], e.g., (1) Estimation of a heterogeneous dose when the collected cells are a mixture of unirradiated and highly irradiated cells, delayed by repair mechanisms resulting in a delayed entry into the cell cycle; (2) accidental exposure to high levels of ionizing radiation, which produces a mitotic delay of unknown duration accompanied by significant apoptotic death; or (3) a very low chronic mitotic index, as in some pathological situations or elderly people.

By combining TC staining with the PCC technique for the analysis of DNA damage, the advantages include: (1) The possibility, for the first time, to visualize and score dicentric chromosomes; (2) determining the nature of acentric breaks; and (3) higher precision to monitor the kinetics of formation of chromosomal aberrations (Figure 6). The combination of these two techniques opens new horizons for the PCC technique, not only for the rapid scoring of DNA damage but also in the application of biological dosimetry into radiation emergency medicine and the automation of the analysis [12,68,70].

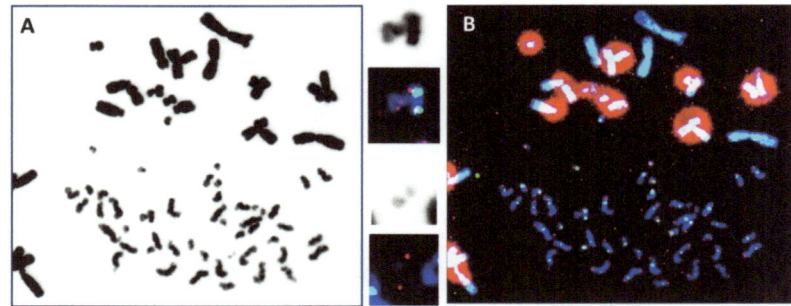

Figure 6. The combination of TC staining with the PCC fusion technique allows the reliable scoring of chromosome fragments and the detection of dicentric chromosomes. (**A**) Conventional DNA staining of PCC permits the scoring of chromosome condensation fragments (63× magnification). (**B**) Simultaneous telomere (red signals) and centromere (green signals) staining permits the detection of dicentric chromosomes (top inserts) and the accurate and consistent detection of acentric chromosomes (bottom inserts). The large red areas represent telomere signals of CHO chromosomes.

5. Automation of Biological Dosimetry Methods

Following considerable development of novel reagents and the standardization of cytogenetic preparations, the quality of cytogenetic slides has increased progressively to levels that make it feasible to automate the search for metaphases and capture slides. The first attempts to automate the scoring of radiation-induced DNA damage began in the 1990s with the automation of the scoring of micronuclei after uniform DNA staining (Giemsa or DAPI) [71]. The first commercially available system was Metafer MNScore from MetaSystems [72].

Spectacular advances have been achieved in recent years in terms of sensitivity and interface after uniform staining using cytogenetic slides or flow cytometers (DAPI) [21,73–75]. However, this automation concerns only the scoring of micronuclei and does not make it possible to differentiate the origin of micronuclei because centromere staining has not yet been implemented. The automation of other DNA damage markers such as anaphase bridges or nuclear buds (NBUDs) is still not relevant despite their crucial importance in biological dosimetry or chromosomal instability fields [76].

The second attempt of automation concerns the scoring of dicentric chromosomes after uniform staining. Reliability had long been hampered by the difficulty of recognizing metaphases by the use of many processors with little software. The first commercially available system was Metafer DCScore from MetaSystems [77–79]. A spectacular improvement was achieved in terms of sensitivity, which is essentially due to the introduction of TC staining [11,80,81] and the marketing of more advanced software.

The automation of PCC–CHO following uniform staining [66] and subsequent TC staining [12] has now been initiated; however, the implementation of this technique and its current use requires further technical development.

The automation of the scoring of translocation has not been undertaken so far. However, ongoing work using machine learning approaches after TC staining followed by M-FISH should make it possible to achieve high efficiency in the automation process.

6. Application of Cytogenetic Tools in a Wider Spectrum of Fields in Medicine and Biology

Cytogenetic biodosimetry is not limited to ionizing radiation and the follow-up of exposed populations. It is, in fact, applicable in the assessment of the effect of any genotoxic agent as well as that of inherent spontaneous genome instability in, e.g., cancer patients. The need to improve cytogenetic biodosimetry assays has been driven by the need to transfer technology to all cytogenetic laboratories to achieve high sample throughput for the processing of large cohorts of exposed populations as well as in medical settings [17,18,82].

The multiplex (M-FISH) technique is the latest evolution of FISH, which stains sex chromosomes and each pair of autosomes with different colors (1986). However, M-FISH has not been used intensively due to the complexity of the analysis. Recently, some studies started to use this technique [83–88]; however, the resolution of chromosomes to identify complex rearrangements can be vastly improved when TC staining with M-FISH [17,18,89].

TC staining followed by multiplex FISH (M-FISH), termed (TC+M-FISH), allows the reliable analysis of both unstable and stable chromosomal aberrations in a single-step analysis (Figure 7). In addition, this approach makes it possible to obtain an accurate karyotype in cases of genome heterogeneity and clonal escape.

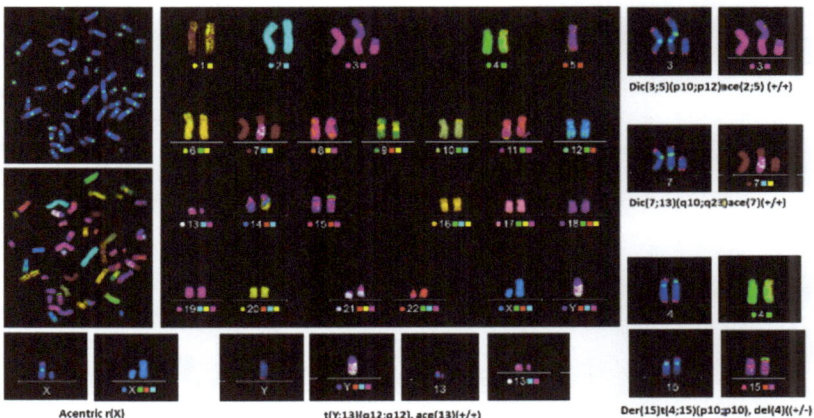

Figure 7. Telomere and centromere staining followed by M-FISH offers the sensitive and accurate detection of all chromosome aberrations, both stable and unstable ones. This approach permits the reliable identification of breakpoints and the assessment of the presence of complex clonal aberrations (63× magnification).

The employment of the TC+M-FISH approach in the analysis of the transmission of unstable chromosomal aberrations through multiple cell divisions has permitted not only the reevaluation of the transmission of dicentric chromosomes but also, for the first time, the documentation of the transmission of an acentric chromosome and the involvement of centromere breakpoints in this transmission [44]. Moreover, we have been able to demonstrate the persistence of specific configurations of dicentric chromosomes with both centromeres in close proximity during cell division [44]. Such dicentric chromosome configurations can easily be mistaken for translocation when only using the M-FISH technique because centromeric regions are not visible in the M-FISH assay.

Recently, we demonstrated the clinical utility of the TC+M-FISH technique for the detection of chromosomal aberrations in cancer patients in general, and of dicentric chromosomes in particular [17]. Today, the latter is considered the best cytological biomarker of chromosomal instability in cancer patients [90].

The TC+M-FISH approach permits the establishment of reliable and accurate karyotypes for cancer diagnosis [17,18]. Thus, the application of TC+M-FISH has revealed a much higher frequency of dicentric chromosomes with a specific configuration (two centromeres in close proximity) than has been observed previously by using conventional and molecular cytogenetics.

Moreover, the TC+M-FISH technique makes it possible to detect both stable and unstable aberrations, allowing accurate identification with high sensitivity of all chromosomal aberrations in addition to the putative progress of clonal escape and chromosomal instability. This approach will improve our knowledge not only of the biological effects of chemotherapy or low doses of irradiation but also of the underlying mechanisms of the formation of chromosomal aberrations. It could also be applied, with advantage, in the follow-up of exposed populations with a high risk of developing secondary cancer or late complications after exposure to genotoxic agents.

7. Advantages and Limitations of Current Cytogenetic Biomarkers of Ionizing Radiation

Most of the cytogenetic markers that have been used routinely for the past 50 years are primarily indicators of structural or functional damage to cellular components. However, despite their well-documented advantages, several challenges remain to be addressed and solved.

7.1. Specificity of Cytogenetic Biodosimetry Markers

It should be borne in mind that none of the chromosomal biomarkers described above are specific for monitoring exposure to ionizing radiation. In fact, they may also reflect the combinatory influence of other stressors such as the prior health status of the individual and genotoxic contamination by pollutants or chemicals that may create severe and long-lasting pathophysiological damage. Consequently, these markers constitute valuable indicators of the stress status of an individual (e.g., DNA repair, chromosome instability, and carcinogenesis). At low and medium doses of ionizing radiation, they may also reflect the subtle association between different additive effects of ionizing radiation such as radiation sensitivity, adaptation, and bystander effect, the consequences of which are not fully understood.

7.2. Challenges in Dose Estimation

1. The spontaneous rate of chromosomal aberrations in the general population is an important factor in cytogenetic biodosimetry because it can influence the interpretation of data. Thus, DNA damage can also be induced by occupational activities, lifestyle, and environmental factors [91]. Furthermore, there are variations in natural, terrestrial, and cosmic radioactivity, which differ from region to region and from country to country [92]. Finally, the worldwide increase in exposure to magnetic fields such as the use of mobile phones and the multiplicity of the employment of ionizing radiation in industry and medicine may have contributed to significant variations [93]. The latest evaluation of the frequencies of spontaneous chromosome aberrations dates back several decades. Since then, a vast amount of insight has accumulated into the causes and frequencies of chromosome aberrations. Moreover, significant technical improvements in their detection have been achieved. Therefore, the re-examination of the frequency of spontaneous chromosomal aberrations in the general population is urgently needed. For that purpose, an automated TC+M-FISH approach would be most relevant.
2. The distribution of aberrations according to age and sex is not clear and differs from one study to another. Recently, several studies have demonstrated the difference in genotoxic stress response according to sex [94–96]. Notably, the used dose-response curves did not take into account the age or sex of the exposed population.
3. The interpretation of complex chromosomal rearrangements in the estimation of the absorbed dose has always been challenging in biological dosimetry. A significant correlation has been found between the formation of complex chromosomal rearrangements and the clinical outcome of patients treated with radiotherapy [97,98]. The presence of these kinds of aberrations has also been correlated with interindividual radiation sensitivity and genomic instability [99]. The lack of analysis of complex chromosomal rearrangement in a large cohort of an exposed population using a sensitive technique did not make it possible to advance our knowledge regarding their formations and their interpretations.

4. The interpretation of "Rogue cells" in the analysis of chromosomal aberrations and the estimation of the dose after exposure is still unclear. "Rogue cells" are cells with multiple and complex chromosomal aberrations (e.g., dicentric, tricentric, translocations, insertions, deletions, and acentric chromosomes) related to the activation of viral infection [100,101]. A significant increase in induced chromosomal aberrations has been detected in the presence of rogue cells [102–105]. Further studies are needed to investigate the role of viral infection in the formation of radiation-induced chromosomal aberrations.

7.3. Relevant Questions for Cytogenetic Biological Dosimetry Assays

Although research over the last 50 years on cytogenetic biomarkers in biodosimetry has sufficiently covered their operational capacities, there still persist some gray areas that need to be addressed and resolved to improve the assessment of potential genotoxic exposures [52,106]:

- How can we validly relate lymphocyte lifetime and (re)circulation to partial exposure and thus introduce useful correction factors in the estimation of an absorbed dose of ionizing radiation?
- What value can be attributed to translocation analysis in the concept of dose, especially decades or years after a potential exposure?
- How do we coordinate all of the biological and biophysical markers available to the dosimetrist into a coherent entity, integrating the concept of multiparameter analyses?
- How do we integrate new developments (genomics, proteomics, and transcriptomics) that, without renovating the current biotechnological landscape, make it possible to associate physiopathology more globally with genomic instability?
- How do we integrate modulation phenomena, such as cellular and tissue radiosensitivity, radiation adaptation, and abscopal or bystander effects, that are still incompletely understood?

7.4. Internal Exposure

The internal exposure to ionizing radiation, particularly that due to contamination, is classically considered in three specific contexts: (*i*) environmental, to which all people are naturally subject; (*ii*) occupational, concerning certain categories of workers, and finally, (*iii*) iatrogenic, the consequences of which evolve with the level of health care [107]. Biological indicators could be very useful to characterize the occurrence and type of effects observed, as well as the intracellular and intercellular processes activated in response to internal exposure. The first interest is the clinical and epidemiological study of cancers developed by humans after exposure to a radio-contaminant; the second interest is related to clinical treatment and the histological characterization of treated cancers after induction of vectorized radioimmunotherapy.

8. New Challenges for the Use of Biological Dosimetry in Detecting Carcinogenesis Susceptibility

The accurate detection of DNA damage is not restricted to cytogenetic biodosimetry after accidental, professional, or medical exposure to ionizing radiation [108]. Personalized medicine also needs this approach for the development of new biomarkers of DNA repair deficiency in order to propose a specific treatment for individual patients. The clinical utility of these techniques—particularly the need for sensitive and specific biomarkers—is justified by the stratification of patients regarding the deleterious consequence of chromosomal instability [108,109]. The introduction of TC staining in the cytogenetic biological dosimetry approach and the automation of the scoring of all chromosomal aberrations must lead to the creation of databases allowing sensitive and specific stratification of exposed populations and/or patients.

The second challenge is related to the impact of low-dose effects on chromosome instability. Improved detection of DNA damage by introducing TC staining makes it possible to reveal genetic consequences for doses below 0.1 Gy. Their application, including telomere analysis to the field of low-dose exposures, could add significant advantages to our understanding of such effects.

The third challenge is paradoxically to have the best-standardized response for various types of irradiation, dose rate, and genetic parameters in any laboratory practicing biological dosimetry assessment. This apparently simple feature, although required for better efficiency, is not always obtainable—and the reasons for that are not always obvious. The introduction of TC staining in the automatic scoring of DNA damage has rendered the analysis independent of the level of expertise of the operator. In addition, high reproducibility of the scoring has been achieved. The systematic use of this technique instead of the classical scoring of chromosome aberrations could greatly improve the respective standardizations.

Finally, the possible fusion between the "gold standard" technique (dicentric chromosome), FISH or M-FISH technique (translocation), and CBMN assay (micronuclei) will represent an important technical challenge that will surely lead to wider applications for sensitive and reliable dose estimation [110,111].

While biodosimetry using traditional cytogenetic assays is useful for dose assessments following accidental exposure to ionizing radiation, the field of biodosimetry has advanced significantly with expansion into the fields of genomics, proteomics, metabolomics, and transcriptomics [112–115]. However, advances in the assessment of radiation exposure using those approaches have more relevance to clinical applications for patients undergoing radiation therapy. The information derived from radiation responses may advance personalized care and could help alleviate the damage to normal tissue [116].

9. Conclusions

For more than 50 years cytogenetic biodosimetry has been routinely and successfully practiced worldwide by a few specialized laboratories for assessing individual exposure to ionizing radiation, and international networks have been established in preparation for a potential nuclear catastrophe. However, all of the classical techniques applied for these purposes suffer from several limitations: they are unnecessarily time-consuming, their sensitivity and specificity are untimely limited, and they require highly skilled personnel that may be in shortage in the event of a major nuclear catastrophe. By including TC staining together with M-FISH, several of these obstacles may be overcome. Moreover, importantly, the automation of these novel techniques adds to the major achievements provided by the inclusion of TC staining in the current cytogenetic assays. We also propose their use in the general assessment of DNA damage and chromosome instability which are largely underestimated in many diseases. Last but not the least, wider potentials exploiting these techniques are emerging for their application in identifying prognostic biomarkers and guides for the better triage and management of medical patients. The standardization of cytogenetic biological dosimetry approaches permits the use of a unique dose-response curve. The automation of these approaches opens new horizons in the construction of large databases in exposed populations, allowing the precise estimation of risk associated with radiation exposure. This is the role of official instances such as the AIEA and OMS as well as an international research program for the harmonization and standardization of the process such as the RENEB program. We also need companies to manufacture the kits and for standardization and development of analysis software with the overall aim of automating all of the processes.

Author Contributions: Conceptualization, R.M. and P.V.; investigation, B.C. and E.E.M.; resources, A.D., A.P., L.H. and E.J.; writing—original draft preparation, R.M., P.V. and S.J.; writing—review and editing, R.M., S.J. and P.C. All authors have read and agreed to the published version of the manuscript.

Funding: This research received no external funding.

Institutional Review Board Statement: Not applicable.

Informed Consent Statement: Not applicable.

Data Availability Statement: Not applicable.

Conflicts of Interest: The authors declare no conflict of interest.

References

1. IAEA. *Cytogenetic Dosimetry: Applications in Preparedness for and Response to Radiation Emergencies: A Manual*; IAEA: Vienna, Austria, 2013.
2. Sproull, M.; Camphausen, K. State-of-the-Art Advances in Radiation Biodosimetry for Mass Casualty Events Involving Radiation Exposure. *Radiat. Res.* **2016**, *186*, 423–435. [CrossRef] [PubMed]
3. Sullivan, J.M.; Prasanna, P.G.; Grace, M.B.; Wathen, L.K.; Wallace, R.L.; Koerner, J.F.; Coleman, C.N. Assessment of biodosimetry methods for a mass-casualty radiological incident: Medical response and management considerations. *Health Phys.* **2013**, *105*, 540–554. [CrossRef] [PubMed]
4. Ainsbury, E.A.; Moquet, J. The future of biological dosimetry in mass casualty radiation emergency response, personalized radiation risk estimation and space radiation protection. *Int. J. Radiat. Biol.* **2022**, *98*, 421–427. [CrossRef] [PubMed]
5. Pernot, E.; Hall, J.; Baatout, S.; Benotmane, M.A.; Blanchardon, E.; Bouffler, S.; El Saghire, H.; Gomolka, M.; Guertler, A.; Harms-Ringdahl, M.; et al. Ionizing radiation biomarkers for potential use in epidemiological studies. *Mutat. Res.* **2012**, *751*, 258–286. [CrossRef]
6. Edwards, A.; Voisin, P.; Sorokine-Durm, I.; Maznik, N.; Vinnikov, V.; Mikhalevich, L.; Moquet, J.; Lloyd, D.; Delbos, M.; Durand, V. Biological estimates of dose to inhabitants of Belarus and Ukraine following the Chernobyl accident. *Radiat. Prot. Dosim.* **2004**, *111*, 211–219. [CrossRef]
7. IAEA. Cytogenetic dosimetry applications in preparedness for and response to radiation emergencies. In *EPR-Biodose*; IAEA: Vienna, Austria, 2011.
8. IAEA. Biological Dosimetry: Chromosomal aberration analysis for dose assessment. In *Technical Report series N° 260*; IAEA: Vienna, Austria, 1986.
9. IAEA. Cytogenetic Analysis for Radiation Dose Assessment. In *Technical Report Series*; IAEA: Vienna, Austria, 2001.
10. Shi, L.; Fujioka, K.; Sun, J.; Kinomura, A.; Inaba, T.; Ikura, T.; Ohtaki, M.; Yoshida, M.; Kodama, Y.; Livingston, G.K.; et al. A modified system for analyzing ionizing radiation-induced chromosome abnormalities. *Radiat. Res.* **2012**, *177*, 533–538. [CrossRef] [PubMed]
11. M'Kacher, R.; Maalouf, E.E.; Ricoul, M.; Heidingsfelder, L.; Laplagne, E.; Cuceu, C.; Hempel, W.M.; Colicchio, B.; Dieterlen, A.; Sabatier, L. New tool for biological dosimetry: Reevaluation and automation of the gold standard method following telomere and centromere staining. *Mutat. Res.* **2014**, *770*, 45–53. [CrossRef]
12. M'Kacher, R.; El Maalouf, E.; Terzoudi, G.; Ricoul, M.; Heidingsfelder, L.; Karachristou, I.; Laplagne, E.; Hempel, W.M.; Colicchio, B.; Dieterlen, A.; et al. Detection and automated scoring of dicentric chromosomes in nonstimulated lymphocyte prematurely condensed chromosomes after telomere and centromere staining. *Int. J. Radiat. Oncol. Biol. Phys.* **2015**, *91*, 640–649. [CrossRef]
13. Gotoh, E. G2 Premature Chromosome Condensation/Chromosome Aberration Assay: Drug-Induced Premature Chromosome Condensation (PCC) Protocols and Cytogenetic Approaches in Mitotic Chromosome and Interphase Chromatin for Radiation Biology. *Methods Mol Biol.* **2019**, *1984*, 47–60. [CrossRef]
14. Zaguia, N.; Laplagne, E.; Colicchio, B.; Cariou, O.; Al Jawhari, M.; Heidingsfelder, L.; Hempel, W.M.; Jrad, B.B.H.; Jeandidier, E.; Dieterlen, A.; et al. A new tool for genotoxic risk assessment: Reevaluation of the cytokinesis-block micronucleus assay using semi-automated scoring following telomere and centromere staining. *Mutat. Res./Genet. Toxicol. Environ. Mutagen.* **2020**, *850–851*, 503143. [CrossRef] [PubMed]
15. Soumboundou, M.; Dossou, J.; Kalaga, Y.; Nkengurutse, I.; Faye, I.; Guingani, A.; Gadji, M.; Yameogo, K.J.; Zongo, H.; Mbaye, G.; et al. Is Response to Genotoxic Stress Similar in Populations of African and European Ancestry? A Study of Dose-Response After in vitro Irradiation. *Front. Genet.* **2021**, *12*, 657999. [CrossRef]
16. Soumboundou, M.; Nkengurutse, I.; Dossou, J.; Colicchio, B.; Djebou, C.; Gadji, M.; Houenon, G.; Dem, A.; Dedjan, A.; Diarra, M.; et al. Biological Dosimetry Network in Africa: Establishment of a Dose-Response Curve Using Telomere and Centromere Staining. *Health Phys.* **2019**, *117*, 618–624. [CrossRef]
17. M'Kacher, R.; Colicchio, B.; Borie, C.; Junker, S.; Marquet, V.; Heidingsfelder, L.; Soehnlen, K.; Najar, W.; Hempel, W.M.; Oudrhiri, N.; et al. Telomere and Centromere Staining Followed by M-FISH Improves Diagnosis of Chromosomal Instability and Its Clinical Utility. *Genes* **2020**, *11*, 475. [CrossRef]
18. M'Kacher, R.; Miguet, M.; Maillard, P.Y. A Central Role of Telomere Dysfunction in the Formation of a Unique Translocation within the Sub-Telomere Region Resulting in Duplication and Partial Trisomy. *Genes* **2020**, *13*, 1762. [CrossRef] [PubMed]
19. Chaurasia, R.K.; Bhat, N.N.; Gaur, N.; Shirsath, K.B.; Desai, U.N.; Sapra, B.K. Establishment and multiparametric-cytogenetic validation of (60)Co-gamma-ray induced, phospho-gamma-H2AX calibration curve for rapid biodosimetry and triage management during radiological emergencies. *Mutat. Res. Toxicol. Environ. Mutagen.* **2021**, *866*, 503354. [CrossRef]
20. Blakely, W.F.; Port, M.; Abend, M. Early-response multiple-parameter biodosimetry and dosimetry: Risk predictions. *J. Radiol. Prot. Off. J. Soc. Radiol. Prot.* **2021**, *41*, R152–R175. [CrossRef] [PubMed]

21. Nair, S.; Cairncross, S.; Miles, X.; Engelbrecht, M.; du Plessis, P.; Bolcaen, J.; Fisher, R.; Ndimba, R.; Cunningham, C.; Martínez-López, W.; et al. An Automated Microscopic Scoring Method for the γ-H2AX Foci Assay in Human Peripheral Blood Lymphocytes. *J. Vis. Exp.* **2021**, *178*. [CrossRef]
22. Jakl, L.; Marková, E.; Koláriková, L.; Belyaev, I. Biodosimetry of Low Dose Ionizing Radiation Using DNA Repair Foci in Human Lymphocytes. *Genes* **2020**, *11*, 58. [CrossRef] [PubMed]
23. Raavi, V.; Perumal, V.; Paul, S.F. Potential application of γ-H2AX as a biodosimetry tool for radiation triage. *Mutat. Res. Rev. Mutat. Res.* **2021**, *787*, 108350. [CrossRef]
24. Viau, M.; Testard, I.; Shim, G.; Morat, L.; Normil, M.D.; Hempel, W.M.; Sabatier, L. Global quantification of γH2AX as a triage tool for the rapid estimation of received dose in the event of accidental radiation exposure. *Mutat. Res. Genet. Toxicol. Environ. Mutagen.* **2015**, *793*, 123–131. [CrossRef]
25. Penninckx, S.; Pariset, E.; Cekanaviciute, E. Quantification of radiation-induced DNA double strand break repair foci to evaluate and predict biological responses to ionizing radiation. *NAR Cancer* **2021**, *3*, zcab046. [CrossRef]
26. Moquet, J.; Barnard, S.; Staynova, A.; Lindholm, C.; Monteiro Gil, O.; Martins, V.; Rößler, U.; Vral, A.; Vandevoorde, C.; Wojewódzka, M.; et al. The second gamma-H2AX assay inter-comparison exercise carried out in the framework of the European biodosimetry network (RENEB). *Int. J. Radiat. Biol.* **2017**, *93*, 58–64. [CrossRef] [PubMed]
27. Valdiglesias, V.; Giunta, S.; Fenech, M.; Neri, M.; Bonassi, S. γH2AX as a marker of DNA double strand breaks and genomic instability in human population studies. *Mutat. Res.* **2013**, *753*, 24–40. [CrossRef]
28. Pantelias, G.E.; Maillie, H.D. The measurement of immediate and persistent radiation-induced chromosome damage in rodent primary cells using premature chromosome condensation. *Health Phys.* **1985**, *49*, 425–433. [CrossRef] [PubMed]
29. Hatzi, V.I.; Terzoudi, G.I.; Paraskevopoulou, C.; Makropoulos, V.; Matthopoulos, D.P.; Pantelias, G.E. The use of premature chromosome condensation to study in interphase cells the influence of environmental factors on human genetic material. *Sci. World J.* **2006**, *6*, 1174–1190. [CrossRef]
30. Awa, A.A. Persistent chromosome aberrations in the somatic cells of A-bomb survivors, Hiroshima and Nagasaki. *J. Radiat. Res.* **1991**, *32* (Suppl. S1), 265–274. [CrossRef] [PubMed]
31. van Dorp, W.; Haupt, R.; Anderson, R.A.; Mulder, R.L.; van den Heuvel-Eibrink, M.M.; van Dulmen-den Broeder, E.; Su, H.I.; Winther, J.F.; Hudson, M.M.; Levine, J.M.; et al. Reproductive Function and Outcomes in Female Survivors of Childhood, Adolescent, and Young Adult Cancer: A Review. *J. Clin. Oncol. Off. J. Am. Soc. Clin. Oncol.* **2018**, *36*, 2169–2180. [CrossRef] [PubMed]
32. Ståhl, O.; Boyd, H.A.; Giwercman, A.; Lindholm, M.; Jensen, A.; Kjær, S.K.; Anderson, H.; Cavallin-Ståhl, E.; Rylander, L. Risk of birth abnormalities in the offspring of men with a history of cancer: A cohort study using Danish and Swedish national registries. *J. Natl. Cancer Inst.* **2011**, *103*, 398–406. [CrossRef]
33. Signorello, L.B.; Mulvihill, J.J.; Green, D.M.; Munro, H.M.; Stovall, M.; Weathers, R.E.; Mertens, A.C.; Whitton, J.A.; Robison, L.L.; Boice, J.D., Jr. Congenital anomalies in the children of cancer survivors: A report from the childhood cancer survivor study. *J. Clin. Oncol. Off. J. Am. Soc. Clin. Oncol.* **2012**, *30*, 239–245. [CrossRef]
34. Reulen, R.C.; Zeegers, M.P.; Wallace, W.H.; Frobisher, C.; Taylor, A.J.; Lancashire, E.R.; Winter, D.L.; Hawkins, M.M. Pregnancy outcomes among adult survivors of childhood cancer in the British Childhood Cancer Survivor Study. *Cancer Epidemiol. Biomark. Prev.* **2009**, *18*, 2239–2247. [CrossRef]
35. Little, M.P.; Goodhead, D.T.; Bridges, B.A.; Bouffler, S.D. Evidence relevant to untargeted and transgenerational effects in the offspring of irradiated parents. *Mutat. Res.* **2013**, *753*, 50–67. [CrossRef]
36. Jordan, B.R. The Hiroshima/Nagasaki Survivor Studies: Discrepancies Between Results and General Perception. *Genetics* **2016**, *203*, 1505–1512. [CrossRef]
37. Nomura, T. Transgenerational carcinogenesis: Induction and transmission of genetic alterations and mechanisms of carcinogenesis. *Mutat. Res.* **2003**, *544*, 425–432. [CrossRef] [PubMed]
38. Straume, T. A radiobiological basis for setting neutron radiation safety standards. *Health Phys.* **1985**, *49*, 883–896. [CrossRef]
39. Doloy, M.T.; Malarbet, J.L.; Guedeney, G.; Bourguignon, M.; Leroy, A.; Reillaudou, M.; Masse, R. Use of unstable chromosome aberrations for biological dosimetry after the first postirradiation mitosis. *Radiat. Res.* **1991**, *125*, 141–151. [CrossRef]
40. Guedeney, G.; Rigaud, O.; Duranton, I.; Malarbet, J.L.; Doloy, M.T.; Magdelenat, H. Chromosomal aberrations and DNA repair ability of in vitro irradiated white blood cells of monkeys previously exposed to total body irradiation. *Mutat. Res.* **1989**, *212*, 159–166. [CrossRef]
41. *ISO21243*; Radiation Protection—Performance Criteria for Laboratories Performing Cytogenetic Triage for Assessment of Mass Casualties in Radiological or Nuclear Emergencies-General Principles and Application to Dicentric Assay. ISO: Genève, Switzerland, 2008.
42. *ISO19238*; Radiological Protection-Performance Criteria for Service Laboratories Performing Biological Dosimetry by Cytogenetics. ISO: Geneva, Switzerland, 2014.
43. *ISO17099*; Radiological Protection-Performance Criteria for Laboratories Using the Cytokinesis-Block Micronucleus (CBMN) Assay in Peripheral Blood Lymphocytes for Biological Dosimetry. ISO: Geneva, Switzerland, 2014.
44. Kaddour, A.; Colicchio, B.; Buron, D.; El Maalouf, E.; Laplagne, E.; Borie, C.; Ricoul, M.; Lenain, A.; Hempel, W.M.; Morat, L.; et al. Transmission of Induced Chromosomal Aberrations through Successive Mitotic Divisions in Human Lymphocytes after In Vitro and In Vivo Radiation. *Sci. Rep.* **2017**, *7*, 3291. [CrossRef] [PubMed]

45. Li, Y.; Knoll, J.H.; Wilkins, R.C.; Flegal, F.N.; Rogan, P.K. Automated discrimination of dicentric and monocentric chromosomes by machine learning-based image processing. *Microsc. Res. Tech.* **2016**, *79*, 393–402. [CrossRef]
46. Romm, H.; Ainsbury, E.A.; Barquinero, J.F.; Barrios, L.; Beinke, C.; Cucu, A.; Domene, M.M.; Filippi, S.; Monteiro Gil, O.; Gregoire, E.; et al. Web based scoring is useful for validation and harmonisation of scoring criteria within RENEB. *Int. J. Radiat. Biol.* **2017**, *93*, 110–117. [CrossRef] [PubMed]
47. Shuryak, I.; Royba, E.; Repin, M.; Turner, H.C.; Garty, G.; Deoli, N.; Brenner, D.J. A machine learning method for improving the accuracy of radiation biodosimetry by combining data from the dicentric chromosomes and micronucleus assays. *Sci. Rep.* **2022**, *12*, 21077. [CrossRef]
48. Royba, E.; Repin, M.; Balajee, A.S.; Shuryak, I.; Pampou, S.; Karan, C.; Brenner, D.J.; Garty, G. The RABiT-II DCA in the Rhesus Macaque Model. *Radiat. Res.* **2020**, *196*, 501–509. [CrossRef] [PubMed]
49. Garty, G.; Bigelow, A.W.; Repin, M.; Turner, H.C.; Bian, D.; Balajee, A.S.; Lyulko, O.V.; Taveras, M.; Yao, Y.L.; Brenner, D.J. An automated imaging system for radiation biodosimetry. *Microsc. Res. Tech.* **2015**, *78*, 587–598. [CrossRef] [PubMed]
50. Roukos, V.; Burman, B.; Misteli, T. The cellular etiology of chromosome translocations. *Curr. Opin. Cell Biol.* **2013**, *25*, 357–364. [CrossRef]
51. Tucker, J.D. Reflections on the development and application of FISH whole chromosome painting. *Mutat. Res. Rev. Mutat. Res.* **2015**, *763*, 2–14. [CrossRef] [PubMed]
52. Simon, S.L.; Bailey, S.M.; Beck, H.L.; Boice, J.D.; Bouville, A.; Brill, A.B.; Cornforth, M.N.; Inskip, P.D.; McKenna, M.J.; Mumma, M.T.; et al. Estimation of Radiation Doses to U.S. Military Test Participants from Nuclear Testing: A Comparison of Historical Film-Badge Measurements, Dose Reconstruction and Retrospective Biodosimetry. *Radiat. Res.* **2019**, *191*, 297–310. [CrossRef] [PubMed]
53. Livingston, G.K.; Khvostunov, I.K. Cytogenetic effects of radioiodine therapy: A 20-year follow-up study. *Radiat. Environ. Biophys.* **2016**, *55*, 203–213. [CrossRef] [PubMed]
54. Goh, V.S.T.; Fujishima, Y.; Abe, Y.; Sakai, A.; Yoshida, M.A.; Ariyoshi, K.; Kasai, K.; Wilkins, R.C.; Blakely, W.F.; Miura, T. Construction of fluorescence in situ hybridization (FISH) translocation dose-response calibration curve with multiple donor data sets using R, based on ISO 20046:2019 recommendations. *Int. J. Radiat. Biol.* **2019**, *95*, 1668–1684. [CrossRef]
55. Gregoire, E.; Barquinero, J.F.; Shi, L.; Tashiro, S.; Sotnik, N.V.; Azizova, T.V.; Darroudi, F.; Ainsbury, E.A.; Moquet, J.E.; Fomina, J.; et al. Verification by the FISH translocation assay of historic doses to Mayak workers from external gamma radiation. *Radiat. Environ. Biophys.* **2015**, *54*, 445–451.
56. Andreassi, M.G.; Little, M.P.; Wakeford, R.; Hatch, M.; Ainsbury, E.A.; Tawn, E.J. Chromosome Aberrations in a Group of People Exposed to Radioactive Releases from the Three Mile Island Nuclear Accident and Inferences for Radiation Effects. *Int. J. Mol. Sci.* **2021**, *22*, 7504. [CrossRef]
57. Sorokine-Durm, I.; Durand, V.; Le Roy, A.; Paillole, N.; Roy, L.; Voisin, P. Is FISH painting an appropriate biological marker for dose estimates of suspected accidental radiation overexposure? A review of cases investigated in France from 1995 to 1996. *Environ. Health Perspect.* **1997**, *105* (Suppl. S6), 1427–1432. [CrossRef]
58. Buckton, K.E.; Jacobs, P.A.; Court Brown, W.M.; Doll, R. A study of the chromosome damage persisting after x-ray therapy for ankylosing spondylitis. *Lancet* **1962**, *2*, 676–682. [CrossRef]
59. Fenech, M.; Knasmueller, S.; Bolognesi, C.; Holland, N.; Bonassi, S.; Kirsch-Volders, M. Micronuclei as biomarkers of DNA damage, aneuploidy, inducers of chromosomal hypermutation and as sources of pro-inflammatory DNA in humans. *Mutat. Res. Rev. Mutat. Res.* **2020**, *786*, 108342. [CrossRef] [PubMed]
60. Fenech, M.; Bonassi, S. The effect of age, gender, diet and lifestyle on DNA damage measured using micronucleus frequency in human peripheral blood lymphocytes. *Mutagenesis* **2011**, *26*, 43–49. [CrossRef] [PubMed]
61. Fenech, M.; Morley, A.A. Measurement of micronuclei in lymphocytes. *Mutat. Res.* **1985**, *147*, 29–36. [CrossRef] [PubMed]
62. Fenech, M. Micronuclei and their association with sperm abnormalities, infertility, pregnancy loss, pre-eclampsia and intra-uterine growth restriction in humans. *Mutagenesis* **2011**, *26*, 63–67. [CrossRef] [PubMed]
63. Vral, A.; Fenech, M.; Thierens, H. The micronucleus assay as a biological dosimeter of in vivo ionising radiation exposure. *Mutagenesis* **2011**, *26*, 11–17. [CrossRef]
64. Depuydt, J.; Baert, A.; Vandersickel, V.; Thierens, H.; Vral, A. Relative biological effectiveness of mammography X-rays at the level of DNA and chromosomes in lymphocytes. *Int. J. Radiat. Biol.* **2013**, *89*, 532–538. [CrossRef]
65. Vral, A.; Decorte, V.; Depuydt, J.; Wambersie, A.; Thierens, H. A semi-automated FISH-based micronucleus-centromere assay for biomonitoring of hospital workers exposed to low doses of ionizing radiation. *Mol. Med. Rep.* **2016**, *14*, 103–110. [CrossRef]
66. Pantelias, A.; Terzoudi, G.I. Development of an automatable micro-PCC biodosimetry assay for rapid individualized risk assessment in large-scale radiological emergencies. *Mutat. Res. Genet. Toxicol. Environ. Mutagen.* **2018**, *836*, 65–71. [CrossRef]
67. Sun, M.; Moquet, J.; Barnard, S.; Lloyd, D.; Ainsbury, E. A Simplified Calyculin A-Induced Premature Chromosome Condensation (PCC) Protocol for the Biodosimetric Analysis of High-Dose Exposure to Gamma Radiation. *Radiat. Res.* **2020**, *193*, 560–568. [CrossRef]
68. Puig, R.; Barrios, L.; Pujol, M.; Caballín, M.R.; Barquinero, J.F. Suitability of scoring PCC rings and fragments for dose assessment after high-dose exposures to ionizing radiation. *Mutat. Res.* **2013**, *757*, 1–7. [CrossRef]
69. Durante, M.; George, K.; Yang, T.C. Biodosimetry of ionizing radiation by selective painting of prematurely condensed chromosomes in human lymphocytes. *Radiat. Res.* **1997**, *148*, S45–S50. [CrossRef]

70. Karachristou, I.; Karakosta, M.; Pantelias, A.; Hatzi, V.I.; Karaiskos, P.; Dimitriou, P.; Pantelias, G.; Terzoudi, G.I. Triage biodosimetry using centromeric/telomeric PNA probes and Giemsa staining to score dicentrics or excess fragments in non-stimulated lymphocyte prematurely condensed chromosomes. *Mutat. Res. Genet. Toxicol. Environ. Mutagen.* **2015**, *793*, 107–114. [CrossRef]
71. Fenech, M.; Kirsch-Volders, M.; Rossnerova, A.; Sram, R.; Romm, H.; Bolognesi, C.; Ramakumar, A.; Soussaline, F.; Schunck, C.; Elhajouji, A.; et al. HUMN project initiative and review of validation, quality control and prospects for further development of automated micronucleus assays using image cytometry systems. *Int. J. Hyg. Environ. Health* **2013**, *216*, 541–552. [CrossRef]
72. Schunck, C.; Johannes, T.; Varga, D.; Lörch, T.; Plesch, A. New developments in automated cytogenetic imaging: Unattended scoring of dicentric chromosomes, micronuclei, single cell gel electrophoresis, and fluorescence signals. *Cytogenet. Genome Res.* **2004**, *104*, 383–389. [CrossRef]
73. Wang, Q.; Rodrigues, M.A.; Repin, M.; Pampou, S.; Beaton-Green, L.A.; Perrier, J.; Garty, G.; Brenner, D.J.; Turner, H.C.; Wilkins, R.C. Automated Triage Radiation Biodosimetry: Integrating Imaging Flow Cytometry with High-Throughput Robotics to Perform the Cytokinesis-Block Micronucleus Assay. *Radiat. Res.* **2019**, *191*, 342–351. [CrossRef] [PubMed]
74. Capaccio, C.; Perrier, J.R.; Cunha, L.; Mahnke, R.C.; Lörch, T.; Porter, M.; Smith, C.L.; Damer, K.; Bourland, J.D.; Frizzell, B.; et al. CytoRADx: A High-Throughput, Standardized Biodosimetry Diagnostic System Based on the Cytokinesis-Block Micronucleus Assay. *Radiat. Res.* **2021**, *196*, 523–534. [CrossRef]
75. Repin, M.; Pampou, S.; Karan, C.; Brenner, D.J.; Garty, G. RABiT-II: Implementation of a High-Throughput Micronucleus Biodosimetry Assay on Commercial Biotech Robotic Systems. *Radiat. Res.* **2017**, *187*, 492–498. [CrossRef] [PubMed]
76. Fenech, M. Cytokinesis-Block Micronucleus Cytome Assay Evolution into a More Comprehensive Method to Measure Chromosomal Instability. *Genes* **2020**, *11*, 1203. [CrossRef] [PubMed]
77. Romm, H.; Ainsbury, E.; Barnard, S.; Barrios, L.; Barquinero, J.F.; Beinke, C.; Deperas, M.; Gregoire, E.; Koivistoinen, A.; Lindholm, C.; et al. Automatic scoring of dicentric chromosomes as a tool in large scale radiation accidents. *Mutat. Res.* **2013**, *756*, 174–183. [CrossRef]
78. Alsbeih, G.A.; Al-Hadyan, K.S.; Al-Harbi, N.M.; Bin Judia, S.S.; Moftah, B.A. Establishing a Reference Dose-Response Calibration Curve for Dicentric Chromosome Aberrations to Assess Accidental Radiation Exposure in Saudi Arabia. *Front. Public Health* **2020**, *8*, 599194. [CrossRef]
79. Oestreicher, U.; Samaga, D.; Ainsbury, E.; Antunes, A.C.; Baeyens, A.; Barrios, L.; Beinke, C.; Beukes, P.; Blakely, W.F.; Cucu, A.; et al. RENEB intercomparisons applying the conventional Dicentric Chromosome Assay (DCA). *Int. J. Radiat. Biol.* **2017**, *93*, 20–29. [CrossRef]
80. Royba, E.; Repin, M.; Pampou, S.; Karan, C.; Brenner, D.J.; Garty, G. RABiT-II-DCA: A Fully-automated Dicentric Chromosome Assay in Multiwell Plates. *Radiat. Res.* **2019**, *192*, 311–323. [CrossRef] [PubMed]
81. Herate, C.; Brochard, P.; De Vathaire, F.; Ricoul, M.; Martins, B.; Laurier, L.; Deverre, J.R.; Thirion, B.; Hertz-Pannier, L.; Sabatier, L. The effects of repeated brain MRI on chromosomal damage. *Eur. Radiol. Exp.* **2022**, *6*, 12. [CrossRef] [PubMed]
82. Oudrhiri, N.; M'Kacher, R. Patient-Derived iPSCs Reveal Evidence of Telomere Instability and DNA Repair Deficiency in Coats Plus Syndrome. *Genes* **2022**, *13*, 1395. [CrossRef]
83. Sumption, N.; Goodhead, D.T.; Anderson, R.M. Alpha-Particle-Induced Complex Chromosome Exchanges Transmitted through Extra-Thymic Lymphopoiesis In Vitro Show Evidence of Emerging Genomic Instability. *PLoS ONE* **2015**, *10*, e0134046. [CrossRef]
84. Nieri, D.; Berardinelli, F.; Antoccia, A.; Tanzarella, C.; Sgura, A. Comparison between two FISH techniques in the in vitro study of cytogenetic markers for low-dose X-ray exposure in human primary fibroblasts. *Front. Genet.* **2013**, *4*, 141. [CrossRef]
85. Kohda, A.; Toyokawa, T.; Umino, T.; Ayabe, Y.; Tanaka, I.B.; Komura, J.I. Frequencies of Chromosome Aberrations are Lower in Splenic Lymphocytes from Mice Continuously Exposed to Very Low-Dose-Rate Gamma Rays Compared with Non-Irradiated Control Mice. *Radiat. Res.* **2022**, *198*, 639–645. [CrossRef] [PubMed]
86. Foster, H.A.; Estrada-Girona, G.; Themis, M.; Garimberti, E.; Hill, M.A.; Bridger, J.M.; Anderson, R.M. Relative proximity of chromosome territories influences chromosome exchange partners in radiation-induced chromosome rearrangements in primary human bronchial epithelial cells. *Mutat. Res.* **2013**, *756*, 66–77. [CrossRef] [PubMed]
87. Bastiani, I.; McMahon, S.J.; Turner, P.; Redmond, K.M.; McGarry, C.K.; Cole, A.; O'Sullivan, J.M.; Prise, K.M.; Ainsbury, L.; Anderson, R. Dose estimation after a mixed field exposure: Radium-223 and intensity modulated radiotherapy. *Nucl. Med. Biol.* **2022**, *106–107*, 10–20. [CrossRef] [PubMed]
88. Balajee, A.S.; Bertucci, A.; Taveras, M.; Brenner, D.J. Multicolour FISH analysis of ionising radiation induced micronucleus formation in human lymphocytes. *Mutagenesis* **2014**, *29*, 447–455. [CrossRef] [PubMed]
89. Cuceu, C.; Colicchio, B.; Jeandidier, E. Independent Mechanisms Lead to Genomic Instability in Hodgkin Lymphoma: Microsatellite or Chromosomal Instability (dagger). *Cancers* **2018**, *10*, 233. [CrossRef]
90. Gascoigne, K.E.; Cheeseman, I.M. Induced dicentric chromosome formation promotes genomic rearrangements and tumorigenesis. *Chromosome Res. Int. J. Mol. Supramol. Evol. Asp. Chromosome Biol.* **2013**, *21*, 407–418. [CrossRef]
91. Vaurijoux, A.; Gruel, G.; Pouzoulet, F.; Grégoire, E.; Martin, C.; Roch-Lefèvre, S.; Voisin, P.; Voisin, P.; Roy, L. Strategy for population triage based on dicentric analysis. *Radiat. Res.* **2009**, *171*, 541–548. [CrossRef] [PubMed]
92. Bauchinger, M. Quantification of low-level radiation exposure by conventional chromosome aberration analysis. *Mutat. Res.* **1995**, *339*, 177–189. [CrossRef]

93. Lopes, J.; Baudin, C.; Leuraud, K.; Klokov, D.; Bernier, M.O. Ionizing radiation exposure during adulthood and risk of developing central nervous system tumors: Systematic review and meta-analysis. *Sci. Rep.* **2022**, *12*, 16209. [CrossRef]
94. Sengupta, P.; Dutta, S.; Slama, P.; Roychoudhury, S. COVID-19, oxidative stress, and male reproductive dysfunctions: Is vitamin C a potential remedy? *Physiol. Res.* **2022**, *71*, 47–54. [CrossRef] [PubMed]
95. Ng, M.; Hazrati, L.N. Evidence of sex differences in cellular senescence. *Neurobiol. Aging* **2022**, *120*, 88–104. [CrossRef]
96. Kananen, L.; Hurme, M.; Bürkle, A.; Moreno-Villanueva, M.; Bernhardt, J.; Debacq-Chainiaux, F.; Grubeck-Loebenstein, B.; Malavolta, M.; Basso, A.; Piacenza, F.; et al. Circulating cell-free DNA in health and disease-the relationship to health behaviours, ageing phenotypes and metabolomics. *GeroScience* **2023**, *45*, 85–103. [CrossRef]
97. M'Kacher, R.; Bennaceur-Griscelli, A.; Girinsky, T.; Koscielny, S.; Delhommeau, F.; Dossou, J.; Violot, D.; Leclercq, E.; Courtier, M.H.; Beron-Gaillard, N.; et al. Telomere shortening and associated chromosomal instability in peripheral blood lymphocytes of patients with Hodgkin's lymphoma prior to any treatment are predictive of second cancers. *Int. J. Radiat. Oncol. Biol. Phys.* **2007**, *68*, 465–471. [CrossRef]
98. M'Kacher, R.; Girinsky, T.; Koscielny, S.; Dossou, J.; Violot, D.; Beron-Gaillard, N.; Ribrag, V.; Bourhis, J.; Bernheim, A.; Parmentier, C.; et al. Baseline and treatment-induced chromosomal abnormalities in peripheral blood lymphocytes of Hodgkin's lymphoma patients. *Int. J. Radiat. Oncol. Biol. Phys.* **2003**, *57*, 321–326. [CrossRef] [PubMed]
99. Mavragani, I.V.; Nikitaki, Z.; Souli, M.P.; Aziz, A.; Nowsheen, S.; Aziz, K.; Rogakou, E.; Georgakilas, A.G. Complex DNA Damage: A Route to Radiation-Induced Genomic Instability and Carcinogenesis. *Cancers* **2017**, *9*, 91. [CrossRef] [PubMed]
100. Lazutka, J.R.; Neel, J.V.; Major, E.O.; Dedonyte, V.; Mierauskine, J.; Slapsyte, G.; Kesminiene, A. High titers of antibodies to two human polyomaviruses, JCV and BKV, correlate with increased frequency of chromosomal damage in human lymphocytes. *Cancer Lett.* **1996**, *109*, 177–183. [CrossRef] [PubMed]
101. Neel, J.V.; Major, E.O.; Awa, A.A.; Glover, T.; Burgess, A.; Traub, R.; Curfman, B.; Satoh, C. Hypothesis: "Rogue cell"-type chromosomal damage in lymphocytes is associated with infection with the JC human polyoma virus and has implications for oncopenesis. *Proc. Natl. Acad. Sci. USA* **1996**, *93*, 2690–2695. [CrossRef]
102. Neel, J.V. An association, in adult Japanese, between the occurrence of rogue cells among cultured lymphocytes (JC virus activity) and the frequency of "simple" chromosomal damage among the lymphocytes of persons exhibiting these rogue cells. *Am. J. Hum. Genet.* **1998**, *63*, 489–497. [CrossRef] [PubMed]
103. M'Kacher, R.; Andreoletti, L.; Flamant, S.; Milliat, F.; Girinsky, T.; Dossou, J.; Violot, D.; Assaf, E.; Clausse, B.; Koscielny, S.; et al. JC human polyomavirus is associated to chromosomal instability in peripheral blood lymphocytes of Hodgkin's lymphoma patients and poor clinical outcome. *Ann. Oncol. Off. J. Eur. Soc. Med. Oncol.* **2010**, *21*, 826–832. [CrossRef]
104. Testard, I.; Ricoul, M.; Hoffschir, F.; Flury-Herard, A.; Dutrillaux, B.; Fedorenko, B.; Gerasimenko, V.; Sabatier, L. Radiation-induced chromosome damage in astronauts' lymphocytes. *Int. J. Radiat. Biol.* **1996**, *70*, 403–411. [CrossRef]
105. Mustonen, R.; Lindholm, C.; Tawn, E.J.; Sabatier, L.; Salomaa, S. The incidence of cytogenetically abnormal rogue cells in peripheral blood. *Int. J. Radiat. Biol.* **1998**, *74*, 781–785. [CrossRef]
106. Pujol-Canadell, M.; Perrier, J.R.; Cunha, L.; Shuryak, I.; Harken, A.; Garty, G.; Brenner, D.J. Cytogenetically-based biodosimetry after high doses of radiation. *PLoS ONE* **2020**, *15*, e0228350. [CrossRef]
107. Abend, M.; Pfeiffer, R.M.; Port, M.; Hatch, M.; Bogdanova, T.; Tronko, M.D.; Mabuchi, K.; Azizova, T.; Unger, K.; Braselmann, H.; et al. Utility of gene expression studies in relation to radiation exposure and clinical outcomes: Thyroid cancer in the Ukrainian-American cohort and late health effects in a MAYAK worker cohort. *Int. J. Radiat. Biol.* **2021**, *97*, 12–18. [CrossRef]
108. Tichy, A.; Kabacik, S.; O'Brien, G.; Pejchal, J.; Sinkorova, Z.; Kmochova, A.; Sirak, I.; Malkova, A.; Beltran, C.G.; Gonzalez, J.R.; et al. The first in vivo multiparametric comparison of different radiation exposure biomarkers in human blood. *PLoS ONE* **2018**, *13*, e0193412. [CrossRef] [PubMed]
109. Moquet, J.; Higueras, M.; Donovan, E.; Boyle, S.; Barnard, S.; Bricknell, C.; Sun, M.; Gothard, L.; O'Brien, G.; Cruz-Garcia, L.; et al. Dicentric Dose Estimates for Patients Undergoing Radiotherapy in the RTGene Study to Assess Blood Dosimetric Models and the New Bayesian Method for Gradient Exposure. *Radiat. Res.* **2018**, *190*, 596–604. [CrossRef]
110. Cruz-Garcia, L.; O'Brien, G.; Donovan, E.; Gothard, L.; Boyle, S.; Laval, A.; Testard, I.; Ponge, L.; Woźniak, G.; Miszczyk, L.; et al. Influence of Confounding Factors on Radiation Dose Estimation Using In Vivo Validated Transcriptional Biomarkers. *Int. J. Radiat. Biol.* **2018**, *115*, 90–101. [CrossRef] [PubMed]
111. Testa, A.; Palma, V.; Patrono, C. A Novel Biological Dosimetry Assay as a Potential Tool for Triage Dose Assessment in Case of Large-Scale Radiological Emergency. *Radiat. Prot. Dosim.* **2019**, *186*, 9–11. [CrossRef] [PubMed]
112. Testa, A.; Palma, V.; Patrono, C. Dicentric Chromosome Assay (DCA) and Cytokinesis-Block Micronucleus (CBMN) Assay in the Field of Biological Dosimetry. *Methods Mol. Biol. (Clifton N.J.)* **2019**, *2031*, 105–119. [CrossRef]
113. Moquet, J.; Ellender, M.; Boufller, S.; Badie, C.; Baldwin-Cleland, R.; Monahan, K.; Latchford, A.; Lloyd, D.; Clark, S.; Anyamene, N.A.; et al. Transcriptional Dynamics of DNA Damage Responsive Genes in Circulating Leukocytes during Radiotherapy. *Fam. Cancer* **2022**, *14*, 2649. [CrossRef]
114. Cruz-Garcia, L.; Badie, C.; Anbalagan, S.; Moquet, J.; Gothard, L.; O'Brien, G.; Somaiah, N.; Ainsbury, E.A. An ionising radiation-induced specific transcriptional signature of inflammation-associated genes in whole blood from radiotherapy patients: A pilot study. *Radiat. Oncol.* **2021**, *16*, 83. [CrossRef]

115. Abend, M.; Amundson, S.A.; Badie, C.; Brzoska, K.; Hargitai, R.; Kriehuber, R.; Schüle, S.; Kis, E.; Ghandhi, S.A.; Lumniczky, K.; et al. Inter-laboratory comparison of gene expression biodosimetry for protracted radiation exposures as part of the RENEB and EURADOS WG10 2019 exercise. *Cancers* **2021**, *11*, 9756. [CrossRef]
116. Tichy, A.; Ricobonno, D.; Cary, L.H.; Badie, C. Editorial: Recent advances in radiation medical countermeasures. *Front. Pharmacol.* **2022**, *13*, 983702. [CrossRef]

Disclaimer/Publisher's Note: The statements, opinions and data contained in all publications are solely those of the individual author(s) and contributor(s) and not of MDPI and/or the editor(s). MDPI and/or the editor(s) disclaim responsibility for any injury to people or property resulting from any ideas, methods, instructions or products referred to in the content.

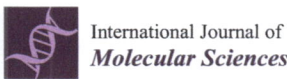

Article

Transcriptome-Based Traits of Radioresistant Sublines of Non-Small Cell Lung Cancer Cells

Margarita Pustovalova [1], Philipp Malakhov [1], Anastasia Guryanova [1], Maxim Sorokin [1,2], Maria Suntsova [2], Anton Buzdin [1,2,3], Andreyan N. Osipov [1,4,5,*] and Sergey Leonov [1,6]

1. School of Biological and Medical Physics, Moscow Institute of Physics and Technology, 141700 Dolgoprudny, Russia
2. World-Class Research Center "Digital Biodesign and Personalized Healthcare", Sechenov First Moscow State Medical University, 119435 Moscow, Russia
3. Shemyakin-Ovchinnikov Institute of Bioorganic Chemistry, 117997 Moscow, Russia
4. State Research Center-Burnasyan Federal Medical Biophysical Center of Federal Medical Biological Agency (SRC-FMBC), 123098 Moscow, Russia
5. N.N. Semenov Research Center of Chemical Physics, Russian Academy of Sciences, 117977 Moscow, Russia
6. Institute of Cell Biophysics, Russian Academy of Sciences, 142290 Pushchino, Russia
* Correspondence: aosipov@fmbcfmba.ru

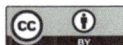

Abstract: Radioresistance is a major obstacle for the successful therapy of many cancers, including non-small cell lung cancer (NSCLC). To elucidate the mechanism of radioresistance of NSCLC cells and to identify key molecules conferring radioresistance, the radioresistant subclones of p53 wild-type A549 and p53-deficient H1299 cell cultures were established. The transcriptional changes between parental and radioresistant NSCLC cells were investigated by RNA-seq. In total, expression levels of 36,596 genes were measured. Changes in the activation of intracellular molecular pathways of cells surviving irradiation relative to parental cells were quantified using the Oncobox bioinformatics platform. Following 30 rounds of 2 Gy irradiation, a total of 322 genes were differentially expressed between p53 wild-type radioresistant A549IR and parental A549 cells. For the p53-deficient (H1299) NSCLC cells, the parental and irradiated populations differed in the expression of 1528 genes and 1616 pathways. The expression of genes associated with radioresistance reflects the complex biological processes involved in clinical cancer cell eradication and might serve as a potential biomarker and therapeutic target for NSCLC treatment.

Keywords: non-small cell lung cancer; DNA repair; radioresistance; ionizing radiation; transcriptomics; gene expression

1. Introduction

Lung cancer is the leading cause of cancer-related deaths worldwide [1], with non-small cell lung cancer (NSCLC) accounting for ~85% of all cases [2]. Radiotherapy is a critical choice in the curative management of patients with inoperable NSCLC; however, the prognosis remains poor due to radioresistance of cancer cells present in heterogeneous tumor populations [3]. Radioresistance is linked to both intrinsic (cancer stem cells, mutational status, epithelial–mesenchymal transition (EMT) process) and extrinsic (hypoxia, tumor microenvironment) mechanisms [4] in which cancer cells accumulate genetic changes allowing them to survive harsh treatment conditions and repopulate. In this case, understanding the changes in gene expression profiles and signal molecular pathways of radioresistant cells is important for the selection of new treatment options and therapeutic schemes for NSCLC patients.

With the development of Next-Generation Sequencing, RNA expression profiles can improve our understanding of the molecular mechanisms responsible for cancer radioresistance. In addition, combining expression data of single gene products with a molecular pathway activation level (PAL) can lead to the development of more robust biomarkers, as shown in both experiment [5,6] and theory [7]. Thus, RNA-seq profiles can be used as potent predictors of tumor radioresistance and might serve as potential biomarkers for therapeutic targets.

We previously generated radioresistant sublines of NSCLC from p53 wild-type A549 and p53-deficient H1299 cells [8,9]. We used Illumina NextSeq 550 to sequence the transcriptomes of parental (A549 and H1299) cells and their radioresistant sublines (A549IR and H1299IR) to expand and improve the data.

Here, we present the changes in gene expression profiles and molecular pathway activation levels of radioresistant NSCLC sublines in relation to their p53 status.

2. Results

2.1. Establishment of the Radioresistant NSCLC Cells

We obtained radioresistant NSCLC sublines using fractionated X-ray irradiation at a total dose of 60 Gy; their survival curves have been previously published [10]. We performed both conventional clonogenic test and the soft agar colony formation assay for assessing cellular radiosensitivity (Figure 1). Both A549IR (wild-type p53) and H1299IR (p53-deficient) cells showed reduced radiosensitivity compared to parental cells growing on a solid surface (Figure 1a). To elucidate further the ability of cells to grow independently of a solid surface, we performed the soft agar colony formation assay (Figure 1b). While A549IR cells showed a statistically significant reduction in radiosensitivity only after exposure to 2 Gy, H1299IR cells showed an overall reduction in radiosensitivity compared to parental H1299 cells (Figure 1b), suggesting their ability to escape from anoikis. Thus, our results demonstrate the overall p53-independent decrease in radiosensitivity of NSCLC cells surviving multifractionated X-ray irradiation.

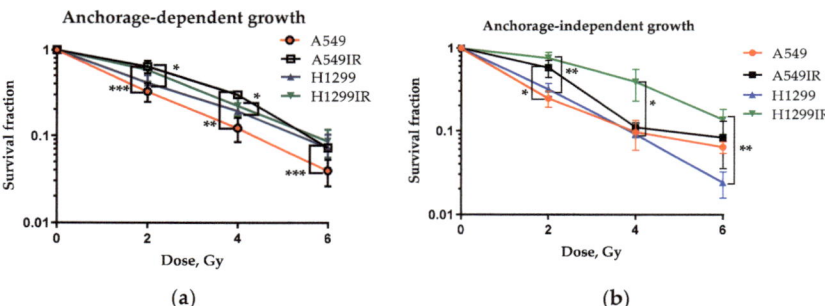

Figure 1. Radiosensitivity of parental and radioresistant NSCLC cells growing in (**a**) anchorage-dependent (solid surface) and in (**b**) anchorage-independent (soft agar) conditions. * $p < 0.05$, ** $p < 0.01$, *** $p < 0.001$. Data are means ± SEM for more than three independent experiments (published previously [10]).

2.2. Differential Gene Expression of NSCLC Cells

To evaluate gene expression changes of radioresistant sublines compared to parental ones, we performed RNA sequencing using the Illumina Nextseq 550 System. The results demonstrated differential expression of 322 genes ($\log10(\text{control}) > 1$, $|\log2FC| > 1$) in p53 wild-type radioresistant compared to parental A549 cells. Among them, 164 genes were up-regulated, while 158 genes were down-regulated (Supplementary Table S1). In p53-deficient NSCLC cells, 1628 genes were expressed differentially ($\log10(\text{control}) > 1$, $|\log2FC| > 1$) in radioresistant vs. parental cells: 808 genes were up-regulated, while 820 genes were down-regulated (Supplementary Table S1). Radioresistant sublines demonstrated seven common up-regulated genes (*ATRNL1, CA2, CNR1, FAM189A1, GFRA1, RASGRP1, RGL3*); however, no statistically significant enrichment was found (Figure 2a). The nine down-regulated genes that were common between A549IR and H1299IR cells included *ADGRF1, EPHA7, LOX, LY6G5C, NSUN7, SLC22A31, SNAI2, TNFRSF11B* and *ZNF233* ($p = 0.0105$) (Figure 2b).

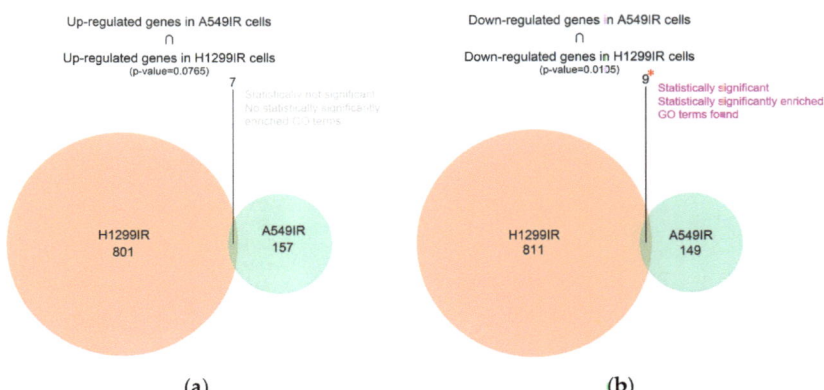

Figure 2. Differential gene intersection showing: (**a**) up-regulated genes in A549IR cells ∩ H1299IR cells; (**b**) down-regulated genes in A549IR cells ∩ H1299IR cells. Red asterisk indicate statistical significance * $p < 0.05$.

Within the obtained gene sets, Gene Ontology (GO)-based functional analysis provides statistically enriched GO terms that show gene relationships according to three ontology categories and described gene products. These categories are biological process, molecular function and cellular component [11]. We then identified significantly enriched GO terms and characterized radioresistant vs. parental A549 and H1299 cells. In total, enriched GO terms were found in 80 subcategories under biological process, three subcategories under cellular component, and seven subcategories under molecular function. In biological process ontology, the results indicated that desmosome organization, regulation of vitamin D biosynthesis and metabolic process, negative regulation of DNA damage response and signal transduction by p53 class mediator, negative regulation of anoikis, apoptosis, regulation of cell adhesion mediated by integrin and regulation of cell morphogenesis were mainly associated with radioresistant A549IR and H1299IR cells. Significant GO enrichment profiles in the biological process (BP) (only the first 30 out of 80 BPs p-value less than 0.01) are summarized in Table 1. Enriched GO molecular function terms in radioresistant A549IR and H1299IR cells were oxidoreductase activity, transmembrane-ephrin receptor activity, chemorepellent activity and E-box binding. Through GO analysis, we found that overrepresented GO terms in our radioresponsive gene sets were closely linked to such cellular components as hippocampal mossy fiber to CA3 synapse, integral and intrinsic components of postsynaptic density membrane.

Table 1. Differential genes intersection for biological process ontology for common down-regulated genes in A549IR cells ∩ H1299IR cells.

ID	Description	p-Value Adjusted	Genes
GO:0002934	desmosome organization	0.019522	SNAI2
GO:0030656	regulation of vitamin metabolic process	0.019522	SNAI2
GO:0042368	vitamin D biosynthetic process	0.019522	SNAI2
GO:0048251	elastic fiber assembly	0.019522	LOX
GO:0048755	branching morphogenesis of a nerve	0.019522	EPHA7
GO:0070561	vitamin D receptor signaling pathway	0.019522	SNAI2
GO:0072178	nephric duct morphogenesis	0.019522	EPHA7
GO:1905809	negative regulation of synapse organization	0.019522	EPHA7

Table 1. *Cont.*

ID	Description	p-Value Adjusted	Genes
GO:0061314	Notch signaling involved in heart development	0.019522	SNAI2
GO:0033629	negative regulation of cell adhesion mediated by integrin	0.019522	SNAI2
GO:0042362	fat-soluble vitamin biosynthetic process	0.019522	SNAI2
GO:0072176	nephric duct development	0.019522	EPHA7
GO:0018158	protein oxidation	0.019522	LOX
GO:0035791	platelet-derived growth factor receptor-beta signaling pathway	0.019522	LOX
GO:0010839	negative regulation of keratinocyte proliferation	0.019522	SNAI2
GO:0042481	regulation of odontogenesis	0.019522	TNFRSF11B
GO:0043518	negative regulation of DNA damage response, signal transduction by p53 class mediator	0.019522	SNAI2
GO:0003198	epithelial to mesenchymal transition involved in endocardial cushion formation	0.019522	SNAI2
GO:0045779	negative regulation of bone resorption	0.019522	TNFRSF11B
GO:0048670	regulation of collateral sprouting	0.019522	EPHA7
GO:2000811	negative regulation of anoikis	0.019522	SNAI2
GO:0032026	response to magnesium ion	0.019522	TNFRSF11B
GO:0046851	negative regulation of bone remodeling	0.019522	TNFRSF11B
GO:0060973	cell migration involved in heart development	0.019522	SNAI2
GO:0009110	vitamin biosynthetic process	0.019522	SNAI2
GO:0031290	retinal ganglion cell axon guidance	0.019522	EPHA7
GO:0032793	positive regulation of CREB transcription factor activity	0.019522	ADGRF1
GO:0034104	negative regulation of tissue remodeling	0.019522	TNFRSF11B
GO:0046716	muscle cell cellular homeostasis	0.019522	LOX
GO:0150146	cell junction disassembly	0.019522	SNAI2

2.3. Radiation-Induced Transcriptome Alteration in Radioresistant NSCLC Cells through Pathway Activation Level (PAL) Analysis

Pathway Activation Level (PAL) is an integral parameter, which serves as an accurate qualitative measure of pathway activation [12]. The PAL analysis was performed for functional analysis of our radioresponsive gene sets acquired from the RNA-seq of radioresistant sublines relative to their parental cells using data from Reactome [13], NCI Pathway Interaction [14], Biocarta, KEGG Adjusted, Metabolism and Primary databases. As a result, we found 420 differential pathways (Benjamini Hochberg adjusted p-value < 0.05) between radioresistant A549IR and parental A549 cells. A total of 230 pathways were up-regulated in radioresistant A549IR cells (PAL > 0) and 190 pathways were down-regulated in A549IR cells (PAL < 0). Here, we present the top 10 up-regulated and down-regulated pathways associated with the radioresistance-related transcriptome alteration in A549IR sublines (p-value less than 0.05) (Figure 3a,b). Based on the results of the PAL analysis, we first identified demannosylation ("Progressive trimming of alpha-1,2-linked mannose residues from Man9/8/7GlcNAc2 to produce Man5GlcNAc2"), interleukin 12 biosynthesis, c-Kit pathways and BCR signaling, proposing metabolical, immunological/inflammatory responses, cell migration and actin filament polymerization as pathways that could be meaningfully associated with radiation tolerance of A549IR cells. Among the top 10 down-regulated pathways with lowest PAL-score, Anthrax toxin pathways involving apoptosis, inflammatory responses, necrosis, negative regulation of macrophage activation and phagocytosis were involved in A549IR radioresistance (Figure 3a).

We found 1616 differential pathways (Benjamini Hochberg adjusted p-value < 0.05) between radioresistant and parental H1299 cells: 917 pathways were up-regulated (PAL > 0), while 699 pathways were down-regulated (PAL < 0) (Figure 3). The most significantly up-regulated pathways (p-value less than 0.001) associated with H1299IR radioresistance are shown in Figure 3b. Significant up-regulation of T cell proliferation and differentiation points to a link between immunological responses and radiation tolerance in H1299IR cells. In addition, the high-scoring functions in the pathways were the insulin-like growth factor 1 receptor (IGF1R) and the diabetes mellitus pathway with subsequent inhibition of the PI3K/Akt pathway involved in glucose import (Figure 3b). The latter was among the top 10 scoring down-regulated pathways considerably involved in H1299IR radioresistance.

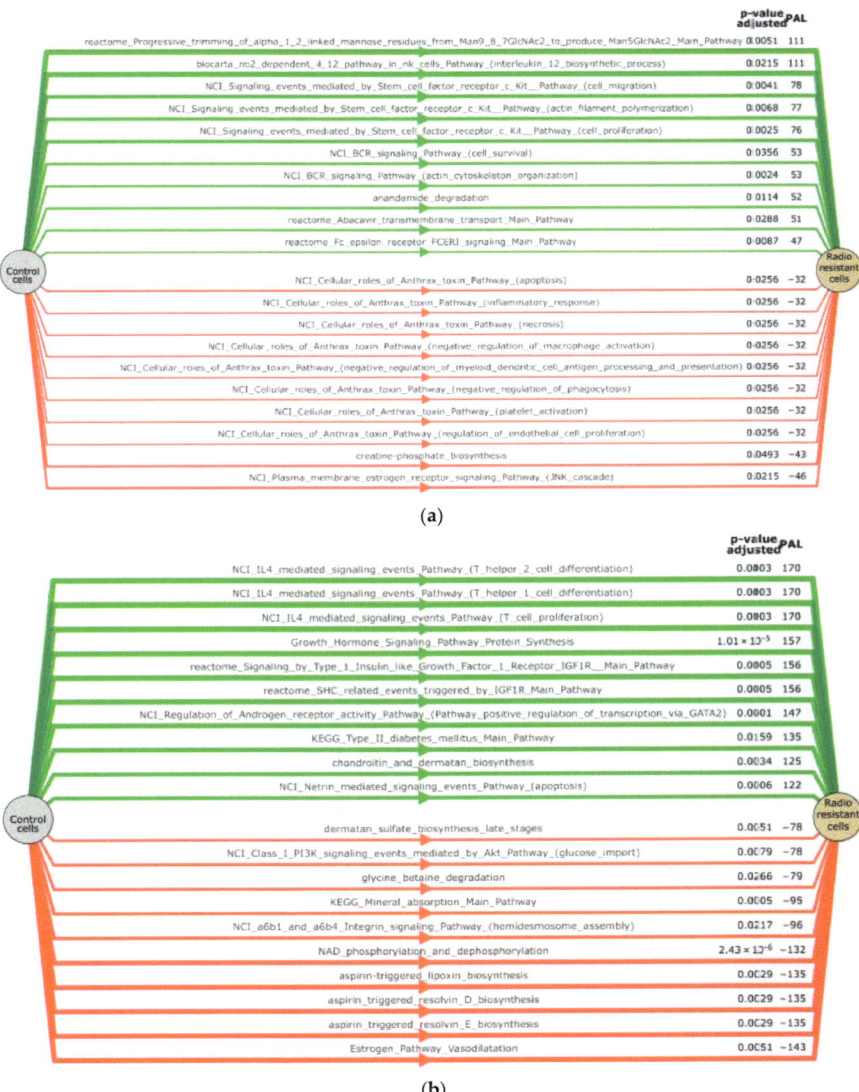

Figure 3. PAL chart of A549 and H1299 cells: (**a**) Top 10 up- and down-regulated pathways in A549IR and (**b**) H1299IR cells, Benjamini Hochberg adjusted p-value < 0.05 (only pathways containing 10 and more genes).

The overlap between A549IR and H1299IR up-regulated and down-regulated pathways contained 142 common differential molecular pathways (Supplementary Table S2).

Eighty-two pathways were activated and 59 were inhibited. This suggests non-random overlap between the differential pathways in both comparisons, $p < 0.05$ (Figure 4).

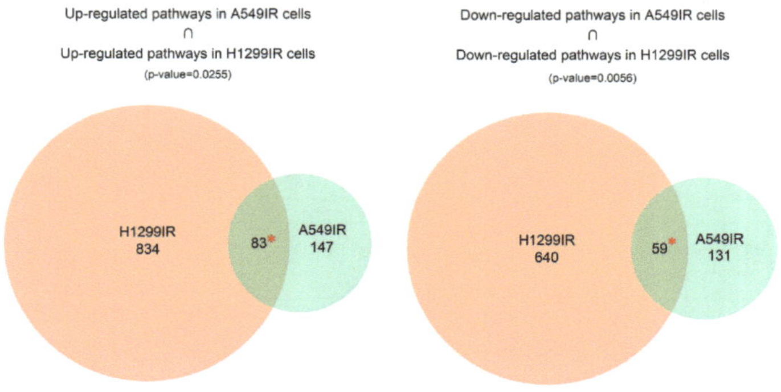

Figure 4. Overlap between differentially regulated molecular pathways between A549IR and H1299IR cells. Overlap of significantly (**a**) up-regulated (PAL > 0) and (**b**) down-regulated (PAL < 0) molecular pathways between A549IR and H1299IR cells are shown; * denotes significance at $p < 0.05$ for the overlaps obtained in perturbation.

2.4. Differential Pathway Changes in NSCLC Cells

A main factor related to radioresistance is the presence of cancer stem cells (CSC) inside tumors, which are responsible for metastases, relapses, radiation therapy failure, and a poor prognosis in cancer patients. The Wnt signaling is one of the key cascades regulating maintenance of CSCs, metastasis and immune control of many cancers including NSCLC [15]. We further analyzed the expression of key signaling pathways involved in cancer radioresistance, including Wnt, p53, Hippo, NF-kB, Akt, FOXO, etc. (22 pathways in total) (Figure 5). Heatmap analysis revealed slight up-regulation of beta1 integrin (Alpha9 beta1 integrin signaling events), Wnt (Wnt ligand biogenesis and trafficking, WNT5A-dependent internalization of FZD4) and NF-κB signaling for both A549IR and H1299IR cells (Figure 5, red rectangle). Among pathways of interest, p53, HSF, Cyclin D1, and FOXO almost did not show any change in radioresistant cells over their parental cell lines.

Interestingly, H1299IR cells demonstrated a significant increase in Wnt signaling over parental level, compared to A549IR subline. "NCI Wnt signaling network Main Pathway" and "NCI FOXA2 and FOXA3 transcription factor networks Main Pathway" were almost 50-fold up-regulated in H1299IR over parental cells, suggesting their role in radioresistance of p53-deficient NSCLC. The level of the main Wnt signaling pathway and Wnt target genes, as well as the "Regulation of HSF1-mediated heat shock response", "Regulation of retinoblastoma protein" and "FOXM1 transcription factor network", were significantly up-regulated in H1299IR compared to A549IR cells (Figure 5), suggesting the role of genotype in radioresistance-associated pathway profiles. In contrast, the down-regulation of "Inactivation of Gsk-3 by Akt Causes Accumulation of B-Catenin in Alveolar Macrophages", "KEGG Hippo signaling pathway" and "Akt phosphorylates targets in the cytosol" were more significantly down-regulated pathways in H1299IR than in A549IR subline.

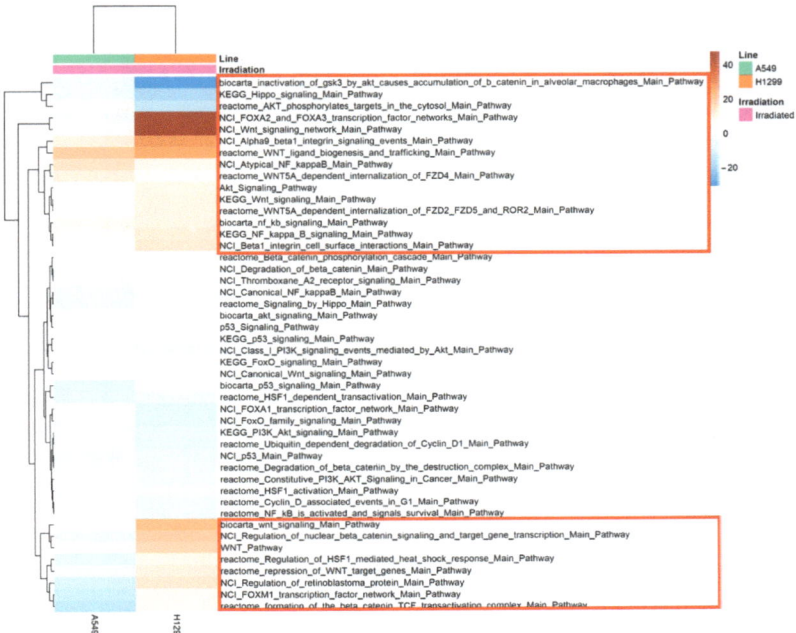

Figure 5. Heat map of RNA-Seq transcriptome analysis for 22 selected pathways in A549IR and H1299IR cells. The most significant differences between H1299IR and A549IR sublines are highlighted in red. Benjamini Hochberg adjusted p-value < 0.05.

2.5. Charachteristics of Senescence-Associated Radioresistance in NSCLC Cells

It is becoming increasingly clear that acute and chronic senescence are characterized by distinct senescence-associated secretory phenotype (SASP) factors involved in tumor progression. A positive correlation between radioresistance and early induction of head-and-neck squamous cell carcinoma (HNSCC) cell senescence accompanied by NF-κB-dependent production of distinct senescence-associated cytokines was identified by Schoetz et al. [16]. Hence, despite the subtle up-regulation of NF-κB signalling (Figure 5), we attempted to further elucidate the transcription of NF-κB-regulated genes encoding key secretory proteins of SASP. Based on the Chien analysis [17] of 263 genes involved in H-RasV12-induced senescence in IMR-90 normal lung fibroblasts, a well-characterized system of cellular senescence, we analyzed changes in the expression of select NF-κB-regulated genes that encode secretory proteins in our radioresistant sublines. In total, we analyzed the expression of 13 genes (Table 2). Only H1299IR showed significant up-regulation of *CXCL8*, a gene coding IL8, a ligand for the chemokine receptor *CXCR2*, and *TGFB2*, the gene encoding a secreted ligand of the TGF-β (transforming growth factor-beta) superfamily of proteins. Both A549IR and H1299IR sublines demonstrated significant increase in the expression of *IL6*.

Table 2. Differential gene expression of NF-κB-regulated secretory proteins in A549IR and H1299IR cells (statistically significantly up-regulated genes shown in green, down-regulated genes shown in red).

Genes	A549IR LFC	A549IR p-Value	H1299IR LFC	H1299IR p-Value
CCL20	−1.325	0.246	−0.085	0.791
CCL3	0.079	0.810	−0.085	0.791
CXCL1	0.043	0.895	0.739	0.134
CXCL2	−0.448	0.348	−0.037	0.917

Table 2. Cont.

Genes	A549IR LFC	A549IR p-Value	H1299IR LFC	H1299IR p-Value
CXCL3	−0.247	0.348	0.054	0.924
CXCL5	0.513	0.119	−0.085	0.791
CXCL8	−0.299	0.424	3.544	0.000
FGF2	−0.066	0.760	−0.194	0.560
IL1A	0.773	0.354	−0.085	0.791
IL1B	0.299	0.582	0.283	0.738
IL6	1.494	0.006	1.500	0.004
NRG1	−0.322	0.212	−2.212	0.009
TGFB2	−0.037	0.863	1.579	0.003

However, the expression of *IL6* alone was not accompanied by the increase in the proportion of SA-β-Gal positive cells in A549IR vs. A549 (Figure 6). In contrast, H1299IR cells had a significantly higher (**** $p < 0.001$) fraction of SA-β-Gal positive cells compared to the parental subline. Collectively, our findings emphasize the emerging role of secreted factors (IL8, IL6, TGF-β and Neuregulin 1) in regulating senescence through paracrine and/or autocrine mechanisms conferring radioresistance in NSCLC cell lines.

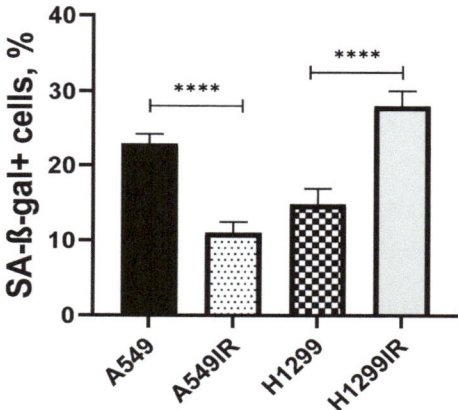

Figure 6. Changes in the proportion of SA-β-Gal positive cells in A549IR and H1299IR. Data are means ± SEM for more than three independent experiments. **** $p < 0.0001$.

3. Discussion

The present study used whole-genome expression profiles to characterize the radioresistance of A549IR and H1299IR NSCLC cells. The integrative analysis of the expression RNA profiles revealed deregulated biological processes or pathways that may serve as predictors of radiosensitivity and future prospective therapeutic targets. To investigate the gene expression profiles and molecular pathway activation levels, two NSCLC radioresistant sublines (A549IR and H1299IR) with different p53 status were established by fractionated irradiation in a total dose of 60 Gy. We previously reported the activation of pro-survival signaling DNA repair pathways in A549IR and H1299IR cells, including G2/M cell cycle progression, BRCA1 pathway, ATR and DNA double-strand breaks repair by homologous recombination and non-homologous end joining [10]. The key molecular and cellular characteristics of radioresistant cells, including DNA repair, proliferation, epithelial-to-mesenchymal transition, etc., were confirmed and characterized in our previous studies [8,9,18,19].

Recent studies using transcriptomic analysis suggested the role of lncRNAs, such as H19 [20], circRNAs, such as ZNF208 [21], whole-genome miRNA and mRNA [22] in determining NSCLC radioresistance. This demonstrates that transcriptomics is a valuable readout for evaluating outcomes in NSCLC patients undergoing radiotherapy [23]. Here, we interrogated the gene expression profiles obtained by sequencing of total RNA isolated from parental (A549 and H1299) and radioresistant (A549IR and H1299IR) NSCLC cells differing in their p53 status.

We observed up-regulation of 164 and 808 genes in radioresistant A549IR and H1299IR cells, respectively. Aiming to identify potent common biomarkers of NSCLC radioresistance, we observed seven common up-regulated genes (*ATRNL1, CA2, CNR1, FAM189A1, GFRA1, RASGRP1, RGL3*) and nine common down-regulated genes (*ADGRF1, EPHA7, LOX, LY6G5C, NSUN7, SLC22A31, SNAI2, TNFRSF11B* and *ZNF233*) between the two cell lines. Among them, several up-regulated genes are known to be involved in the formation of tumor microenvironments (Carbonic anhydrase 2 (*CA2*)) [24,25], cancer chemoresistance (Cannabinoid receptor 1 (*CNR1*) [26], *GFRA1* [27]) and cancer recurrence after therapy (*RGL3*) [27,28]. Interestingly, some of the common down-regulated genes, such as *EPHA7* and *NSUN7*, are known for both their tumor suppressing and promoting roles, or are associated with overall survival (OS) (*SLC22A31*) [29–32], while others have clear pro-tumorigenic roles (*ADGRF1, LOX, LY6G5C, SNAI2, TNFRSF11B, ZNF233*) [30,33–36]. This may suggest a differential role of many potent pro-tumorigenic genes in cancer aggressiveness and in sustaining radioresistant phenotypes of NSCLC cells during normal culture conditions. However, this notion warrants further investigation and the role of each up-regulated and down-regulated gene in NSCLC radioresistance must be confirmed individually.

High-throughput gene expression data allows calculating pathway activity levels (PAL) associated with cancer radioresistance. In A549IR cells, one of the most activated pathways included progressive trimming of alpha-1,2-linked mannose residues from Man9/8/7GlcNAc2 to produce Man5GlcNAc2 (Figure 4a). N-glycan demannosylation is a highly conserved mechanism allowing cells to avoid protein misfolding and subsequent functional deficiency and cellular toxicity [37]. This process occurs in the Golgi apparatus and forces irreparable misfolded glycoproteins into the Endoplasmic Reticulum-Associated Degradation (ERAD) pathway, where they can be destroyed [38]. Our results demonstrate for the first time the association of the Man-trimming pathway with NSCLC radioresistance.

Surprisingly, we observed the NO2-dependent IL-12 Pathway in NK cells (Figure 4a) as the second most activated pathway in A549IR cells. The IL-12 is a cytokine that activates the large granular lymphocytes or natural killer cells (NK) and is considered a strong candidate for immunotherapy-based tumor cell killing [39]. At the same time, Single Nucleotide Polymorphisms (SNPs) in the IL-12 gene have been associated with the risk of NSCLC [40,41] and breast cancer [42].

The overall effect of senescence on cancer progression and cancer cell resistance to X-ray radiation is still not fully understood and remains controversial. Senescence is a state where cells neither function normally nor die. Cells that are damaged or old may enter this suspended state. In this state, they do not reproduce, but are able to communicate with the tumor microenvironment (TME) through senescence-associated secretory phenotype (SASP) in a paracrine fashion [43]. Albeit stress-induced senescence is generally considered to be a tumor-suppressive mechanism [44], long-term treatment-induced senescence of cells may be harmful. Long-term induction of senescence will produce TME that promotes inflammation and immunosuppression [45]. Hence, induction of cancer cell senescence as a recently suggested new therapeutic strategy against cancer [46–49] should be context-dependent and evaluated carefully based on the cancer stage. Additionally, it seems to be possible to develop new therapeutic strategies to combine priming (immunization) with IR-induced senescent patient-derived cancer cells with IR treatments. In this regard, our study provides new add-in transcriptomic information about activation of SASP-related genes and signaling pathways in response to certain IR stress-inducing insults of different duration.

Interleukins as secretory proteins are involved in SASP-related radioresistance [50]. Previously reported positive correlation between radioresistance of human HNSCC cell senescence accompanied by NF-κB-dependent production of distinct senescence-associated cytokines [16], together with the up-regulation of NF-κB signaling observed in our study, allowed us to assume their potent role in NSCLC radioresistance. The results of the differential gene expression analysis of NF-κB-regulated secretory proteins revealed the association of *CXCL8*, *IL6* and *TGFB2* up-regulation and *NRG1* down-regulation with the increase in the proportion of SA-β-Gal positive cells in H1299IR subline (Table 2). Notably, *CXCR2/IL8* activation is associated with both NSCLC lymph node metastasis and unfavorable prognosis for patients with NSCLC [51]. TGF-β1 causes a switch from cohesive to single cell motility and intravasation that are essential for blood-borne metastasis in breast cancer [52]. It also mediated neutrophil recruitment that drives NOTCH1 signaling-mediated metastasis in colorectal cancer [53]. In H1299IR cells, *NRG1*, Neuregulin 1 coding gene, was significantly down-regulated (Table 2). Importantly, *MUC1* and NRG1 are controlled by the Eukaryotic Translation Initiation Factor 4 Gamma 1 (EIF4G1) for NSCLC survival and tumorigenesis with clinical relevance [54], while *NRG1* is the major tumor suppressor gene postulated to be on 8p: it is in the correct location, is antiproliferative and is silenced in many breast cancers [55]. Last, but not least, the up-regulation of *IL6* alone seemed to be insufficient to induce senescence, as can be seen by the low SA-β-Gal-positive fraction of A549IR cell subline (Figure 6). Our findings suggest that the CXCR2/ligand-axis activation can be pivotal in driving radiotherapy-induced senescence in NSCLC.

Among other pathways involved in cell migration, proliferation and survival, we observed the up-regulation of anandamide degradation pathways in the A549IR subline. Anandamide is an endocannabinoid, part of a family of biologically active lipids that bind to and activate cannabinoid receptors and play a role in biological activities of both the central and periphery nervous systems [56,57]. Anandamide can be transported into the cell where it is metabolized by cyclooxygenase 2 (COX-2) to prostaglandin-ethanolamines (PG-EAs) [58]. The PGs, for example PGE2, are likely to mediate some of the tumour-promoting effects of COX-2, such as immune response, angiogenesis and cell proliferation [59,60]. An IR-induced increase in *COX-2* expression was previously observed in radioresistant A549 cells [61]. Moreover, targeting COX-2 inhibited malignant proliferation of A549 cells in vivo and in vitro [62]. Thus, our results support previously published data on anandamide degradation pathways in radioresistance.

Most of the down-regulated pathways in A549IR cells contained the Anthrax toxin (Figure 4a). Tumor endothelial marker 8 (TEM8), also known as anthrax toxin receptor 1 (ANTXR1), is highly expressed in cancers. Its expression level was associated with tumor size, primary tumor stage and a poor prognosis in patients with lung adenocarcinoma [63]. The ANTXR1 is expressed on metastatic breast cancer stem cells (CSCs) and functions in collagen signaling, as well as Wnt signaling, ZEB1 expression, and CSC self-renewal, invasion, tumorigenicity, and metastasis [64]. The ANTXR1 was identified as a functional biomarker of triple-negative breast CSCs, and pancreatic ductal adenocarcinoma (PDAC) patients stratified based on the ANTXR1 expression level showed increased mortality and enrichment of pathways known to be necessary for CSC biology, including TGF-β, NOTCH, Wnt/β-catenin, and IL-6/JAK/STAT3 signaling and epithelial to mesenchymal transition, suggesting that ANTXR1 may represent a putative CSC marker [65]. However, based on our data, the ANTXR1 pathway does not play a role in NSCLC radioresistance.

In H1299IR cells, radioresistance was associated with deregulation of metabolism including PI3K/Akt signaling pathway involved in the development of obesity and type 2 diabetes mellitus (DM) [66]. The DM has been shown to be associated with NSCLC progression, suggesting that pre-existing diabetes is an independent prognostic factor for overall survival (OS) among patients with both diabetes and lung squamous cell lung carcinoma who receive standard treatments [67–69]. Women with lung cancer and diabetes had significantly increased risk of overall mortality (HR = 1.27, 95% CI: 1.07–1.50) compared to those without diabetes [70]. However, it is still unclear whether the DM is a risk factor for developing NSCLC or vice versa. Here we demonstrate significant up-regulation of Type 2 diabetes mellitus pathways in H1299IR cells through overexpression of IGF-1R and down-regulation of the PI3K/Akt signaling pathway (Figure 3b). The IGF-1R may activate two major signaling pathways, the PI3K/Akt and MAPK pathways [71]. The activated form of Akt, phosphorylated Akt (p-Akt), may inhibit several proapoptotic factors including glycogen synthase kinase-3 beta (GSK3β) [72], which in turn mediates insulin resistance and human type 2 diabetes [73]. Thus, it is tempting to speculate that up-regulation of DM pathways in H1299IR cells serve as a prognostic biomarker of DM in patients with NSCLC, suggesting that pre-existing NSCLC is a potent inducer of DM leading to a worse prognosis. However, this notion warrants further investigation.

Unlike A549IR, H1299IR cells demonstrated significant up-regulation of the IL-4 signaling pathway (Figure 3b). The IL-4 plays a role in T cell activation, differentiation, proliferation, and survival [74] and, together with its receptor complex (IL4R), has been studied for their role in epithelial cancer progression, including enhanced migration, invasion, survival, and proliferation [75]. Recently, T cell marker genes were proposed as novel prognostic signatures for lung squamous cell carcinoma (LUSC) patients [76].

We observed significant 50-fold up-regulation of Wnt signaling in H1299IR cells. Wnt proteins are secreted glyco-lipoproteins that participate in cell fate determination, proliferation and the control of asymmetric cell division during lung development [77]. It has been suggested that Wnt signaling is also involved in the regulation of cancer stem cells [78] and thus, plays an important role in lung carcinogenesis [79]. The major (canonical) Wnt pathway signals through β-catenin [80]. In the absence of Wnt, β-catenin undergoes proteolytic degradation by β-catenin destruction complex consisting of axis inhibition protein (AX-IN), adenomatous polyposis coli (APC), and glycogen synthase kinase 3 beta (GSK3β) phosphorylates β-catenin [78]. In the presence of Wnt, cytoplasmic levels of β-catenin rise and it migrates to the nucleus where it activates the expression of various target genes, including cyclin D1 [81], c-Myc [82] and survivin [83].

To elucidate whether Wnt pathway contributes to radioresistance in NSCLC, we further evaluated the Wnt pathway activation. We observed significant up-regulation of canonical (Wnt/β-catenin) pathway in radioresistant H1299IR cells, but not in A549IR cells (Figure 5). Moreover, this process was accompanied by down-regulation of inactivation of GSK3 by Akt, which can cause accumulation of β-catenin in alveolar macrophages pathway. A GSK3β inactivation influences β-catenin, leading to increases in cell motility and migration. The phosphorylation of GSK3β by Akt results in its inactivation. The down-regulation of this process leads to the presence of activated, non-phosphorylated GSK3β, which in turn can phosphorylate β-catenin at Ser33/37. This results in the proteasomal degradation of β-catenin. In colon cancer cells with hyperactivated canonical Wnt signaling, pharmacological inhibition of the PI3K-Akt signaling leads to a nuclear accumulation of β-catenin and FOXO3a, and subsequently increased cell scattering and metastasis [84]. The FOXA2 and FOXA3 transcription factor networks were also up-regulated in H1299IR cells (Figure 5). In A549IR cells, down-regulation of the Wnt signaling pathway might be associated with upregulation of the *MCC* gene which can suppress cell proliferation and the Wnt/β-catenin pathway in colorectal cancer cells (Supplementary Table S1) [85].

The genes and signaling pathways identified in this study provide new important insights into the mechanisms underlying radioresistance in NSCLC cells. The observed whole genome expression profiles can be linked to molecular and cellular characteristics of radioresistant cells, including decreased radiosensitivity, resistance to cell death, enhanced cell proliferation and migration, and raise interest as potential biomarkers and therapeutic targets for NSCLC treatment.

4. Materials and Methods
4.1. Cell Cultures and Irradiation

The A549 (p53 wild-type) and H1299 (p53-deficient cells) cell cultures and their isogenic radioresistant sublines A549IR and H1299IR were cultured in RPMI-1640 medium (Gibco, Thermo Fisher Scientific, Waltham, MA, USA) containing 10% fetal bovine serum (Gibco, Thermo Fisher Scientific, Waltham, MA, USA) supplemented with L-glutamine and antibiotics under standard conditions (37 °C, 5% CO_2).

The radioresistant sublines were established after 30 fractions of 2 Gy X-ray exposure using 200 kV X-ray RUB RUST-M1 X-irradiator facility (0.85 Gy/min, 2 × 5 mA, 1.5 mm Al filter, JSC "Ruselectronics", Moscow, Russia). Cells were irradiated five days a week at room temperature. After reaching a total dose of 60 Gy, cells were cultured at 37 °C in a humidified atmosphere with 5% CO_2 for up to 3 weeks to recover. The radioresistence was previously confirmed using clonogenic assay [19].

4.2. Clonogenic Test and Soft Agar Colony Formation

The A549, A549IR, H1299, and H1299IR cells were subjected to single X-ray irradiation at doses of 2 Gy, 4 Gy, and 6 Gy, removed from the plastic surface immediately after irradiation, and plated on Petri dishes 60 mm in diameter in the amount of 150, 500, 1000, and 2000 cells/well, respectively. Petri dishes were incubated at 37 °C in a humid atmosphere with 5% CO_2 for two weeks to form colonies. After that, the cells were fixed with 100% methanol for 15 min at room temperature, followed by Giemsa staining for 15 min. Only colonies containing more than 50 cells were counted. Seeding efficiency (PE) and survival rate (SF) were calculated using the following equations:

$$PE = \text{number of colonies formed/number of cells seeded} \times 100\% \quad (1)$$

$$SF = \text{number of colonies formed/(number of cells seeded} \times PE) \quad (2)$$

The ancorage-independent soft agar colony formation assay was performed according to the procedure described Borowicz et al. [86]. Exponentially growing A549, A549IR, H1299, and H1299IR cells were X-rayed at doses of 0 Gy, 2 Gy, 4 Gy, and 6 Gy. Collected by trypsin treatment, cells were mixed with 0.6% purified agar. Cell/agar mixtures were added to 6 well plates pre-coated with 1.0% purified agar in complete medium (1.5 mL agar per well) and allowed to solidify for 30 min at room temperature before being placed in a humidified cell culture incubator at 37 °C. Twice a week, 100 μL of culture medium was added to the wells to prevent the agar from desiccation. After colonies formed (~21 days), they were stained with 0.05% crystal violet and counted manually.

4.3. Transcriptomic Analysis

The gene expression level was evaluated by RNA-seq analyses of three biological replicates of each cell line. The InnuPREP RNA Mini Kit 2.0 together with innuPREP DNase I Digest (Analytik Jena, Berlin, Germany) were used to isolate total RNA. To measure RNA concentration, we used the Qubit 4 Fluorometer with Qubit RNA Assay kit. The RNA integrity number (RIN) was measured by TapeStation with RNA ScreenTape reagents (Agilent, Santa Clara, CA, USA). For depletion of ribosomal RNA and library construction, the KAPA RNA HyperPrep Kit with the RiboErase (HMR) kit were used. The KAPA UDI Primer Mixes were used for sample barcoding to allow their multiplexing in a single sequencing run. Library concentrations were measured using the Qubit 4 Fluorometer with the Qubit dsDNA HS Assay kit (Life Technologies, Waltham, MA, USA) and TapeStation with High Sensitivity D1000 reagents (Agilent). The RNA sequencing was performed on the Illumina Nextseq 550 System with reagents for single-end sequencing and read length of 75 bp.

4.4. Bioinformatics Analysis

FASTQ read files were analyzed using the STAR software [87] in "GeneCounts" mode using transcriptome annotation from Ensembl (GRCh38 genome assembly and GRCh38.89 transcriptome annotation). In total, expression levels of 36,596 genes were measured. The data was normalized using DESeq2 [88].

Changes in the activation of intracellular molecular pathways of IR-survived cells compared to parental cells were quantified using the Oncobox bioinformatics platform [89]. A total of 38 molecular pathways associated with DNA repair were used for analysis [90].

Pathway activation level (PAL) for each molecular pathway was calculated using the formula:

$$\text{PAL}_p = \sum_n ARR_{np} \times \ln CNR_n \div \sum_n |ARR_n|, \qquad (3)$$

where PAL_p is the level of activation of the molecular pathway p; CNR_n (case-to-normal ratio)—the ratio of gene n expression level in a tumor sample under study to an average level for the control group; 'ln' is the natural logarithm; the discrete ARR_{np} value (role of activator/repressor) of gene n product in the p pathway is determined as follows: ARR_{np} is -1 if gene product n inhibits pathway p; 1 if n activates pathway p; 0 if n has ambiguous or unclear role in a pathway p; 0.5 or -0.5 if n is rather an activator of a pathway or its inhibitor, respectively.

4.5. Gene Ontology (GO) Analysis

The GO analysis is a commonly applied method for functional studies of large-scale genomic or transcriptomic data [11]. Function enrichGO from the clusterProfiler package was used to identify significantly enriched GO terms among the given list of genes that are differentially expressed in radioresistant and parental cells [PMID: 22455463]. Statistically overrepresented GO categories with p-value < 0.05 were considered significant.

4.6. Analysis of Senescence-Associated β-Galactosidase (SA-β-Gal) Positive Cells

The "Cellular Senescence Assay" commercial kit (EMD Millipore, Burlington, MA, USA, Catalog Number: KAA002) was used for quantification of senescence-associated β-galactosidase (SA-β-Gal) positive cells. The cells were stained according to the manufacturer's protocol. The stained cells were visualized using EVOS® FL Auto Imaging System (Fisher Scientific, Pittsburgh, PA, USA) with 20× objective. The proportion of SA-β-Gal positive cells was calculated manually.

4.7. Statistics

Statistics were performed using GraphPad Prism 9.0.2.161 software (GraphPad Software, San Diego, CA, USA). Statistical significance was tested using the Student t-test. The results are represented as means ± SEM of more than three independent experiments. Significance levels were denoted by asterisks: * $p < 0.05$, ** $p < 0.01$, *** $p < 0.001$, **** $p < 0.0001$.

5. Conclusions

For the first time, we investigated the transcriptome profile of radioresistant NSCLC sublines of A549 and H1299 cells through RNA-seq and bioinformatic functional analysis. Our research with this new methodological approach may provide a useful guideline for the experimental design of gene expression studies and for exploring novel routes to uncover the complete regulatory network involved in radioresistance. In the present study, we used only two radioresistant NSCLC cell sublines derived from parental A549 and H1299 cells. However, it will be worth investigating the differences of the same set of differentially expressed genes in other tumor cell lines and primary cells isolated from lung tumor tissue. Some of the identified novel targets could be potentially interesting in further studies for sensitization of tumor cells to improve radiation effects. Our research could help to interpret the complicated molecular mechanisms leading to radioresistance. Furthermore, it might contribute to the identification of other target genes for predictive biomarkers, improving radiotherapy.

Supplementary Materials: The following supporting information can be downloaded at: https://www.mdpi.com/article/10.3390/ijms24033042/s1.

Author Contributions: Conceptualization, M.P., S.L. and A.N.O.; software, M.S. (Maxim Sorokin); formal analysis, M.S. (Maxim Sorokin); research, M.S. (Maria Suntsova), A.G. and P.M.; writing—original draft preparation, M.P.; writing—review and editing, S.L., A.N.O and A.B.; visualization,

M.S. (Maxim Sorokin) and M.P.; project administration, M.P.; funding acquisition, M.P. All authors have read and agreed to the published version of the manuscript.

Funding: This research was funded by the strategic academic leadership program 'Priority 2030' (Agreement 075-02-2021-1316, 30 September 2021).

Institutional Review Board Statement: Not applicable.

Informed Consent Statement: Not applicable.

Data Availability Statement: The materials and data are available from the corresponding authors.

Conflicts of Interest: The authors declare no conflict of interest.

References

1. Thandra, K.C.; Barsouk, A.; Saginala, K.; Aluru, J.S.; Barsouk, A. Epidemiology of lung cancer. *Contemp. Oncol.* **2021**, *25*, 45–52. [CrossRef]
2. Herbst, R.S.; Morgensztern, D.; Boshoff, C. The biology and management of non-small cell lung cancer. *Nature* **2018**, *553*, 446–454. [CrossRef] [PubMed]
3. Prabavathy, D.; Swarnalatha, Y.; Ramadoss, N. Lung cancer stem cells—Origin, characteristics and therapy. *Stem Cell Investig.* **2018**, *5*, 6. [CrossRef] [PubMed]
4. Césaire, M.; Montanari, J.; Curcio, H.; Lerouge, D.; Gervais, R.; Demontrond, P.; Balosso, J.; Chevalier, F. Radioresistance of Non-Small Cell Lung Cancers and Therapeutic Perspectives. *Cancers* **2022**, *14*, 2829. [CrossRef]
5. Borisov, N.M.; Terekhanova, N.V.; Aliper, A.M.; Venkova, L.S.; Smirnov, P.Y.; Roumiantsev, S.; Korzinkin, M.B.; Zhavoronkov, A.A.; Buzdin, A.A. Signaling pathways activation profiles make better markers of cancer than expression of individual genes. *Oncotarget* **2014**, *5*, 10198–10205. [CrossRef]
6. Kamashev, D.; Sorokin, M.; Kochergina, I.; Drobyshev, A.; Vladimirova, U.; Zolotovskaia, M.; Vorotnikov, I.; Shaban, N.; Raevskiy, M.; Kuzmin, D.; et al. Human blood serum can donor-specifically antagonize effects of EGFR-targeted drugs on squamous carcinoma cell growth. *Heliyon* **2021**, *7*, e06394. [CrossRef]
7. Crispo, F.; Notarangelo, T.; Pietrafesa, M.; Lettini, G.; Storto, G.; Sgambato, A.; Maddalena, F.; Landriscina, M. BRAF Inhibitors in Thyroid Cancer: Clinical Impact, Mechanisms of Resistance and Future Perspectives. *Cancers* **2019**, *11*, 1388. [CrossRef]
8. Pustovalova, M.; Alhaddad, L.; Smetanina, N.; Chigasova, A.; Blokhina, T.; Chuprov-Netochin, R.; Osipov, A.N.; Leonov, S. The p53–53BP1-Related Survival of A549 and H1299 Human Lung Cancer Cells after Multifractionated Radiotherapy Demonstrated Different Response to Additional Acute X-ray Exposure. *Int. J. Mol. Sci.* **2020**, *21*, 3342. [CrossRef]
9. Pustovalova, M.; Alhaddad, L.; Blokhina, T.; Smetanina, N.; Chigasova, A.; Chuprov-Netochin, R.; Eremin, P.; Gilmutdinova, I.; Osipov, A.; Leonov, S. The CD44high Subpopulation of Multifraction Irradiation-Surviving NSCLC Cells Exhibits Partial EMT-Program Activation and DNA Damage Response Depending on Their p53 Status. *Int. J. Mol. Sci.* **2021**, *22*, 2369. [CrossRef]
10. Pustovalova, M.V.; Guryanova, A.A.; Sorokin, M.I.; Suntsova, M.V.; Buzdin, A.A.; Alhaddad, L.; Osipov, A.N.; Leonov, S.V. Transcriptomic Analysis of DNA Repair Pathways in Human Non-Small Cell Lung Cancer Cells Surviving Multifraction X-ray Irradiation. *Bull. Exp. Biol. Med.* **2022**, *173*, 454–458. [CrossRef]
11. Zheng, Q.; Wang, X.-J. GOEAST: A web-based software toolkit for Gene Ontology enrichment analysis. *Nucleic Acids Res.* **2008**, *36*, W358–W363. [CrossRef]
12. Borisov, N.; Sorokin, M.; Garazha, A.; Buzdin, A. Quantitation of Molecular Pathway Activation Using RNA Sequencing Data. In *Nucleic Acid Detection and Structural Investigations*; Humana: New York, NY, USA, 2019; Volume 2063, pp. 189–206. [CrossRef]
13. Croft, D.; Mundo, A.F.; Haw, R.; Milacic, M.; Weiser, J.; Wu, G.; Caudy, M.; Garapati, P.; Gillespie, M.; Kamdar, M.R.; et al. The Reactome pathway knowledgebase. *Nucleic Acids Res.* **2013**, *42*, D472–D477. [CrossRef]
14. Schaefer, C.F.; Anthony, K.; Krupa, S.; Buchoff, J.; Day, M.; Hannay, T.; Buetow, K.H. PID: The Pathway Interaction Database. *Nucleic Acids Res.* **2008**, *37*, D674–D679. [CrossRef]
15. Zhu, W.; Wang, H.; Zhu, D. Wnt/β-catenin signaling pathway in lung cancer. *Med. Drug Discov.* **2021**, *13*, 100113. [CrossRef]
16. Schoetz, U.; Klein, D.; Hess, J.; Shnayien, S.; Spoerl, S.; Orth, M.; Mutlu, S.; Hennel, R.; Sieber, A.; Ganswindt, U.; et al. Early senescence and production of senescence-associated cytokines are major determinants of radioresistance in head-and-neck squamous cell carcinoma. *Cell Death Dis.* **2021**, *12*, 1162. [CrossRef]
17. Chien, Y.; Scuoppo, C.; Wang, X.; Fang, X.; Balgley, B.; Bolden, J.E.; Premsrirut, P.; Luo, W.; Chicas, A.; Lee, C.S.; et al. Control of the senescence-associated secretory phenotype by NF-κB promotes senescence and enhances chemosensitivity. *Genes Dev.* **2011**, *25*, 2125–2136. [CrossRef]
18. Pustovalova, M.; Blokhina, T.; Alhaddad, L.; Chigasova, A.; Chuprov-Netochin, R.; Veviorskiy, A.; Filkov, G.; Osipov, A.N.; Leonov, S. CD44+ and CD133+ Non-Small Cell Lung Cancer Cells Exhibit DNA Damage Response Pathways and Dormant Polyploid Giant Cancer Cell Enrichment Relating to Their p53 Status. *Int. J. Mol. Sci.* **2022**, *23*, 4922. [CrossRef]
19. Alhaddad, L.; Pustovalova, M.; Blokhina, T.; Chuprov-Netochin, R.; Osipov, A.; Leonov, S. IR-Surviving NSCLC Cells Exhibit Different Patterns of Molecular and Cellular Reactions Relating to the Multifraction Irradiation Regimen and p53-Family Proteins Expression. *Cancers* **2021**, *13*, 2669. [CrossRef]

20. Zhao, X.; Jin, X.; Zhang, Q.; Liu, R.; Luo, H.; Yang, Z.; Geng, Y.; Feng, S.; Li, C.; Wang, L.; et al. Silencing of the lncRNA H19 enhances sensitivity to X-ray and carbon-ions through the miR-130a-3p /WNK3 signaling axis in NSCLC cells. *Cancer Cell Int.* **2021**, *21*, 644. [CrossRef]
21. Liu, B.; Li, H.; Liu, X.; Li, F.; Chen, W.; Kuang, Y.; Zhao, X.; Li, L.; Yu, B.; Jin, X.; et al. CircZNF208 enhances the sensitivity to X-rays instead of carbon-ions through the miR-7-5p /SNCA signal axis in non-small-cell lung cancer cells. *Cell. Signal.* **2021**, *84*, 110012. [CrossRef]
22. Guo, W.; Xie, L.; Zhao, L.; Zhao, Y. mRNA and microRNA expression profiles of radioresistant NCI-H520 non-small cell lung cancer cells. *Mol. Med. Rep.* **2015**, *12*, 1857–1867. [CrossRef] [PubMed]
23. Fan, L.; Cao, Q.; Ding, X.; Gao, D.; Yang, Q.; Li, B. Radiotranscriptomics signature-based predictive nomograms for radiotherapy response in patients with nonsmall cell lung cancer: Combination and association of CT features and serum miRNAs levels. *Cancer Med.* **2020**, *9*, 5065–5074. [CrossRef] [PubMed]
24. Mboge, M.Y.; Mahon, B.P.; McKenna, R.; Frost, S.C. Carbonic Anhydrases: Role in pH Control and Cancer. *Metabolites* **2018**, *8*, 19. [CrossRef] [PubMed]
25. Annan, D.A.; Maishi, N.; Soga, T.; Dawood, R.; Li, C.; Kikuchi, H.; Hojo, T.; Morimoto, M.; Kitamura, T.; Alam, M.T.; et al. Carbonic anhydrase 2 (CAII) supports tumor blood endothelial cell survival under lactic acidosis in the tumor microenvironment. *Cell Commun. Signal.* **2019**, *17*, 169. [CrossRef]
26. Hermawan, A.; Putri, H. Integrative bioinformatics analysis reveals miR-494 and its target genes as predictive biomarkers of trastuzumab-resistant breast cancer. *J. Egypt. Natl. Cancer Inst.* **2020**, *32*, 16. [CrossRef]
27. Kim, M.; Kim, D.J. GFRA1: A Novel Molecular Target for the Prevention of Osteosarcoma Chemoresistance. *Int. J. Mol. Sci.* **2018**, *19*, 1078. [CrossRef]
28. Wang, L.; Shen, X.; Wang, Z.; Xiao, X.; Wei, P.; Wang, Q.; Ren, F.; Wang, Y.; Liu, Z.; Sheng, W.; et al. A molecular signature for the prediction of recurrence in colorectal cancer. *Mol. Cancer* **2015**, *14*, 22. [CrossRef]
29. Liu, J.; Yu, N.; Feng, R.; He, Y.; Lv, K.; Zhu, H.; Wang, J. Loss of EphA7 Expression in Basal Cell Carcinoma by Hypermethylation of CpG Islands in the Promoter Region. *Anal. Cell. Pathol.* **2022**, *2022*, 4220786. [CrossRef]
30. Wang, T.-H.; Hsia, S.-M.; Shieh, T.-M. Lysyl Oxidase and the Tumor Microenvironment. *Int. J. Mol. Sci.* **2016**, *18*, 62. [CrossRef]
31. Abdulkareem, N.M.; Bhat, R.; Qin, L.; Vasaikar, S.; Gopinathan, A.; Mitchell, T.; Shea, M.J.; Nanda, S.; Thangavel, H.; Zhang, B.; et al. A novel role of ADGRF1 (GPR110) in promoting cellular quiescence and chemoresistance in human epidermal growth factor receptor 2-positive breast cancer. *FASEB J.* **2021**, *35*, e21719. [CrossRef]
32. Zhong, L.; Gan, X.; Deng, X.; Shen, F.; Feng, J.; Cai, W.; Liu, Q.; Miao, J.; Zheng, B.; Xu, B. Potential five-mRNA signature model for the prediction of prognosis in patients with papillary thyroid carcinoma. *Oncol. Lett.* **2020**, *20*, 2302–2310. [CrossRef]
33. Upadhyay, G. Emerging Role of Lymphocyte Antigen-6 Family of Genes in Cancer and Immune Cells. *Front. Immunol.* **2019**, *10*, 819. [CrossRef]
34. Alves, C.L.; Elias, D.; Lyng, M.B.; Bak, M.; Ditzel, H.J. SNAI2 upregulation is associated with an aggressive phenotype in fulvestrant-resistant breast cancer cells and is an indicator of poor response to endocrine therapy in estrogen receptor-positive metastatic breast cancer. *Breast Cancer Res.* **2018**, *20*, 60. [CrossRef]
35. Luan, F.; Li, X.; Cheng, X.; Huangfu, L.; Han, J.; Guo, T.; Du, H.; Wen, X.; Ji, J. TNFRSF11B activates Wnt/β-catenin signaling and promotes gastric cancer progression. *Int. J. Biol. Sci.* **2020**, *16*, 1956–1971. [CrossRef]
36. Xie, W.; Qiao, X.; Shang, L.; Dou, J.; Yang, X.; Qiao, S.; Wu, Y. Knockdown of ZNF233 suppresses hepatocellular carcinoma cell proliferation and tumorigenesis. *Gene* **2018**, *679*, 179–185. [CrossRef]
37. Tepedelen, B.E.; Kirmizibayrak, P.B. Endoplasmic Reticulum-Associated Degradation (ERAD). In *Endoplasmic Reticulum*; IntechOpen: London, UK, 2019. [CrossRef]
38. Zhang, J.; Wu, J.; Liu, L.; Li, J. The Crucial Role of Demannosylating Asparagine-Linked Glycans in ERADicating Misfolded Glycoproteins in the Endoplasmic Reticulum. *Front. Plant Sci.* **2021**, *11*, 625033. [CrossRef]
39. Habiba, U.; Rafiq, M.; Khawar, M.B.; Nazir, B.; Haider, G.; Nazir, N. The multifaceted role of IL-12 in cancer. *Adv. Cancer Biol.-Metastasis* **2022**, *5*, 100053. [CrossRef]
40. Wu, M.-F.; Wang, Y.-C.; Li, H.-T.; Chen, W.-C.; Liao, C.-H.; Shih, T.-C.; Chang, W.-S.; Tsai, C.-W.; Hsia, T.-C.; Bau, D.-T. The Contribution of Interleukin-12 Genetic Variations to Taiwanese Lung Cancer. *Anticancer Res.* **2018**, *38*, 6321–6327. [CrossRef]
41. Zhang, W.; Dang, S.; Zhang, G.; He, H.; Wen, X. Genetic polymorphisms of IL-10, IL-18 and IL12B are associated with risk of non-small cell lung cancer in a Chinese Han population. *Int. Immunopharmacol.* **2019**, *77*, 105938. [CrossRef]
42. Núñez-Marrero, A.; Arroyo, N.; Godoy-Munoz, L.; Rahman, M.Z.; Matta, J.L.; Dutil, J. SNPs in the interleukin-12 signaling pathway are associated with breast cancer risk in Puerto Rican women. *Oncotarget* **2020**, *11*, 3420–3431. [CrossRef]
43. Herranz, N.; Gil, J. Mechanisms and functions of cellular senescence. *J. Clin. Investig.* **2018**, *128*, 1238–1246. [CrossRef] [PubMed]
44. Wang, L.; Lankhorst, L.; Bernards, R. Exploiting senescence for the treatment of cancer. *Nat. Rev. Cancer* **2022**, *22*, 340–355. [CrossRef] [PubMed]
45. Ruhland, M.K.; Loza, A.J.; Capietto, A.-H.; Luo, X.; Knolhoff, B.L.; Flanagan, K.C.; Belt, B.A.; Alspach, E.; Leahy, K.; Luo, J.; et al. Stromal senescence establishes an immunosuppressive microenvironment that drives tumorigenesis. *Nat. Commun.* **2016**, *7*, 11762. [CrossRef] [PubMed]

46. Marin, I.; Boix, O.; Garcia-Garijo, A.; Sirois, I.; Caballe, A.; Zarzuela, E.; Ruano, I.; Stephan-Otto Attolini, C.; Prats, N.; Lopez-Dominguez, J.A.; et al. Cellular senescence is immunogenic and promotes anti-tumor immunity. *Cancer Discov* **2022**, *12*, 2154115. [CrossRef]
47. Hu, X.; Guo, L.; Liu, G.; Dai, Z.; Wang, L.; Zhang, J.; Wang, J. Novel cellular senescence-related risk model identified as the prognostic biomarkers for lung squamous cell carcinoma. *Front. Oncol.* **2022**, *12*, 997702. [CrossRef]
48. Xiong, J.; Jiang, P.; Zhong, L.; Wang, Y. The Novel Tumor Suppressor Gene ZNF24 Induces THCA Cells Senescence by Regulating Wnt Signaling Pathway, Resulting in Inhibition of THCA Tumorigenesis and Invasion. *Front. Oncol.* **2021**, *11*, 646511. [CrossRef]
49. Pang, B.; Wang, Y.; Chang, X. A Novel Tumor Suppressor Gene, ZNF24, Inhibits the Development of NSCLC by Inhibiting the WNT Signaling Pathway to Induce Cell Senescence. *Front. Oncol.* **2021**, *11*, 664369. [CrossRef]
50. Cuollo, L.; Antonangeli, F.; Santoni, A.; Soriani, A. The Senescence-Associated Secretory Phenotype (SASP) in the Challenging Future of Cancer Therapy and Age-Related Diseases. *Biology* **2020**, *9*, 485. [CrossRef]
51. Cong, L.; Qiu, Z.-Y.; Zhao, Y.; Wang, W.-B.; Wang, C.-X.; Shen, H.-C.; Han, J.-Q. Loss of β-arrestin-2 and Activation of CXCR2 Correlate with Lymph Node Metastasis in Non-small Cell Lung Cancer. *J. Cancer* **2017**, *8*, 2785–2792. [CrossRef]
52. Giampieri, S.; Manning, C.; Hooper, S.; Jones, L.; Hill, C.; Sahai, E. Localized and reversible TGFβ signalling switches breast cancer cells from cohesive to single cell motility. *Nature* **2009**, *11*, 1287–1296. [CrossRef]
53. Jackstadt, R.; van Hooff, S.R.; Leach, J.D.; Cortes-Lavaud, X.; Lohuis, J.O.; Ridgway, R.A.; Wouters, V.M.; Roper, J.; Kendall, T.J.; Roxburgh, C.S.; et al. Epithelial NOTCH Signaling Rewires the Tumor Microenvironment of Colorectal Cancer to Drive Poor-Prognosis Subtypes and Metastasis. *Cancer Cell* **2019**, *36*, 319–336. [CrossRef]
54. Del Valle, L.; Dai, L.; Lin, H.; Lin, Z.; Chen, J.; Post, S.R.; Qin, Z. Role of EIF4G1 network in non-small cell lung cancers (NSCLC) cell survival and disease progression. *J. Cell. Mol. Med.* **2021**, *25*, 2795–2805. [CrossRef]
55. Chua, Y.L.; Ito, Y.; Pole, J.C.M.; Newman, S.; Chin, S.F.; Stein, R.C.; Ellis, I.O.; Caldas, C.; O'Hare, M.J.; Murrell, A.; et al. The NRG1 gene is frequently silenced by methylation in breast cancers and is a strong candidate for the 8p tumour suppressor gene. *Oncogene* **2009**, *28*, 4041–4052. [CrossRef]
56. Piomelli, D. Endocannabinoids. In *Encyclopedia of Biological Chemistry*; Academic Press: Cambridge, MA, USA, 2013; pp. 194–196. [CrossRef]
57. Maccarrone, M. Metabolism of the Endocannabinoid Anandamide: Open Questions after 25 Years. *Front. Mol. Neurosci.* **2017**, *10*, 166. [CrossRef]
58. Kozak, K.R.; Crews, B.C.; Morrow, J.D.; Wang, L.-H.; Ma, Y.H.; Weinander, R.; Jakobsson, P.-J.; Marnett, L.J. Metabolism of the Endocannabinoids, 2-Arachidonylglycerol and Anandamide, into Prostaglandin, Thromboxane, and Prostacyclin Glycerol Esters and Ethanolamides. *J. Biol. Chem.* **2002**, *277*, 44877–44885. [CrossRef]
59. Qiao, L.; Kozoni, V.; Tsioulias, G.J.; Koutsos, M.I.; Hanif, R.; Shiff, S.J.; Rigas, B. Selected eicosanoids increase the proliferation rate of human colon carcinoma cell lines and mouse colonocytes in vivo. *Biochim. Biophys. Acta BBA Lipids Lipid Metab.* **1995**, *1258*, 215–223. [CrossRef]
60. Tsujii, M.; Kawano, S.; Tsuji, S.; Sawaoka, H.; Hori, M.; DuBois, R.N. Cyclooxygenase Regulates Angiogenesis Induced by Colon Cancer Cells. *Cell* **1998**, *93*, 705–716. [CrossRef]
61. Yang, H.J.; Kim, N.; Seong, K.M.; Youn, H.; Youn, B. Investigation of Radiation-induced Transcriptome Profile of Radioresistant Non-small Cell Lung Cancer A549 Cells Using RNA-seq. *PLoS ONE* **2013**, *8*, e59319. [CrossRef]
62. Li, W.; Yue, W.; Zhang, L.; Zhao, X.; Ma, L.; Yang, X.; Zhang, Y.; Wang, Y.; Gu, M. COX-2 silencing inhibits cell proliferation in A549 cell. *Chin.-Ger. J. Clin. Oncol.* **2011**, *10*, 423–427. [CrossRef]
63. Ding, C.; Liu, J.; Zhang, J.; Wan, Y.; Hu, L.; Charwudzi, A.; Zhan, H.; Meng, Y.; Zheng, H.; Wang, H.; et al. Tumor Endothelial Marker 8 Promotes Proliferation and Metastasis via the Wnt/β-Catenin Signaling Pathway in Lung Adenocarcinoma. *Front. Oncol.* **2021**, *11*, 712371. [CrossRef]
64. Chen, D.; Bhat-Nakshatri, P.; Goswami, C.; Badve, S.; Nakshatri, H. ANTXR1, a Stem Cell-Enriched Functional Biomarker, Connects Collagen Signaling to Cancer Stem-like Cells and Metastasis in Breast Cancer. *Cancer Res* **2013**, *73*, 5821–5833. [CrossRef] [PubMed]
65. Alcalá, S.; Martinelli, P.; Hermann, P.C.; Heeschen, C.; Sainz, B. The Anthrax Toxin Receptor 1 (ANTXR1) Is Enriched in Pancreatic Cancer Stem Cells Derived from Primary Tumor Cultures. *Stem Cells Int.* **2019**, *2019*, 1378639. [CrossRef] [PubMed]
66. Huang, X.; Liu, G.; Guo, J.; Su, Z. The PI3K/AKT pathway in obesity and type 2 diabetes. *Int. J. Biol. Sci.* **2018**, *14*, 1483–1496. [CrossRef] [PubMed]
67. Shen, Y.; Li, J.; Qiang, H.; Lei, Y.; Chang, Q.; Zhong, R.; Stella, G.M.; Gelsomino, F.; Kim, Y.W.; Abed, A.; et al. A retrospective study for prognostic significance of type II diabetes mellitus and hemoglobin A1c levels in non-small cell lung cancer patients treated with pembrolizumab. *Transl. Lung Cancer Res.* **2021**, *11*, 1619–1630. [CrossRef] [PubMed]
68. Su, C.-H.; Chen, W.-M.; Chen, M.; Shia, B.-C.; Wu, S.-Y. Association of Diabetes Severity and Mortality with Lung Squamous Cell Carcinoma. *Cancers* **2022**, *14*, 2553. [CrossRef]
69. Zhu, L.; Cao, H.; Zhang, T.; Shen, H.; Dong, W.; Wang, L.; Du, J. The Effect of Diabetes Mellitus on Lung Cancer Prognosis: A PRISMA-compliant meta-analysis of cohort studies. *Medicine* **2016**, *95*, e3528. [CrossRef]
70. Luo, J.; Hendryx, M.; Qi, L.; Ho, G.Y.; Margolis, K. Pre-existing diabetes and lung cancer prognosis. *Br. J. Cancer* **2016**, *115*, 76–79. [CrossRef]

71. Ma, X.; Bai, Y. IGF-1 activates the P13K/AKT signaling pathway via upregulation of secretory clusterin. *Mol. Med. Rep.* **2012**, *6*, 1433–1437. [CrossRef]
72. Vafopoulou, X.; Steel, C.G. Insulin-like and testis ecdysiotropin neuropeptides are regulated by the circadian timing system in the brain during larval–adult development in the insect *Rhodnius prolixus* (Hemiptera). *Gen. Comp. Endocrinol.* **2012**, *179*, 277–288. [CrossRef]
73. Henriksen, E.J.; Dokken, B.B. Role of glycogen synthase kinase-3 in insulin resistance and type 2 diabetes. *Curr. Drug Targets* **2006**, *7*, 1435–1441. [CrossRef]
74. Silva-Filho, J.L.; Caruso-Neves, C.; Pinheiro, A.A.S. IL-4: An important cytokine in determining the fate of T cells. *Biophys. Rev.* **2014**, *6*, 111–118. [CrossRef]
75. Bankaitis, K.V.; Fingleton, B. Targeting IL4/IL4R for the treatment of epithelial cancer metastasis. *Clin. Exp. Metastasis* **2015**, *32*, 847–856. [CrossRef]
76. Shi, X.; Dong, A.; Jia, X.; Zheng, G.; Wang, N.; Wang, Y.; Yang, C.; Lu, J.; Yang, Y. Integrated analysis of single-cell and bulk RNA-sequencing identifies a signature based on T-cell marker genes to predict prognosis and therapeutic response in lung squamous cell carcinoma. *Front. Immunol.* **2022**, *13*, 992990. [CrossRef]
77. Rapp, J.; Jaromi, L.; Kvell, K.; Miskei, G.; Pongracz, J.E. WNT signaling—Lung cancer is no exception. *Respir. Res.* **2017**, *18*, 167. [CrossRef]
78. Takahashi-Yanaga, F.; Kahn, M. Targeting Wnt Signaling: Can We Safely Eradicate Cancer Stem Cells? *Clin. Cancer Res.* **2010**, *16*, 3153–3162. [CrossRef]
79. Stewart, D.J. Wnt Signaling Pathway in Non-Small Cell Lung Cancer. *JNCI J. Natl. Cancer Inst.* **2014**, *106*, djt356. [CrossRef]
80. Nalbantoglu, B.; Durmu, S.; Ülgen, K.Ö. Wnt Signaling Network in Homo Sapiens. In *Cell Metabolism—Cell Homeostasis and Stress Response*; IntechOpen: London, UK, 2012. [CrossRef]
81. Teng, Y.; Wang, X.; Wang, Y.; Ma, D. Wnt/β-catenin signaling regulates cancer stem cells in lung cancer A549 cells. *Biochem. Biophys. Res. Commun.* **2010**, *392*, 373–379. [CrossRef]
82. Mazieres, J.; He, B.; You, L.; Xu, Z.; Jablons, D.M. Wnt signaling in lung cancer. *Cancer Lett.* **2005**, *222*, 1–10. [CrossRef]
83. Jaiswal, P.K.; Goel, A.; Mittal, R.D. Survivin: A molecular biomarker in cancer. *Indian J. Med. Res.* **2015**, *141*, 389–397. [CrossRef]
84. Tenbaum, S.P.; Ordóñez-Morán, P.; Puig, I.; Chicote, I.; Arqués, O.; Landolfi, S.; Fernández, Y.; Herance, J.R.; Gispert, J.D.; Mendizabal, L.; et al. β-catenin confers resistance to PI3K and AKT inhibitors and subverts FOXO3a to promote metastasis in colon cancer. *Nat. Med.* **2012**, *18*, 892–901. [CrossRef]
85. Pangon, L.; Mladenova, D.; Watkins, L.; Van Kralingen, C.; Currey, N.; Al-Sohaily, S.; Lecine, P.; Borg, J.-P.; Kohonen-Corish, M.R. MCC inhibits β-catenin transcriptional activity by sequestering DBC1 in the cytoplasm. *Int. J. Cancer* **2014**, *136*, 55–64. [CrossRef] [PubMed]
86. Borowicz, S.; Van Scoyk, M.; Avasarala, S.; Karuppusamy Rathinam, M.K.; Tauler, J.; Bikkavilli, R.K.; Winn, R.A. The soft agar colony formation assay. *JoVE J. Vis. Exp.* **2014**, *92*, e51998. [CrossRef]
87. Dobin, A.; Davis, C.A.; Schlesinger, F.; Drenkow, J.; Zaleski, C.; Jha, S.; Batut, P.; Chaisson, M.; Gingeras, T.R. STAR: Ultrafast universal RNA-seq aligner. *Bioinformatics* **2013**, *29*, 15–21. [CrossRef] [PubMed]
88. Love, M.I.; Huber, W.; Anders, S. Moderated estimation of fold change and dispersion for RNA-seq data with DESeq. *Genome Biol.* **2014**, *15*, 550. [CrossRef]
89. Sorokin, M.; Kholodenko, R.; Suntsova, M.; Malakhova, G.; Garazha, A.; Kholodenko, I.; Poddubskaya, E.; Lantsov, D.; Stilidi, I.; Arhiri, P.; et al. Oncobox Bioinformatical Platform for Selecting Potentially Effective Combinations of Target Cancer Drugs Using High-Throughput Gene Expression Data. *Cancers* **2018**, *10*, 365. [CrossRef]
90. Sorokin, M.; Borisov, N.; Kuzmin, D.; Gudkov, A.; Zolotovskaia, M.; Garazha, A.; Buzdin, A. Algorithmic Annotation of Functional Roles for Components of 3044 Human Molecular Pathways. *Front. Genet.* **2021**, *12*, 617059. [CrossRef]

Disclaimer/Publisher's Note: The statements, opinions and data contained in all publications are solely those of the individual author(s) and contributor(s) and not of MDPI and/or the editor(s). MDPI and/or the editor(s) disclaim responsibility for any injury to people or property resulting from any ideas, methods, instructions or products referred to in the content.

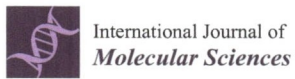

Article

Long-Term Cultured Human Glioblastoma Multiforme Cells Demonstrate Increased Radiosensitivity and Senescence-Associated Secretory Phenotype in Response to Irradiation

Lina Alhaddad [1,2,†], Zain Nofal [1,†], Margarita Pustovalova [1,3], Andreyan N. Osipov [1,3,4,*] and Sergey Leonov [1,5]

1. School of Biological and Medical Physics, Moscow Institute of Physics and Technology (National Research University), 141701 Dolgoprudny, Russia
2. Department of Environmental Sciences, Faculty of Sciences, Damascus University, Damascus P.O. Box 30621, Syria
3. State Research Center—Burnasyan Federal Medical Biophysical Center of Federal Medical Biological Agency (SRC-FMBC), 123098 Moscow, Russia
4. N.N. Semenov Federal Research Center for Chemical Physics, Russian Academy of Sciences, 119991 Moscow, Russia
5. Institute of Cell Biophysics, Russian Academy of Sciences, 142290 Pushchino, Russia
* Correspondence: aosipov@fmbcfmba.ru
† These authors contributed equally to this work.

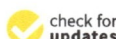

Citation: Alhaddad, L.; Nofal, Z.; Pustovalova, M.; Osipov, A.N.; Leonov, S. Long-Term Cultured Human Glioblastoma Multiforme Cells Demonstrate Increased Radiosensitivity and Senescence-Associated Secretory Phenotype in Response to Irradiation. *Int. J. Mol. Sci.* **2023**, *24*, 2002. https://doi.org/10.3390/ijms24032002

Academic Editor: François Chevalier

Received: 15 December 2022
Revised: 14 January 2023
Accepted: 17 January 2023
Published: 19 January 2023

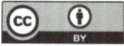

Copyright: © 2023 by the authors. Licensee MDPI, Basel, Switzerland. This article is an open access article distributed under the terms and conditions of the Creative Commons Attribution (CC BY) license (https://creativecommons.org/licenses/by/4.0/).

Abstract: The overall effect of senescence on cancer progression and cancer cell resistance to X-ray radiation (IR) is still not fully understood and remains controversial. How to induce tumor cell senescence and which senescent cell characteristics will ensure the safest therapeutic strategy for cancer treatment are under extensive investigation. While the evidence for passage number-related effects on malignant primary cells or cell lines is compelling, much less is known about how the changes affect safety and Senescence-Associated Secretory Phenotype (SASP), both of which are needed for the senescence cell-based vaccine to be effective against cancer. The present study aimed to investigate the effects of repeated passaging on the biological (self-renewal capacity and radioresistance) and functional (senescence) characteristics of the different populations of short- and long-term passaging glioblastoma multiforme (GBM) cells responding to senescence-inducing DNA-damaging IR stress. For this purpose, we compared radiobiological effects of X-ray exposure on two isogenic human U87 cell lines: U87L, minimally cultured cells (<15 passages after obtaining from the ATCC) and U87H, long-term cultured cells (>3 years of continuous culturing after obtaining from the ATCC). U87L cells displayed IR dose-related changes in the signs of IR stress-induced premature senescence. These included an increase in the proportion of senescence-associated β-galactosidase (SA-β-Gal)-positive cells, and concomitant decrease in the proportion of Ki67-positive cells and metabolically active cells. However, reproductive survival of irradiated short-term cultured U87L cells was higher compared to long-term cultured U87H cells, as the clonogenic activity results demonstrated. In contrast, the irradiated long-term cultured U87H cells possessed dose-related increases in the proportion of multinucleated giant cancer cells (MGCCs), while demonstrating higher radiosensitivity (lower self-renewal) and a significantly reduced fraction of DNA-replicating cells compared to short-term cultured U87L cells. Conditioned culture medium from U87H cells induced a significant rise of SA-β-Gal staining in U87L cells in a paracrine manner suggesting inherent SASP. Our data suggested that low-dose irradiated long-term cultured GBM cells might be a safer candidate for a recently proposed senescence cell-based vaccine against cancer.

Keywords: glioblastoma multiforme; multinucleated giant cancer cell; senescent tumor cells (STC); stress-induced premature senescence (SIPS); senescence-associated secretory phenotype (SASP)

1. Introduction

Glioblastoma multiforme (GBM) is one of the most aggressive and most common malignant primary brain tumors in adults and often occurs in patients over 65 years of age [1,2]. Radiotherapy is still a treatment of choice for patients with GBM. However, its efficacy is limited by the dose that can be safely administered without eliciting serious side-effects, especially in elderly and debilitated patients, as well as the fact that recurrence, metastasis and radioresistance are common in GBM [3]. Radiotherapy can cause cancer cells to enter a state of stress-induced premature senescence (SIPS), thereby slowing down the cell cycle and further proliferation and allowing cancer cells to escape the DNA-damaging effects of X-rays. It is believed that SIPS rather than apoptosis, is preferentially induced in GBM cells after radio-and chemotherapy. Cancer cell senescence inhibits cancer growth by halting massive proliferation and increasing chances of immune clearance [4].

While the evidence for passage number-related effects on malignant primary cells or cell lines is compelling, much less is known about how the changes affect safety and SASP, both of which are needed for a recently proposed senescence cell-based vaccine to be effective against cancer. Indeed, it was discovered that senescent tumor cells induce a bigger immune response than dead cancer cells [5]. Inducing tumor formation in mice previously injected with senescent tumor cells led to the development of fewer tumors, with some developing none. Albeit the injection was less effective against pre-existing tumors, this research suggests that a potential senescent cell cancer vaccine could show promise.

The quality and the reproducibility of anti-cancer effects of senescence cell-based vaccines depends on the quality and safety of the tumor cells used to make the vaccine. In turn, these characteristics of tumor cells seem to depend not least on the degree of subcultivation of cancer cells. The effects of passage number are usually long lasting. Transformed and diseased cell lines are of special concern, since they represent abnormal starting populations. Over time, they may change both their genotypic and their phenotypic traits. In these cell types, one or all of the typical cellular checkpoint genes, such as p16/INK4a, pRB and p53, have been altered whereby the cells have become "eternal". These alterations are often in parallel with other cellular mutations, and the continual subculture of these cell lines exacerbates genomic and phenotypic instability [6]. For example, reduced cancer stem cell characteristics in a side population (SP) of late-passage non-small cell lung cancer (NSCLC) cells was reported. These include increased frequency of tumor-initiating and self-renewal capacity, and resistance to DNA-damaging agent doxorubicin and ionizing radiation [7]. The discovery that the SP from long-term passage NSCLC cells was not consistently enriched for stem cell-like cancer cells in the cancer stem cell research field leads to the recommendation to use only low-passage cell lines.

Further complicating matters is that a passage level considered "high" for one cell line may not give rise to any significant passage effects in another. To prevent passage-related effects from affecting experiments, it is important to know how many experiments can be performed in a given set of cells at the same time, and how many there are.

How to induce tumor cell senescence to serve as a therapeutic strategy for cancer treatment is under extensive investigation. Thus, studies of the molecular mechanisms of cancer cell senescence and cancer cells' escape from senescence will provide a new perspective on how cancer can be treated safely.

The overall effect of senescence on cancer progression and cancer cell resistance to X-ray radiation (IR) is still not fully understood and remains controversial. Senescence is a state where cells neither function normally nor die. Cells that are damaged or old may enter this suspended state. In this state, they do not reproduce, but they still communicate with the tumor microenvironment through SASP in a paracrine fashion [8]. Albeit stress-induced senescence is generally considered to be a tumor-suppressive mechanism [9], long-term treatment-induced senescence of cells may be harmful. Long-term induction of senescence will produce a tumor microenvironment that promotes inflammation and immunosuppression [10]. Hence, induction of cancer cell senescence as a recently suggested new therapeutic strategies against cancer [5,11–13] should be context-dependent and evaluated carefully based on the cancer age. Additionally, it is possible to develop new therapeutic strategies to combine priming (immunization) with IR-induced senescent patient-derived cancer cells with IR treatments [14].

Based on all these findings, we thought be worth investigating the effects of repeated passaging on the biological (self-renewal capacity and radioresistance) and functional (senescence) characteristics of different populations of short- and long-term cultivated GBM cells responding to senescence-inducing DNA-damaging IR stress. We compared U87 cell lines that differ significantly in the culture duration after receiving from the ATCC: low passage number U87 cell lines (U87L) that have undergone up to 15 passages and high passage number U87 cell lines (U87H) that have undergone more than 3 years of continuous passaging. Our results demonstrate that long-term cultivation may sensitize GBM cells to IR, while possessing the safest phenotype, including constitutive highest SASP and lowest self-renewal capacities. In contrast, the short-term cultivated GBM cells sustained higher reproductive survival possibly through an IR dose-related increase in the proportion of SA-β-Gal-positive cells (both MGCCs and non-MGCCs) that might ultimately lead to GBM radioresistance.

2. Results

2.1. Long-Term Cultivation Leads to a Decrease in Clonogenic Growth of GBM Cell Line after Irradiation

Clonogenic assay or colony formation assay is an in vitro cell survival assay based on the ability of a single adherent cell to grow into a colony and is a "gold standard" for assessing cancer cells' radiosensitivity [15]. The number of colonies originating from single cells is expressed by plating efficiency (PE), an index which has emerged for normalization of surviving fractions based on the major premise that under untreated conditions the relation between the number of seeded cells and the number of resulting colonies is linear. PE is often used for determining the effects of growth factors and toxicity testing. We aimed to evaluate PE alteration of IR exposed minimally cultured (U87L) and long-term cultured (U87H) GBM cells. We observed that 2 Gy IR significantly increases PE of U87L cells (by 1.45 times, $p < 0.01$) and decreases its value after 6 Gy exposure (by 2.71 times, $p < 0.001$) compared to non-irradiated cells (Figure 1a). In contrast, U87H cells displayed a dose-dependent decrease in the PE by 1.55 times ($p < 0.01$) and by 3.67 times ($p < 0.001$) after irradiation at doses of 2 and 6 Gy, respectively (Figure 1b). Despite the PE results, U87L cells had higher survival fractions (SF) compared to U87H after irradiation at a dose of 6 Gy ($p < 0.01$) (Figure 1c), indicating their higher radioresistance growing under anchorage-dependent conditions.

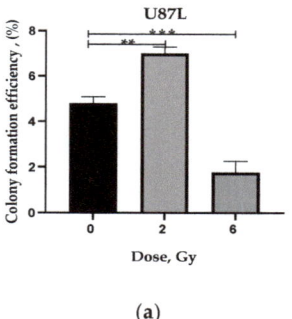
(a)

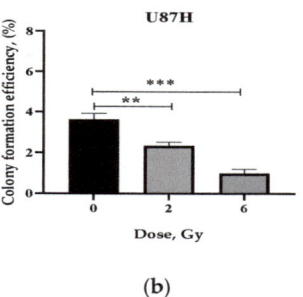
(b)

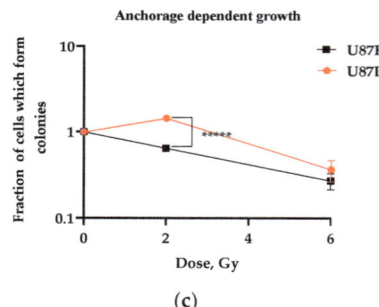
(c)

Figure 1. Cont.

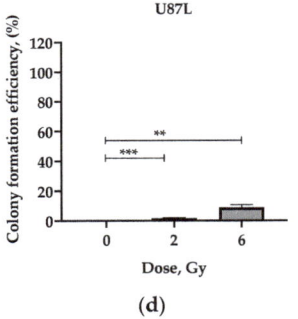 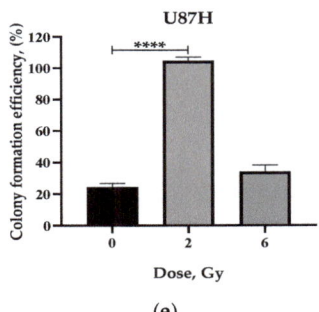 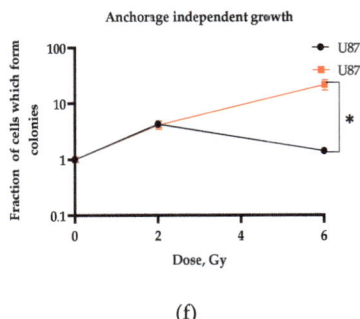

(d)   (e)   (f)

Figure 1. Plating efficiency of U87L (**a**) and U87H (**b**) cells after exposure to 2 and 6 Gy IR. Colony formation efficiency in soft agar of U87L (**d**) and U87H (**e**) cells after exposure to the same doses of IR. Reproductive survival of GBM cell lines was analyzed using survival fraction of cells grown under both anchorage-dependent (**c**) and anchorage-independent conditions (**f**). * $p < 0.05$; ** $p < 0.01$; *** $p < 0.001$; **** $p < 0.0001$; ***** $p < 0.00001$.

Anchorage-independent growth is the ability of transformed cells to grow independently of the attachment to a solid surface, and is a hallmark of carcinogenesis, anoikis resistance and propensity to tumor metastasis [16]. To evaluate whether the long-term culturing affects the anoikis resistance of two isogenic U87 cell sublines, we assessed their reproductive survival using anchorage-independent soft agar colony formation assay. Whereas U87L cells demonstrated increased ability to grow and to form colonies under non-adherent conditions (Figure 1d), the long-term cultured U87H cells had a significantly reduced ability (Figure 1e) both with and without IR exposure. Consequently, the survival fraction of U87L cells significantly exceeded that of U87H cells (Figure 1f) supporting the notion that long-term culturing leads to decreases in reproductive survival of the GBM U87H cell subline in response to IR-induced stress.

2.2. Influence of Preceding Cultivation Length on Metabolism of GBM Cells after Irradiation

To understand the underlying mechanisms of the discovered clonogenic effect of long culturing of malignant cells, we evaluated the metabolic changes in cells of two U87 sublines forming the colonies in soft agar. Alamar Blue test has been widely used for cytotoxicity and viability assays based on the ability of NADPH oxidoreductases to reduce the oxidized, non-fluorescent, blue state of the compound to a fluorescent, pink state [17]. The significant increase (by 1.25 times, $p < 0.01$) and decrease by 2.83 times ($p < 0.00001$) in metabolic activity of U87L cells in response to IR at 2 and 6 Gy, respectively (Figure 2a), correlates well with the dynamics in their colony formation efficacy (Figure 1d) after IR exposure at the same doses. At the same time, irradiation did not lead to a change in metabolic activity of colony-forming long-term cultured cells of U87H subline (Figure 2b). Taken together, our results demonstrate that the retained ability of the U87L cell subline to modulate its own activity of NADPH oxidoreductases may underlie the high reproductive survival in response to IR-induced stress.

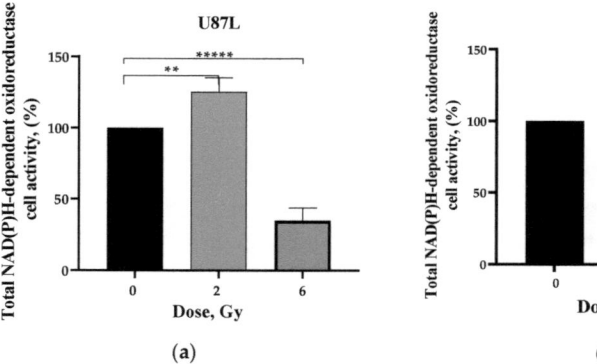

Figure 2. Assessment of the metabolic activity of U87L (**a**) and U87H (**b**) cells 7 days after irradiation at doses of 2 and 6 Gy using the Alamar Blue test in soft agar. ** $p < 0.01$; ***** $p < 0.00001$.

2.3. IR Increases the Proportion of Senescent MGCCs in the Short-Term, but Not in the Long-Term Cultivated GBM Cell Line

Advanced age is a major risk factor for the development of GBM [18]. At the same time, MGCCs arise in response to ionizing radiation in many tumors and contribute to cancer relapse by first entering a state of dormancy which is often accompanied by the stress-induced premature senescence (SIPS) phenotype and ultimately giving rise to cell progeny with stem-like properties [19]. We found that the proportion of MGCCs in response to irradiation at single therapeutically relevant doses of 2 and 6 Gy differs for U87 cell sublines depending on the duration of their preceding cultivation. We observed an increase in the proportion of MGCCs in U87L cells by 1.5 times (from 7.2% in non-irradiated cells to 10.5%, $p = 0.006$) 24 h after irradiation at a dose of 6 Gy (Figure 3b). For U87H cells, this effect was more pronounced: there was a statistically significant increase in the proportion of MGCCs by 2.2 times (from 5% in non-irradiated cells up to 11.2%, $p = 0.0095$) and 3.77 times (up to 18.8%, $p = 0.0002$) at 24 h after irradiation at doses of 2 and 6 Gy, respectively (Figure 3c).

As the stress-induced premature senescence (SIPS) phenotype is typically identified by senescence-associated β-galactosidase (SA-β-Gal) staining, we further aimed to compare the proportion of SA-β-Gal+ cells in the MGCCs and non-MGCCs populations of two GBM cell lines.

The basal proportion of SA-β-Gal+ cells in the non-MNGCs population of non-irradiated U87H cells (27.9%) was almost the same as in the U87L cell line (28.5%) (Figure 3d,e). Ionizing irradiation of U87L cell lines caused significant increase in SA-β-Gal+ cells up to 31.3% ($p = 0.07$) and 42% ($p = 0.0008$) at 2 Gy and 6 Gy, respectively (Figure 3d). In contrast, the same populations of irradiated U87H cells did not change significantly, reaching 27.2% ($p = 0.6$) and 29.7% ($p = 0, 7$) at 2 Gy and 6 Gy, respectively (Figure 3e).

The proportion of SA-β-Gal+ MGCC population in U87L cell lines increased up to 3% ($p = 0.2$) and 4.5% ($p = 0.014$) in response to irradiation doses of 2 and 6 Gy (Figure 3d), while the proportion of SA-β-Gal+ MGCCs in the U87H cell line was statistically indistinguishable (Figure 3e). Consequently, the proportion of SA-β-Gal+ MGCCs in the U87L cell lines after irradiation increased from 31.5% (non-irradiated cells) up to 45% and 43% of total MGCC population irradiated at 2 Gy and 6 Gy, respectively. The SA-β-Gal+ MGCC proportion in U87H cell lines decreased from 52% (non-irradiated cells) down to 23% of total MGCC population after irradiation at doses of 2 and 6 Gy.

Thus, irradiation triggered an increase in the proportion of both SA-β-Gal-positive MGCCs and non-MGCC populations in U87L cell lines, leaving unchanged the level of this senescence marker in the U87H cell line.

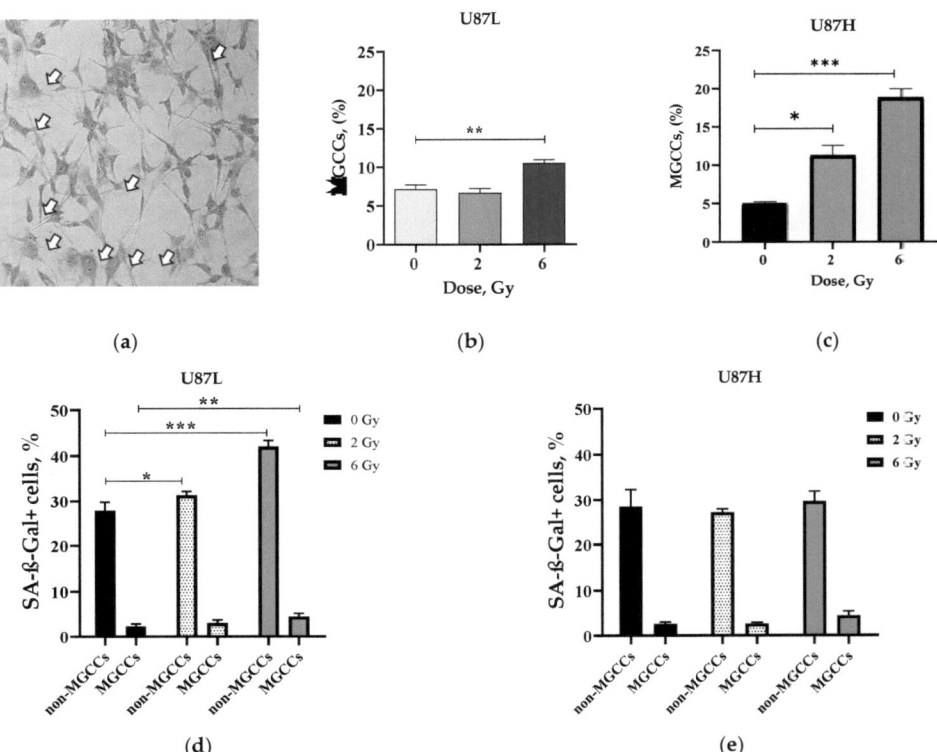

Figure 3. MGCCs formation in minimally-cultured and long-term cultivated GBM upon irradiation. Representative picture of MGCCs (indicated by arrows) (**a**). Change in the proportion (%) of MGCCs in U87L (**b**) and in U87H (**c**) cell lines 24 h after irradiation. Changes in the proportion (%) of SA-β-Gal+ populations in U87L (**d**) and U87H (**e**) cell lines 24 h after exposure to IR at doses of 2 and 6 Gy. * $p < 0.05$; ** $p < 0.01$, *** $p < 0.001$.

2.4. Proliferative Activity of GBM Cells in Response to a Single Dose Irradiation

While eliminating tumor cells, cancer therapies could also induce a sustained proliferation arrest (treatment-induced dormancy) allowing a significant proportion of dormant cells to remain viable and metabolically active for long times post-treatment. We compared the level of EdU-positive (DNA replicating) cells between U87L and U87H lines using conventional Click-IT™ EdU Alexa Fluor 488 cell proliferation assay. The irradiation did not affect the fraction of DNA-replicating (EdU+) U87L cells (Figure 4a), while it reduced the fraction of proliferating U87H cells (Figure 4b) after 6 Gy by 1.8 times ($p < 0.001$) compared to non-irradiated cells.

The Ki-67 protein is not required for cancer cell proliferation, but is required for all stages of carcinogenesis [20]. As seen from our data, 6 Gy irradiation caused completely opposite changes in Ki-67 expression: there was a more than 3 times increase ($p < 0.0001$) and almost 3 times decrease ($p < 0.0001$) in U87H (Figure 4d) and U87L (Figure 4c) cells, respectively. Thus, increased levels of Ki-67 expression led to an almost 2-fold decrease in the amount of DNA-replicating minimally-cultured U87H cells (Figure 4a), indicating inhibition of proliferation caused by an excess of Ki-67, which is in good agreement with the previous investigations [21]. On the other hand, a significant decrease in the percentage of Ki-67 in U87L cells may evidence a slowdown in their cell cycle without a significant change in the fraction of DNA-replicating cells (Figure 4a).

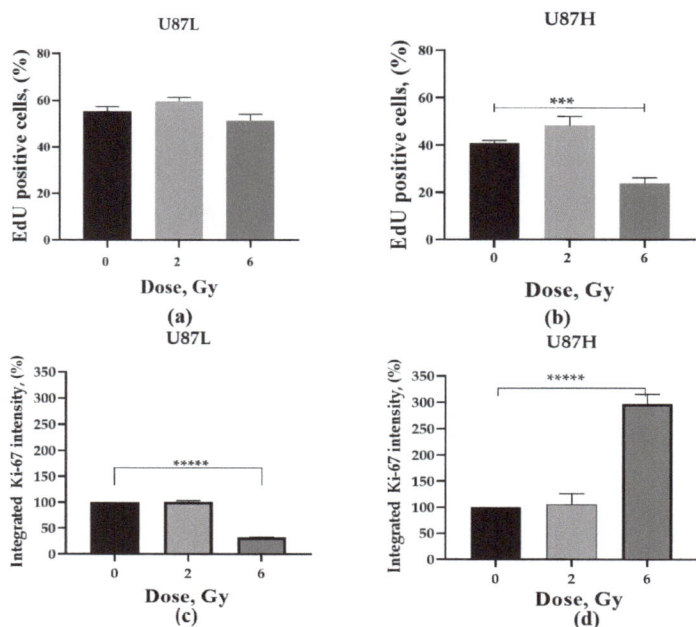

Figure 4. Assessment of the proliferative activity of minimally cultured U87L (**a**,**c**) and long-term cultured U87H cells (**b**,**d**). Change in the percentage of EdU+ cells (**a**,**b**), as well as change in the Ki-67 fluorescence intensity (%) (**c**,**d**) was measured 24 h after irradiation at doses of 2 and 6 Gy. *** $p < 0.001$; ***** $p < 0.00001$.

2.5. Long-Term Cultured U87H Cells Demonstrate Senescence-Associated Secretory Phenotype

To elucidate whether the changes in long-term cultivated U87H line are associated with Senescence-Associated Secretory Phenotype (SASP), we cultivated U87L cells with the condition medium (CM) obtained from U87H cells (Figure 5a). CM obtained from high passaged U87H cells increased the proportion of SA-β-Gal+ U87L cells by 1.6 times compared to control after incubation for 3 days (Figure 5b).

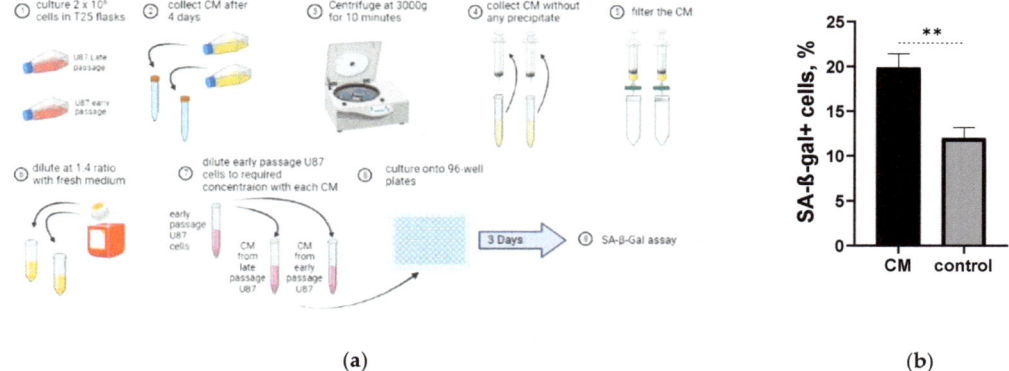

Figure 5. Assessment of the formation of SA-β-Gal positive cells in U87L line cultured in conditioned medium (CM) obtained from U87H cells. Schematic representation of the experiment (**a**). Percentage of SA-b-Gal positive cells formed in U87L cells cultured in CM and in the medium from U87L cell line (control) (**b**). ** $p < 0.01$.

3. Discussion

Cellular senescence emerges in response to multiple extracellular or intracellular stress stimuli, such as telomeric dysfunction resulting from repeated cell division, mitochondrial impairment, oxidative stress, severe or irreparable DNA damage and chromatin disruption, and the expression of certain oncogenes. The senescence program causes permanent cell-cycle arrest, preventing the spread of damage to the next cell generation and precludes potential malignant transformation, which makes it a plausible anticancer mechanism during radiotherapy. However, this state of stable proliferative arrest is accompanied by the Senescence-Associated Secretory Phenotype (SASP), which entails the abundant secretion of pro-inflammatory molecules in the tissue microenvironment and contributes to age-related diseases, including GBM [22]. GBM is a primary brain tumor with a median age of diagnosis of 68–70 years [23]. The incidence rate of GBM increases with age from 1.25 per 100,000 people in adults of 35–44 years of age to 15.13 among older people of 75–84 years of age [24]. The basis for the increased incidence of GBM among elderly people remains poorly understood [18].

In the present study, we demonstrate the comparative analysis of X-ray irradiation exposure on two isogenic GBM cell lines: U87L, minimally cultured cells (<15 passages after obtaining from the ATCC) and U87H, long-term cultured cells (>3 years of continuous culturing after obtaining from the ATCC). During the cultivation period, U87H cells underwent several episodes of neosis—one of the forms of cell division, characterized by atypical karyokinesis through nuclear membrane budding, followed by asymmetric intracellular cytokinesis, producing various amounts of small mononuclear cells called Raju cells, which have an extended mitotic lifespan [25].

Short-term cultured U87L cells further demonstrated reduced radiosensitivity based on the resistance to anoikis assessed by soft agar assay (Figure 1f). Anoikis is the type of apoptotic cell death arising upon loss of attachment to the extracellular matrix and neighboring cells. Cancer cells may acquire resistance to anoikis, which allows them to survive after detachment from the primary sites, disseminate throughout the body and repopulate in secondary sites giving metastases [26]. Recent study demonstrated that clusters of circulating tumor cells were mostly large (≥ 5 µm), exhibited polyploidy and were associated with worse outcomes in non-small cell lung cancer (NSCLC) patients [27]. Here we demonstrate that the radioresistance of short-term cultured GBM cells may be associated with an increase in MGCC formation (Figure 3).

Is the increase solely enough to confer radioresistance of short-term cultivated GBM cell lines? Corroborating the notion that MGCC formation in GBM induces senescence upon irradiation to sustain survival [28], we observed the increase of SA-β-Gal positive cells in U87L cell line. Surprisingly, despite the isogenic U87H cell line producing more MGCC (Figure 3c,b), there was no change in the fraction of SA-β-Gal+ cells in response to IR-induced stress (Figure 3d,e).

To investigate the source of this discrepancy we analyzed the proportion of SA-β-gal-positive cells among MGCC and non-MGCC populations of both isogenic cell lines. In contrast to observations by Kaur et al. [28], we found almost the same significant amount of preexisting MGCC cells, while radiation-induced MGCC formation and senescent marker expression (SA-β-Gal) were different between isogenic cell lines (Figure 3). Indeed, we found for the first time that long-term cultivated cells lost the ability to produce significant amounts of SA-β-Gal+ cells within both MGCC and non-MGCC populations respectively to the doses of IR-induced stress. Thus, sustainably increased SA-β-Gal activity rather than a rise in total MGCC production might play a pivotal role in maintenance of the reproductive survival of the short-term cultivated U87L cell line in response to IR-induced stress.

There are two phenotypes of cell dormancy: senescent cells (SIPS phenotype), in which cell cycle arrest is often irreversible, and resting cells (quiescence phenotype), which can be both non-proliferating, and slowly cycling [29]. While U87L cells demonstrated no change in DNA replication and decreased Ki-67 expression upon 6 Gy irradiation, U87H cells showed decreased DNA replicating activity accompanied by significant increase of

Ki-67 expression (Figure 4). It is important to note that Ki-67 protein is not required for cancer cell proliferation, but rather required for all stages of carcinogenesis. The variability in Ki-67 expression is explained by its regulation through the cell cycle and is linked to heterochromatin packing density [20]. Our data corroborate previous findings that significant up-regulation of Ki-67 expression often down-regulates the DNA-replication in cancer cells [21]. Cancer treatment selects for Ki67− dormant cells, and at the same time, induces both apoptosis and tumor dormancy in Ki67+ tumor cells, resulting in an increased number of Ki67− and Ki67 low dormant cells [30]. Since SA-β-Gal activity can be found in both senescent and quiescent cells, in the present study we could not specify the precise dormancy phenotype of our GBM cell lines, albeit it warrants further investigation.

One of the hallmarks of the activation of cellular senescence is the secretion of a plethora of cytokines, chemokines, and growth factors, which is referred to as SASP [31]. It was demonstrated that oncogene-induced senescence acted to induce senescence in human primary melanocytes through an autocrine/paracrine fashion primarily by the secretion of IGFBP7 [32]. A senescent cell bystander effect was illustrated by Nelson et al., in which replicative senescent fibroblasts induce senescence in young fibroblasts in vitro through junction-mediated cell-cell contact [33]. Later on, it was shown that the senescence phenotype can be transmitted in a paracrine manner from fibroblasts undergoing oncogene-induced senescence to normal human fibroblasts and that the transmitted phenotype is stable [34]. In the present study, we observed that long-term culturing of cells alleviates SASP phenotype enabling induction of senescence marker in short-term cultured U87L cells (Figure 5b). The last, not least, our findings might have important clinical implications. The recent discovery that senescent tumor cells induce a bigger immune response than dead cancer cells [5] suggests that a potential senescent cell cancer vaccine could show promise. It is possible to develop new therapeutic strategies to combine priming (immunization) with IR-induced senescent patient-derived cancer cells with IR treatments [14].

Moreover, other recent studies have also shown that in situ-induced senescent cancer cells cause the adaptive immune system to become active. These cells can be caused by either GATA6 [35] or ZNF24 [12,13] ectopic expressions. Alternatively, cancer cell senescence can be alleviated by HMGCR inhibitor statins [36]. This offers a new strategy for the treatment of pancreatic cancer by suppression of up-stream TFCP2 signaling and induction of senescence.

Now, the question of how senescent cells interact with the adaptive immune system has become a subject of intensive studies. The immune system activation includes dendritic cells and CD8 T-cells recruited by senescent cancer cells producing SASP [37]. These effects were supplemented by inducing the processing and presentation of MHC-I antigens elicited by either X-ray irradiation [38] or doxorubicin [5]. Moreover, senescence related-genes controlling immune cell infiltration of senescence will produce a tumor microenvironment and responses to immune checkpoint blockage (ICB) as a lung cancer therapy [11].

While the evidence for passage number-related effects on malignant primary cells or cell lines is compelling, much less is known about how the changes affect safety and SASP, both of which are needed for the senescence cell-based vaccine to be effective against cancer. In this regard, with some assumptions and reservations, it is possible to consider the U87H cell line as an "aging" subline of U87L cells. Then, short-term cultured U87L cells demonstrated higher reproductive survival compared to their isogenic "aged" counterpart after X-ray radiation exposure. Thus, long-term cultivated GBM cells possess the safest phenotype: highest sensitivity to IR and constitutive highest SASP, while having the lowest self-renewal capacities. Our data provides novel molecular insights into a multistep process of post-radiation reproductive survival in GBM and can be exploited for age-related anti-cancer interventions in the treatment of GBM.

4. Materials and Methods

4.1. Cell Culture

The ATCC human U87 GBM cell lines were used in our study. U87 cell lines were cultured in DMEM (Gibco, Thermo Fisher Scientific, Waltham, MA, USA) supplemented with 10% FBS (BioloT, Saint Petersburg, Russia), 1% L-glutamine (Gibco, Grand Island, NY, USA), and 1% antibiotics (100 U/mL penicillin, 100 µg/mL streptomycin) (Sigma-Aldrich, St. Louis, MO, USA). U87L cell lines, which have undergone (up to 15 passages) after thawing and culturing of the original ampoule from ATCC, and the U87H cell lines, which have undergone long-term continuous cultivation (more than 3 years) were used. Cell lines were kept in a humidified atmosphere with 5% CO_2.

4.2. Irradiation

Cells were irradiated at room temperature in doses of 2 and 6 Gy using a 200 kV X-ray RUB RUST-M1 biological unit (Ruselectronics, Moscow, Russia). The dose rate was 0.85 Gy/min ± 10%.

4.3. Anchorage-Dependent Growth Assay

After reaching 70–80% confluence, the cells were exposed to X-ray radiation at doses of 2 and 6 Gy. Immediately after irradiation, control cells and cells irradiated at doses of 2 and 6 Gy were harvested using a 0.05% solution of trypsin-EDTA (PanEco, Moscow, Russia) and seeded on Petri dishes (60 mm in diameter) at concentrations of 5×10^2, 8×10^2 and 1×10^3 cells/dish, respectively. Then, Petri dishes were incubated at 37 °C in a humidified atmosphere with 5% CO_2 for 14 days to form colonies. After that, the culture medium was removed by aspiration from each dish, the cells were fixed with 100% methanol for 15 min at room temperature, followed by Giemsa staining for 15 min. Only colonies containing ≥ 50 individual cells were counted manually.

Plating Efficiency (PE) and Fraction of Cells, which form Colonies (FCC), were calculated using the following equations:

$$PE = \text{\# of colonies formed}/\text{\# of cells seeded} \times 100\% \quad (1)$$

$$FCC = \text{\# of colonies formed after irradiation}/[\text{\# of cells seeded} \times PE] \quad (2)$$

4.4. Soft Agar Clonogenic Assay

6-well plates were coated with 0.6% agar-agar (Sigma-Aldrich, St. Louis, MO, USA) pre-warmed to 43 °C in complete medium. Immediately after irradiation, cells were collected and cell concentrations were adjusted to 5×10^2, 8×10^2 and 1×10^3 cells/mL. Cell/0.3% noble agar mixtures were added into each well and allowed to solidify for another 30 min at room temperature before placing into a 37 °C humidified cell culture incubator. Three weeks later, colonies were stained with 5% Crystal Violet solution and their number was counted manually.

4.5. AlamarBlue Cell Viability Assay in Soft Agar

100 µL of 0.3% agar-agar in growth medium was added to a 96-well microculture plate (Sigma-Aldrich, TPP Zellkultur. Testplatte, Trazadingen, Switzerland) and left to solidify at room temperature for 30 min. Immediately after irradiation, cell suspensions were gently mixed with 0.2% agar-agar preheated on water at 43 °C. The final concentration of cells per well was 6×10^2 cells/100 µL. Immediately after solidification, 50 µL of 0.3% agar-agar in growth medium was added to each well as a feeding layer and allowed to solidify for 30 min at room temperature. Cells were incubated under standard CO_2 incubator conditions (5% CO_2, 37 C) for 7 days, after which 10% AlamarBlue reagent (Invitrogen, Frederick, MD, USA) was added to each well and cells were incubated for 2 h at 5% CO_2 and 37 °C. The fluorescence of the AlamarBlue reagent was determined using a CLARIOstar instrument (BMG LABTECH, Ortenberg, Germany) at excitation/emission wavelengths of

530/590 nm. The obtained data were processed using the MARS data analysis software (BMG LABTECH, Ortenberg, Germany).

4.6. Wright-Giemsa Staining and Analysis of MGCCs

Cells were cultured in a 96-well plate (Sigma-Aldrich, TPP Zellkultur. Testplatte, Trazadingen, Switzerland) at a concentration of 5×10^3 cells/0.32 cm^2. 24 h after irradiation, the cells were fixed with absolute methanol for 5 min, after which they were stained using Wright-Giemsa solution diluted 1:10 in 1X PBS (pH 6.6) for 1 h, followed by washing with 1X PBS (pH 6.6) and distilled water. The average number of MGCCs was calculated in five microscopic fields of view at ×100 magnification.

4.7. Senescence Associated β Galactosidase Assay (SA-β-Gal)

Detection of the activity of aging-associated beta-galactosidase (SA-β-Gal) (a marker of the cellular senescence phenotype) was performed using a commercial cell senescence assay kit (EMD Millipore KAA002, CA, USA). The presence of the β-Gal enzyme in cells is determined by the characteristic green staining of the cytoplasm. The cells were stained according to supplemented manufacturer protocol with the following modification: at the final 1X PBS washing step, the cell nuclei were stained with 1 μg/mL Hoechst 33342 (Thermo Scientific, Rockford, IL, USA). Such modification significantly improves the quality of counting of SA-β-Gal-negative cells [39,40]. The stained cells were visualized using an EVOS® FL Auto Imaging System (Fisher Scientific, Pittsburgh, PA, USA) with 20× objective. The proportion of SA-β-Gal-positive cells was calculated manually.

4.8. Click-iT™ EdU Alexa Fluor 488 (Cell Proliferation Assay)

The Click-iT™ EdU Alexa Fluor 488 Imaging kit (Invitrogen, Thermo Fisher Scientific, Waltham, MA, USA) was used to assess cell proliferation. Cells were visualized using an ImageXpress Micro XL automated digital imaging and High Content imaging and Analysis system (Molecular Devices LLC, San Jose, CA, USA).

4.9. Immunofluorescence Analysis of Ki-67

Cells (at a concentration of 2×10^3 cells/0.05 cm^2) were seeded in a 384-well plate for 24 h. Then, cells were washed briefly in 1X PBS (pH 7.4) and fixed with 4% formaldehyde for 15 min, followed by 3 rinses in 1X PBS (pH 7.4). After blocking cells with 6% BSA (bovine serum albumin) in 1X PBS (pH 7.4) for 1 h at room temperature, cells were incubated with mouse monoclonal Ki-67 antibody (5 μg/mL, clone Ki-S5, Sigma-Aldrich, Darmstadt, Germany) diluted in 1X PBS with 1% BSA and 0.3% TritonX-100 for 1 h at room temperature. After 3 rinses in PBS, cells were incubated for 1 h at room temperature with Alexa Fluor 555 goat Anti-mouse secondary antibody (1:500, Merck-Millipore, Burlington, VT, USA) diluted in 1X PBS with 1% BSA and 0.3% Triton X-100. Nuclei were counterstained with Hoechst 33342 Solution (dilution 6 μg/mL, Thermo Scientific, Rockford, IL, USA). Cells were imaged and inner integrated fluorescence intensities of cells were calculated using the ImageXpress XL fluorescence microscopy (Molecular Devices LLC, San Jose, CA, USA).

4.10. Conditioned Medium Experiment

U87H and U87L cells were cultured in T25 flasks with 2×10^6 cells in each and incubated at 37 °C and 5% CO$_2$. The conditioned medium from each flask was collected on the 4th day of incubation and centrifuged at 3000× g for 10 min; then, without collecting any debris from the bottom of the tubes, the conditioned medium from each flask was filtered through 0.22 mm filter and diluted in 1:4 ratio with fresh DMEM medium. U87L cells were later cultured in 6 repeats with the conditioned medium form U87H cells and 6 repeats with the conditioned medium from U87L cells into 96-well plate with seeding density of 3125 cell/cm^2. After 3 days of incubation SA-β-Gal assay was performed.

4.11. Statistical Analysis

Statistical data processing was carried out using statistical software GraphPad Prism 9.0.2.161 (GraphPad Software, San Diego, CA, USA) and EXCEL 2010 Software (Microsoft, Redmond, WA, USA). Data presented as means ± SEM. Significance levels are marked with asterisks: * $p < 0.05$, ** $p < 0.01$, *** $p < 0.001$, **** $p < 0.0001$, ***** $p < 0.00001$.

Author Contributions: Conceptualization, S.L.; methodology, S.L. and A.N.O.; formal analysis, L.A. and Z.N.; irradiation, clonogenic tests, AlamarBlue test, EdU test and ki-67 test, L.A.; MGCCs test and SA-β-Gal test, L.A. and Z.N.; conditioned medium experiment, Z.N.; visualization, L.A. and Z.N.; writing—original draft preparation, L.A.; writing—review and editing, S.L., M.P. and A.N.O.; supervision, S.L. All authors have read and agreed to the published version of the manuscript.

Funding: The studies were supported by Priority 2030 Strategic Academic Leadership Program project # 075-02-2021-1316.

Institutional Review Board Statement: Not applicable.

Informed Consent Statement: Not applicable.

Data Availability Statement: Not applicable.

Conflicts of Interest: The authors declare no conflict of interest.

References

1. Jeon, H.Y.; Kim, J.K.; Ham, S.W.; Oh, S.Y.; Kim, J.; Park, J.B.; Lee, J.Y.; Kim, S.C.; Kim, H. Irradiation induces glioblastoma cell senescence and senescence-associated secretory phenotype. *Tumour Biol.* **2016**, *37*, 5857–5867. [CrossRef]
2. Villa, S.; Balana, C.; Comas, S. Radiation and concomitant chemotherapy for patients with glioblastoma multiforme. *Chin. J. Cancer* **2014**, *33*, 25–31. [CrossRef]
3. Mann, J.; Ramakrishna, R.; Magge, R.; Wernicke, A.G. Advances in Radiotherapy for Glioblastoma. *Front. Neurol.* **2017**, *8*, 748. [CrossRef] [PubMed]
4. Serrano, M.; Lin, A.W.; McCurrach, M.E.; Beach, D.; Lowe, S.W. Oncogenic ras provokes premature cell senescence associated with accumulation of p53 and p16INK4a. *Cell* **1997**, *88*, 593–602. [CrossRef] [PubMed]
5. Marin, I.; Boix, O.; Garcia-Garijo, A.; Sirois, I.; Caballe, A.; Zarzuela, E.; Ruano, I.; Stephan-Otto Attolini, C.; Prats, N.; Lopez-Dominguez, J.A.; et al. Cellular senescence is immunogenic and promotes anti-tumor immunity. *Cancer Discov.* **2022**. [CrossRef] [PubMed]
6. Hynds, R.E.; Vladimirou, E.; Janes, S.M. The secret lives of cancer cell lines. *Dis. Model Mech.* **2018**, *11*, dmm037366. [CrossRef] [PubMed]
7. Gu, H.; Wu, X.Y.; Fan, R.T.; Wang, X.; Guo, Y.Z.; Wang, R. Side population cells from long-term passage non-small cell lung cancer cells display loss of cancer stem cell-like properties and chemoradioresistance. *Oncol. Lett.* **2016**, *12*, 2886–2393. [CrossRef] [PubMed]
8. Herranz, N.; Gil, J. Mechanisms and functions of cellular senescence. *J. Clin. Investig.* **2018**, *128*, 1238–1246. [CrossRef]
9. Wang, L.; Lankhorst, L.; Bernards, R. Exploiting senescence for the treatment of cancer. *Nat. Rev. Cancer* **2022**, *22*, 340–355. [CrossRef]
10. Ruhland, M.K.; Loza, A.J.; Capietto, A.H.; Luo, X.; Knolhoff, B.L.; Flanagan, K.C.; Belt, B.A.; Alspach, E.; Leahy, K.; Luo, J.; et al. Stromal senescence establishes an immunosuppressive microenvironment that drives tumorigenesis. *Nat. Commun.* **2016**, *7*, 11762. [CrossRef]
11. Hu, X.; Guo, L.; Liu, G.; Dai, Z.; Wang, L.; Zhang, J.; Wang, J. Novel cellular senescence-related risk model identified as the prognostic biomarkers for lung squamous cell carcinoma. *Front. Oncol.* **2022**, *12*, 997702. [CrossRef] [PubMed]
12. Xiong, J.; Jiang, P.; Zhong, L.; Wang, Y. The Novel Tumor Suppressor Gene ZNF24 Induces THCA Cells Senescence by Regulating Wnt Signaling Pathway, Resulting in Inhibition of THCA Tumorigenesis and Invasion. *Front. Oncol.* **2021**, *11*, 646511. [CrossRef] [PubMed]
13. Pang, B.; Wang, Y.; Chang, X. A Novel Tumor Suppressor Gene, ZNF24, Inhibits the Development of NSCLC by Inhibiting the WNT Signaling Pathway to Induce Cell Senescence. *Front. Oncol.* **2021**, *11*, 664369. [CrossRef]
14. Meng, Y.; Efimova, E.V.; Hamzeh, K.W.; Darga, T.E.; Mauceri, H.J.; Fu, Y.X.; Kron, S.J.; Weichselbaum, R.R. Radiation-inducible immunotherapy for cancer: Senescent tumor cells as a cancer vaccine. *Mol. Ther.* **2012**, *20*, 1046–1055. [CrossRef]
15. Franken, N.A.; Rodermond, H.M.; Stap, J.; Haveman, J.; van Bree, C. Clonogenic assay of cells in vitro. *Nat. Protoc.* **2006**, *1*, 2315–2319. [CrossRef] [PubMed]
16. Borowicz, S.; Van Scoyk, M.; Avasarala, S.; Karuppusamy Rathinam, M.K.; Tauler, J.; Bikkavilli, R.K.; Winn, R.A. The soft agar colony formation assay. *J. Vis. Exp.* **2014**, *92*, e51998. [CrossRef]
17. Rampersad, S.N. Multiple applications of Alamar Blue as an indicator of metabolic function and cellular health in cell viability bioassays. *Sensors* **2012**, *12*, 12347–12360. [CrossRef]

18. Kim, M.; Ladomersky, E.; Mozny, A.; Kocherginsky, M.; O'Shea, K.; Reinstein, Z.Z.; Zhai, L.; Bell, A.; Lauing, K.L.; Bollu, L.; et al. Glioblastoma as an age-related neurological disorder in adults. *Neurooncol. Adv.* **2021**, *3*, vdab125. [CrossRef]
19. Mirzayans, R.; Andrais, B.; Murray, D. Roles of Polyploid/Multinucleated Giant Cancer Cells in Metastasis and Disease Relapse Following Anticancer Treatment. *Cancers* **2018**, *10*, 118. [CrossRef]
20. Mrouj, K.; Andres-Sanchez, N.; Dubra, G.; Singh, P.; Sobecki, M.; Chahar, D.; Al Ghoul, E.; Aznar, A.B.; Prieto, S.; Pirot, N.; et al. Ki-67 regulates global gene expression and promotes sequential stages of carcinogenesis. *Proc. Natl. Acad. Sci. USA* **2021**, *118*, e2026507118. [CrossRef]
21. Sobecki, M.; Mrouj, K.; Camasses, A.; Parisis, N.; Nicolas, E.; Lleres, D.; Gerbe, F.; Prieto, S.; Krasinska, L.; David, A.; et al. The cell proliferation antigen Ki-67 organises heterochromatin. *eLife* **2016**, *5*, e13722. [CrossRef] [PubMed]
22. Cuollo, L.; Antonangeli, F.; Santoni, A.; Soriani, A. The Senescence-Associated Secretory Phenotype (SASP) in the Challenging Future of Cancer Therapy and Age-Related Diseases. *Biology* **2020**, *9*, 485. [CrossRef] [PubMed]
23. Ostrom, Q.T.; Patil, N.; Cioffi, G.; Waite, K.; Kruchko, C.; Barnholtz-Sloan, J.S. CBTRUS Statistical Report: Primary Brain and Other Central Nervous System Tumors Diagnosed in the United States in 2013–2017. *Neuro-Oncology* **2020**, *22*, iv1–iv96. [CrossRef] [PubMed]
24. Ostrom, Q.T.; Gittleman, H.; Truitt, G.; Boscia, A.; Kruchko, C.; Barnholtz-Sloan, J.S. CBTRUS Statistical Report: Primary Brain and Other Central Nervous System Tumors Diagnosed in the United States in 2011–2015. *Neuro-Oncology* **2018**, *20*, iv1–iv86. [CrossRef]
25. Zhang, Z.; Feng, X.; Deng, Z.; Cheng, J.; Wang, Y.; Zhao, M.; Zhao, Y.; He, S.; Huang, Q. Irradiation-induced polyploid giant cancer cells are involved in tumor cell repopulation via neosis. *Mol. Oncol.* **2021**, *15*, 2219–2234. [CrossRef]
26. Kim, Y.N.; Koo, K.H.; Sung, J.Y.; Yun, U.J.; Kim, H. Anoikis resistance: An essential prerequisite for tumor metastasis. *Int. J. Cell Biol.* **2012**, *2012*, 306879. [CrossRef]
27. Li, Z.; Fan, L.; Wu, Y.; Niu, Y.; Zhang, X.; Wang, B.; Yao, Y.; Chen, C.; Qi, N.; Wang, D.D.; et al. Analysis of the prognostic role and biological characteristics of circulating tumor cell-associated white blood cell clusters in non-small cell lung cancer. *J. Thorac. Dis.* **2022**, *14*, 1544–1555. [CrossRef]
28. Kaur, E.; Rajendra, J.; Jadhav, S.; Shridhar, E.; Goda, J.S.; Moiyadi, A.; Dutt, S. Radiation-induced homotypic cell fusions of innately resistant glioblastoma cells mediate their sustained survival and recurrence. *Carcinogenesis* **2015**, *36*, 685–695. [CrossRef]
29. Gao, X.L.; Zhang, M.; Tang, Y.L.; Liang, X.H. Cancer cell dormancy: Mechanisms and implications of cancer recurrence and metastasis. *Onco Targets Ther.* **2017**, *10*, 5219–5228. [CrossRef]
30. Manjili, M.H. The premise of personalized immunotherapy for cancer dormancy. *Oncogene* **2020**, *39*, 4323–4330. [CrossRef]
31. Gonzalez-Meljem, J.M.; Apps, J.R.; Fraser, H.C.; Martinez-Barbera, J.P. Paracrine roles of cellular senescence in promoting tumourigenesis. *Br. J. Cancer* **2018**, *118*, 1283–1288. [CrossRef]
32. Wajapeyee, N.; Serra, R.W.; Zhu, X.; Mahalingam, M.; Green, M.R. Oncogenic BRAF induces senescence and apoptosis through pathways mediated by the secreted protein IGFBP7. *Cell* **2008**, *132*, 363–374. [CrossRef]
33. Nelson, G.; Wordsworth, J.; Wang, C.; Jurk, D.; Lawless, C.; Martin-Ruiz, C.; von Zglinicki, T. A senescent cell bystander effect: Senescence-induced senescence. *Aging Cell* **2012**, *11*, 345–349. [CrossRef]
34. Acosta, J.C.; Banito, A.; Wuestefeld, T.; Georgilis, A.; Janich, P.; Morton, J.P.; Athineos, D.; Kang, T.W.; Lasitschka, F.; Andrulis, M.; et al. A complex secretory program orchestrated by the inflammasome controls paracrine senescence. *Nat. Cell Biol.* **2013**, *15*, 978–990. [CrossRef]
35. Chen, W.; Chen, Z.; Zhang, M.; Tian, Y.; Liu, L.; Lan, R.; Zeng, G.; Fu, X.; Ru, G.; Liu, W.; et al. GATA6 Exerts Potent Lung Cancer Suppressive Function by Inducing Cell Senescence. *Front. Oncol.* **2020**, *10*, 824. [CrossRef]
36. Zhang, D.; Lu, P.; Zhu, K.; Wu, H.; Dai, Y. TFCP2 Overcomes Senescence by Cooperating with SREBP2 to Activate Cholesterol Synthesis in Pancreatic Cancer. *Front. Oncol.* **2021**, *11*, 724437. [CrossRef]
37. Kang, T.W.; Yevsa, T.; Woller, N.; Hoenicke, L.; Wuestefeld, T.; Dauch, D.; Hohmeyer, A.; Gereke, M.; Rudalska, R.; Potapova, A.; et al. Senescence surveillance of pre-malignant hepatocytes limits liver cancer development. *Nature* **2011**, *479*, 547–551. [CrossRef]
38. Reits, E.A.; Hodge, J.W.; Herberts, C.A.; Groothuis, T.A.; Chakraborty, M.; Wansley, E.K.; Camphausen, K.; Luiten, R.M.; de Ru, A.H.; Neijssen, J.; et al. Radiation modulates the peptide repertoire, enhances MHC class I expression, and induces successful antitumor immunotherapy. *J. Exp. Med.* **2006**, *203*, 1259–1271. [CrossRef]
39. Zorin, V.; Zorina, A.; Smetanina, N.; Kopnin, P.; Ozerov, I.V.; Leonov, S.; Isaev, A.; Klokov, D.; Osipov, A.N. Diffuse colonies of human skin fibroblasts in relation to cellular senescence and proliferation. *Aging* **2017**, *9*, 1404–1413. [CrossRef]
40. Pustovalova, M.; Astrelina, T.A.; Grekhova, A.; Vorobyeva, N.; Tsvetkova, A.; Blokhina, T.; Nikitina, V.; Suchkova, Y.; Usupzhanova, D.; Brunchukov, V.; et al. Residual gammaH2AX foci induced by low dose X-ray radiation in bone marrow mesenchymal stem cells do not cause accelerated senescence in the progeny of irradiated cells. *Aging* **2017**, *9*, 2397–2410. [CrossRef]

Disclaimer/Publisher's Note: The statements, opinions and data contained in all publications are solely those of the individual author(s) and contributor(s) and not of MDPI and/or the editor(s). MDPI and/or the editor(s) disclaim responsibility for any injury to people or property resulting from any ideas, methods, instructions or products referred to in the content.

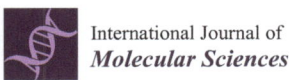

Article

Clustered DNA Damage Patterns after Proton Therapy Beam Irradiation Using Plasmid DNA

Maria P. Souli [1,2], Zacharenia Nikitaki [1,2], Monika Puchalska [1], Kateřina Pachnerová Brabcová [3], Ellas Spyratou [4], Panagiotis Kote [2], Efstathios P. Efstathopoulos [4], Megumi Hada [5], Alexandros G. Georgakilas [2,*] and Lembit Sihver [1,3,*]

1. Atominstitut, Technische Universität Wien, 1020 Vienna, Austria
2. DNA Damage Laboratory, Physics Department, School of Applied Mathematical and Physical Sciences, National Technical University of Athens, 15780 Athens, Greece
3. Nuclear Physics Institute, Czech Academy of Sciences, Na Truhlářce 39/64, 180 86 Prague, Czech Republic
4. 2nd Department of Radiology, Medical School, National and Kapodistrian University of Athens, 11517 Athens, Greece
5. Radiation Institute for Science & Engineering, Prairie View A&M University, Prairie View, TX 77446, USA
* Correspondence: alexg@mail.ntua.gr (A.G.G.); lembit.sihver@tuwien.ac.at (L.S.)

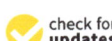

Citation: Souli, M.P.; Nikitaki, Z.; Puchalska, M.; Brabcová, K.P.; Spyratou, E.; Kote, P.; Efstathopoulos, E.P.; Hada, M.; Georgakilas, A.G.; Sihver, L. Clustered DNA Damage Patterns after Proton Therapy Beam Irradiation Using Plasmid DNA. *Int. J. Mol. Sci.* **2022**, *23*, 15606. https://doi.org/10.3390/ijms232415606

Academic Editor: François Chevalier

Received: 13 October 2022
Accepted: 6 December 2022
Published: 9 December 2022

Publisher's Note: MDPI stays neutral with regard to jurisdictional claims in published maps and institutional affiliations.

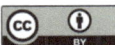

Copyright: © 2022 by the authors. Licensee MDPI, Basel, Switzerland. This article is an open access article distributed under the terms and conditions of the Creative Commons Attribution (CC BY) license (https://creativecommons.org/licenses/by/4.0/).

Abstract: Modeling ionizing radiation interaction with biological matter is a major scientific challenge, especially for protons that are nowadays widely used in cancer treatment. That presupposes a sound understanding of the mechanisms that take place from the early events of the induction of DNA damage. Herein, we present results of irradiation-induced complex DNA damage measurements using plasmid pBR322 along a typical Proton Treatment Plan at the MedAustron proton and carbon beam therapy facility (energy 137–198 MeV and Linear Energy Transfer (LET) range 1–9 keV/μm), by means of Agarose Gel Electrophoresis and DNA fragmentation using Atomic Force Microscopy (AFM). The induction rate $Mbp^{-1} Gy^{-1}$ for each type of damage, single strand breaks (SSBs), double-strand breaks (DSBs), base lesions and non-DSB clusters was measured after irradiations in solutions with varying scavenging capacity containing 2-amino-2-(hydroxymethyl)propane-1,3-diol (Tris) and coumarin-3-carboxylic acid (C3CA) as scavengers. Our combined results reveal the determining role of LET and Reactive Oxygen Species (ROS) in DNA fragmentation. Furthermore, AFM used to measure apparent DNA lengths provided us with insights into the role of increasing LET in the induction of highly complex DNA damage.

Keywords: proton therapy beam; clustered DNA damage; linear energy transfer (LET); Agarose Gel Electrophoresis (AGE); Atomic Force Microscopy (AFM); damage biomarkers; scavenging capacity; biodosimetry

1. Introduction

The radiobiological and physical advantages of highly energetic proton beam therapy result in a ground-gaining field over several types of photon radiotherapy, with many proton treatment facilities—in operation or under construction—around the world. Proton beams transverse biological matter depositing a small amount of energy along the track with a low entrance dose but releasing most of their energy just before they stop at a well-defined space range called Bragg Peak. At the distal fall-off of this peak, the energy deposition stops rapidly. This property is employed in treatment planning systems to design different beam combinations that produce wider peaks, called Spread-Out Bragg Peaks (SOBP), with the desired geometrical characteristics of the tumor volume to be treated. This allows the irradiation of cancers with complicated volumes and/or close to radiosensitive organs while minimizing normal tissue complications and dose to organs at risk.

The excellent dose distribution is the utmost asset of proton beam therapy compared to photon-based modalities, with relative biological effectiveness (RBE) values slightly higher than 1 (1.1–1.4) [1]. For many tumor types, this can reduce radiation-induced long- and short-term side effects in the patients. This is important, especially in reducing the risks of secondary cancer in pediatric cancer treatment.

The most critical target for radiation-induced damage inside a cell is DNA. Ionizing radiation (IR) is known to cause many different lesions in the DNA molecule: single-strand breaks (SSB), double-strand breaks (DSB), base oxidations, abasic sites and DNA protein crosslinks [2]. When these lesions are not randomly distributed along the DNA helix within the cell nucleus volume but are located within an area of 10–20 base pairs of DNA length (few nm), it is defined as complex or clustered DNA damage, which is more complicated and difficult to repair than SSB. These clustered lesions are considered to be responsible for cell death and mutations [3,4]. The DNA repair efficiency in such cases depends on the location, types and number of lesions accumulated in close proximity [5,6]. Although clustered damages are linked to higher cell lethality and mutagenic potential [7], the stochastic formation perplexes its investigation.

Results in experimental radiobiology underline the direct relationship between clustered DNA damage and the interactions of IR with biological matter, especially the ionization cascades created along the tracks inside the target. Linear Energy Transfer (LET)-oriented studies shows, in most cases, an increased amount of clustered damage with increasing LET, leading to increased DNA fragmentation [8–13]. Monte Carlo simulations and multiscale mathematical approaches also agree with these results and suggest that LET (or, more exactly, the ionization density) plays a major role in determining the biological effects [6,14–16]. Therefore, there is a great need for DNA damage biomarkers for a better understanding of the normal tissue damage in proton and particle therapy beams and a deeper understanding of the mechanisms leading to either cell death or other effects [17]. RBE greater than unity is generally accepted to reflect the increased complexity of DNA damage induced by charged particles [1,18]. Several published studies underline the importance of DNA damage experiments using a variety of biological systems (plasmids, mammalian DNA and cells) to help us better understand the intriguing biological responses triggered by particles like protons or carbons [19].

The energy of the IR can either be deposited on the DNA macromolecule or the aqueous environment that surrounds DNA. As a result, DNA damage may occur either due to direct ionization or excitation of the molecule or due to indirect interaction with energetic electrons and products like Reactive Oxygen Species (ROS), created by radiolysis of water, which in their turn react directly/indirectly with the DNA [20,21]. This oxidative environment enhances the probability of induction of non-DSB clusters, often called OCDLs (Oxidative Clustered DNA Lesions) [22]. By adding scavengers in the aqueous environment before irradiation, the production of some of the reactants is eliminated, blocking the subsequent chain reaction and deactivating ROS. The type and the induction rate of DNA damage also depend on the free radical generation, scavenger concentration and DNA characteristics [20,23]. In the presence of radiation, the probability of radiolysis is quite high since water is the most abundant cell component.

The present work is a bottom-up approach to studying DNA damage, primarily induced by proton therapy beams, by employing a system of plasmid DNA in an aqueous solution. This is a simplified model, excluding cell response factors and when irradiated, it becomes a radiation damage detector. DNA molecules of full and known length in supercoiled (SC) form are vitiated by irradiation to a different extent according to radiation parameters and turn to circular (C), linear (L) and fragmented (F) forms. These forms can be detected by rapid electrophoretic methods, easily quantified and translated into a number of strand breaks. On the contrary, the number of short fragments of DNA is more arduous to define and leads to an apparent complex damage decrease, probably due to underestimation. The number of short fragments can either be estimated through mathematical models or by employing more radical molecule visualization methods. The first method used in this study was Agarose Gel Electrophoresis (AGE) combined with the Cowan Model, a "traditional" estimation created to describe plasmid forms transitions and DNA breaks formation, while a second supplementary method used Atomic Force Microscopy (AFM), which could be a powerful but demanding method to detect fragments down to 20 nm long (60 bps) [24–26].

Indirect damage through free radicals has been investigated by the addition of Tris and C3CA ROS-scavengers in the initial plasmid solution before irradiation as a radioprotectant. Tris is a common buffer scavenging solution that generally protects from DNA denaturation and free radical attack. C3CA is a coumarin derivative, and coumarins show high biological activity and low toxicity and are commonly used components in cancer treatment (prostate and renal cancer and leukemia) since they have the ability to counteract the side effects of radiotherapy [27].

2. Results and Discussion
2.1. AGE

The DNA electrophoresis adaptation in this study reveals an easily identified transition between SC, C and L forms of DNA which follows the dose increment and increased fragmentation (Figure 1a). In general, one expects that as the dose increases, the intact SC form is dramatically reduced, i.e., within the first 10 Gy. Of course, this phenomenon is also dependent on the scavenging capacity of the solution, plasmid type and water content, radiation quality and energies of the particles [28]. Simultaneously, the increasing dose of IR produces more breaks recorded as C and L bands (top and middle bands equivalently inside the gel). C is dominant for the first 10 Gy, while the linear DNA production rate (DSB formation) increases after the saturation point of the circular (Figure 1b). For doses higher than 10 Gy, the presence of the SC form is less than 1% and what we detect is the further breakage of C and L plasmid, producing gradually smaller fragments, leading to the formation of smear in the Agarose Gel Electrophoresis (AGE) gels.

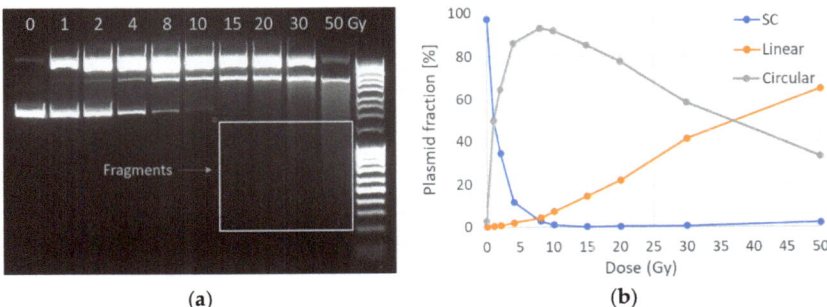

Figure 1. Electrophoretic plasmid analysis: (**a**) gel image of plasmid form transition for 10 different doses from 0 to 50 Gy with DNA ladder also included (right column). The original image has been slightly enhanced by increasing intensity in order to reveal low-intensity bands (small fragments) but not altered in other editing ways; SC, C and L are separated as expected due to their different DNA molecule mobility in the field. The image presented was oversaturated in order to visualize the fragments (smear in the last lanes). (**b**) Three plasmid forms transition with increasing dose as quantified according to gel band intensity.

The above pattern is also followed for samples containing the ROS radioprotectants (scavengers) Tris and C3CA. As shown in Figure 2, an increase in scavengers' concentration results in an overall decrease in SSB formation (which is mainly due to ROS attack). Figure 2a presents proton (entrance)-induced damage detected as the decrease of SC fraction with a dose for different Tris scavenging capacities, from no scavenging (10^5 s^{-1} of residual Tris) to 10^8 s^{-1}, revealing radioprotection of the plasmid integrity up to 90%.

This also proves that a significant amount of the DNA damage is not caused by the initial particle-target interactions, as the most amount of breaks on SC is caused by water radiolysis products. In Figure 2b, the SSB Mbp^{-1} Gy^{-1} versus scavenging capacity for Tris and C3CA for protons 198 MeV at the entrance of the beam proves that both scavengers protect DNA from ROS-mediated fragmentation in a concentration-dependent manner from 55% to 98%.

Table 1. Irradiation parameters along the therapeutic proton SOBP.

Irradiation Position	Depth in PMMA (cm)	LET (keV/μm)	Energy Range (MeV)
A—beam entrance	2	1	198
B—plateau of SOBP	15	3	137–167
C—tail of SOBP	16.8	9	137–167

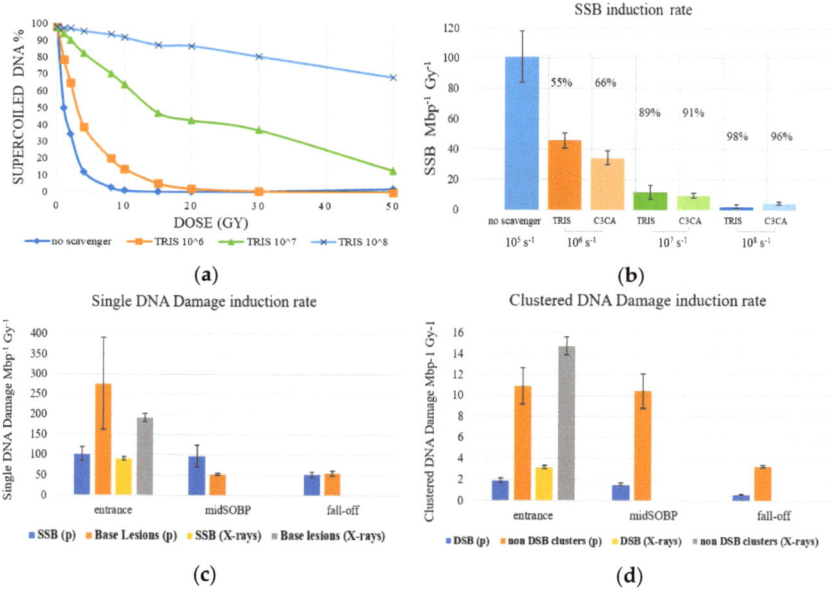

Figure 2. Proton (p) and X-rays−induced DNA damage. (**a**) Proton (entrance)−induced damage revealed as the decrease of SC plasmid with dose for Tris scavenging capacity ranging from no scavenging (10^5 s^{-1} of residual Tris) to 10^8 s^{-1}, revealing the radioprotectant shielding of the plasmid integrity (up to 90%) the highest Tris concentration. (**b**) SSB Mbp^{-1} Gy^{-1} versus scavenging capacity for Tris and C3CA for 198 MeV protons at the entrance of the beam proves concentration-dependent manner. (**c**) Average number of SSB and single base lesions produced along the Proton Treatment Plan or X-rays, respectively. (**d**) Average number of DSB and non−DSB clustered damage produced along the Proton Treatment Plan or X-rays. The positions are the entrance of the beam, the middle of the SOBP plateau (midSOBP) and SOBP fall-off, as seen in Figure 3 and Table 1.

The different positions along the treatment plan (Figure 3), and the subsequent relatively slight difference in LET values (Table 1), are also presented in Figure 2. Both strand breaks and base lesions (breaks deliberately created during post-irradiation treatment by restriction enzymes on sites of oxidized purines and pyrimidines) for protons and X-rays are grouped in SSB (Figure 2c) and DSB (Figure 2d) histograms. SSB is accompanied by a number of single base lesions (Figure 2c) that are 2.7 and 1.1 times the SSB value at beam entrance and SOBP fall-off. This no remarkably different pattern recorded in SSB along the beamline is overturned at the middle of the SOBP position, with base lesions being 0.5 times the SSB. Furthermore, SSB is 29–88 times more than DSB in each case, with the difference between entrance and SOBP within the error range for both SSB and DSB, probably due to similar LET values. Specifically, the mean rates of damage induction at the entrance of the proton beam are:

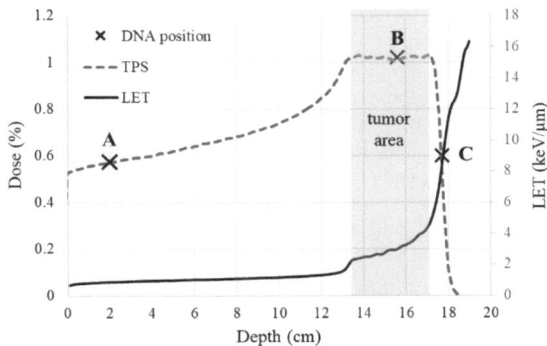

Figure 3. General treatment plan dose distribution: the % dose (dashed line) deposited when irradiating a volume of a hypothetical tumor of 4 cm thickness and approximately 13 cm under the skin (grey tumor area), as exported by TPS and the equivalent LET change over depth in water (solid line). The three positions of DNA irradiation (×) along the treatment plan are also marked: the beam entrance (A), the middle of SOBP plateau (B) and the SOBP fall-off (C).

101.101 ± 16.868 SSB Mbp^{-1}Gy^{-1}, 1.914 ± 0.247 DSB Mbp^{-1}Gy^{-1}, 275.852 ± 114.295 Base Lesions Mbp^{-1}Gy^{-1}, 10.908 ± 1.778 non-DSB Clusters Mbp^{-1}Gy^{-1}, and for the irradiation with X-rays at the same position we record 89.559 ± 4.490 SSB Mbp^{-1}Gy^{-1}, 3.147 ± 0.141 DSB Mbp^{-1}Gy^{-1}, 191.102 ± 10.867 Base Lesions Mbp^{-1}Gy^{-1}, 14.723 ± 0.856 non-DSB Clusters Mbp^{-1}Gy^{-1}. Figure 2d shows that clustered DNA damages produced by X-rays outnumber those created by proton beams at the entrance. This may originate from the very low LET for the protons in the entrance that is similar to that of X-rays (~1 keV/μm); therefore, no major differences are expected in general. Furthermore, the contribution of non-DSB oxidative damages in the clusters measured in the case of X-rays is expected to be high, translated into higher levels of clustered damage. Interestingly enough, previous studies [29–31] support the prevalence of oxidized base damages in the case of low-LET radiations such as X-rays. Considering that a percentage of these non-DSB lesions may almost instantly be converted to DSBs through the lyase/endonuclease enzymatic activity used in the present assays, then this may lead to higher levels of clusters as measured in the electrophoresis. Although clustering induced by X-rays appears to numerically exceed clustering produced by protons at the entrance of the beam, proton radiation is more efficient than X-rays, as evidenced by the ratio of non-DSB clusters to DSB for X-rays (4.7) being higher than that for protons (5.7).

At the middle of the SOBP plateau, the mean damage induction rate recorded is 96.012 ± 27.211 SSB Mbp^{-1}Gy^{-1}, 1.529 ± 0.169 DSB Mbp^{-1}Gy^{-1}, 52.085 ± 2.365 Base Lesions Mbp^{-1}Gy^{-1}, 10.415 ± 1.666 non-DSB Clusters Mbp^{-1}Gy^{-1}. At the fall-off of SOBP, where we expect to have higher LET values, the recorded damages were not greater as estimated by simulations for increased LET values but were not always verified by experimental studies [9]. This may have two interpretations. Considering the steep slope shift in LET and the dose distribution at the end of the beam trajectory (Figure 3), where LET increases abruptly but not critically, lower levels of DNA damage is an astounding proof of the successful use of protons for patient treatment since the healthy tissue area in very close proximity (within a few millimeters) of the tumor is only mildly stressed. Especially the low DSB and clustered damage levels, which are potentially lethal for a cell, imply a relatively safe cell environment. On the other hand, the apparent lower level of DSB and clustered damage recorded at the SOBP fall-off might be a result of underestimation of the damage due to the highly complex and fragmented DNA molecules, as also arises by AFM results. This is probably due to the limitations of the method since, in agarose gel electrophoresis, shorter DNA fragments may escape due to their higher mobility. The values of the mean damage induction rate recorded at the SOBP fall-off are 51.069 ± 6.923 SSB Mbp^{-1}Gy^{-1}, 0.579 ± 0.060 DSB Mbp^{-1}Gy^{-1}, 54.453 ± 6.350 Base Lesions Mbp^{-1}Gy^{-1}, 3.255 ± 0.092 non-DSB Clusters Mbp^{-1}Gy^{-1}.

Experimental results for different scavenging conditions are presented in Figure 4 and for all irradiation positions along the Proton Treatment Plan: proton beam entrance (LET = 1 keV/μm), middle of SOBP plateau (LET = 3 keV/μm) and SOBP fall-off (LET = 9 keV/μm), for Tris and C3CA radioprotectants in all three different values of scavenging capacity (10^6 s^{-1}, 10^7 s^{-1}, 10^8 s^{-1}) and 10^5 s^{-1} of residual TRIS (no scavenger). Overall, we detect a decrease in the induction of proton-induced DNA damage with increasing scavenging capacity of the solutions. Comparing reduction in damage levels, the general trend is that with increasing LET (from the entrance to mid-SOBP and fall-off), the dependency on the antioxidant concentration is reduced.

Figure 5a–d shows our experimental values together with the comparable literature data on the plasmid model. The numerical values of the present radiation conditions and the comparable literature data of the plasmid model can be found in Table 1 (Appendix A), accompanied by all critical radiation and sample parameters. For example, for DSBs in, the entrance reduction between 'no scavenger' to C3CA is ~76% falling to ~65% for the SOBP. Similarly, for non-DSB (base) clusters, from ~75% reduction (entrance), we go to ~60% for the SOBP region.

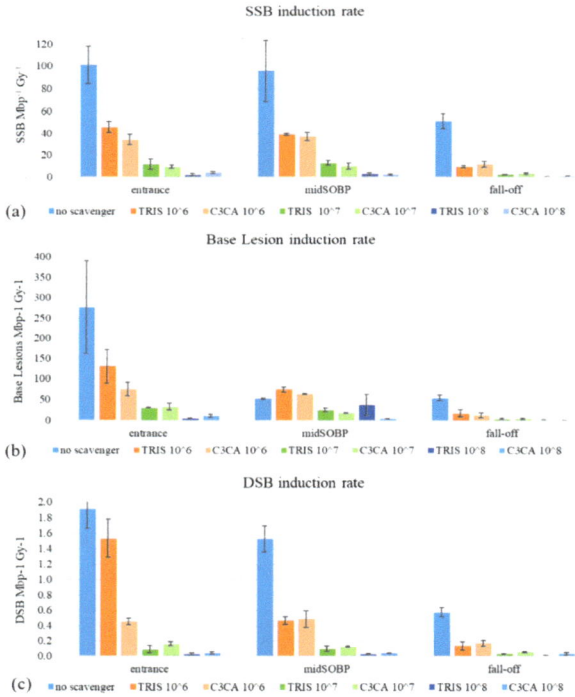

Figure 4. *Cont.*

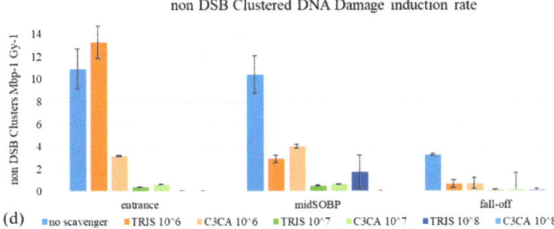

Figure 4. Proton-induced DNA damage: (**a**) Average number of SSB (SSB Mbp^{-1} Gy^{-1}), (**b**) DSB (DSB Mbp^{-1} Gy^{-1}), (**c**) Base Lesion and (**d**) non-DSB Clustered DNA damage induction rate versus increasing the scavenging capacity of Tris and C3CA scavengers (from 10^{-6} to 10^{-8} s^{-1}) for the three irradiation positions: the entrance of the beam (entrance), the middle of the SOBP plateau (midSOBP) and SOBP fall-off (fall-off).

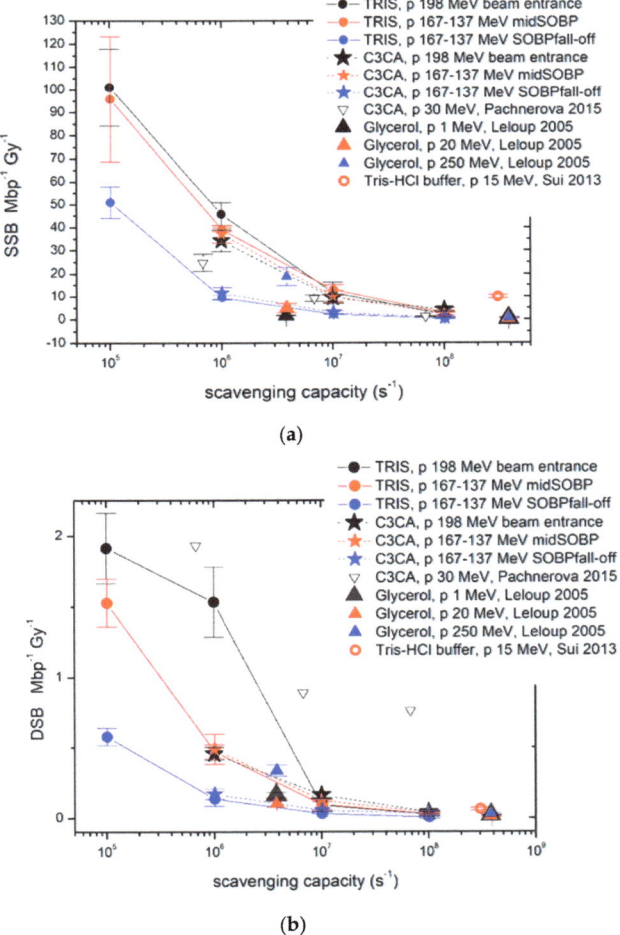

Figure 5. *Cont.*

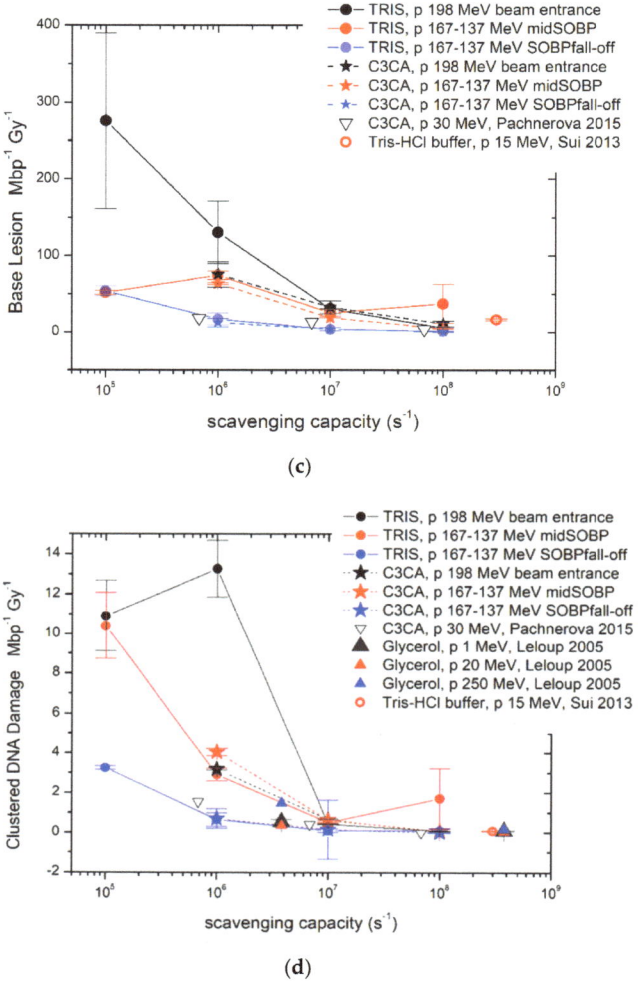

Figure 5. Proton (p)−induced damage yield (Mbp^{-1} Gy^{-1}) versus scavenging capacity (s^{-1}) as calculated in the present study for Tris and C3CA (lines are used as guides to the eyes) and literature values from studies using plasmid models with comparable proton energies and solution scavenging capacity. (**a**) SSB, (**b**) DSB, (**c**) Base Lesion, (**d**) Clustered DNA damage induction rates result from a variety of irradiation conditions, e.g., plasmid in solution or dried, different plasmid concentration and proton energy, details that can be found in Table 1. (see Refs. [28,32–34]).

In Figure 5, we have included cumulative data from different studies using protons of different energies and under different scavenging capacities. Closed circles correspond to the data from the present study, which are in good agreement with the literature data. One general comment is that when reviewing the data from other studies (Table 1), it can be seen that there is a great variety of values and, in some cases, disharmony between our experimental output and the others' data. Of course, as already explained above, these type of irradiation experiments depends on several physical and chemical parameters that may change the overall interaction of protons with DNA. A comparison with results within the scavenging range of the present study (Figure 5a–d) confirms the strong DNA damages elimination by scavengers depicted in Figure 4a–d. Although it is generally believed that 60–70% of the biological effects of low LET IR in mammalian cells are caused by indirect action [35,36], plasmid studies show larger proportions of indirect damage through more efficient scavenging. Plasmid studies testing scavenging high LET carbon ion-induced damage also report results implying 96% of the total SSB amount is attributed to indirect damage [37,38]. The aqueous nature of the plasmid solutions probably enhances such findings due to the high radiolysis probability.

By using the mean rate of DSB induction for protons and dividing by the DSB induction rate for X-rays at the entrance of the beam, we estimated an apparent RBE value of 0.61 at the entrance, 0.49 in the middle of the SOBP plateau and 0.18 at the SOBP fall-off. The reported [39] average RBE values for cell survival are 1.1 at the entrance, 1.15 in the center, 1.35 at the distal edge and up to 1.7 in the distal fall-off of the SOEP. These values are calculated with clonogenic cell survival as an endpoint. It is generally accepted that endpoints other than clonogenic survival produce such diverse results that do not allow to avoid the general statement that the RBE is, on average, in line with a value of ~1.1 [40]. RBE values of the present study are based on a simple DNA system of plasmid in an aqueous solution, which excludes the cell response and their repair mechanisms. This model serves well when the focus is on damage (excluding cell response and repair), and the presented RBE values should be considered as damage-calculated. Comparison with the literature values from cell survival would be unfair, first due to the different complexity of the systems and calculation methods, but also due to the fact that the generally accepted RBE values are under question, given the diversity of the results from different irradiation conditions like cell lines, dose and LET.

2.2. AFM

The results from the AFM length measurements are organized into histograms presenting length distributions in 50-nm-wide bins in the range of 0 to 1550 nm. The relative frequency of calibrated-from-pixel-to-length plasmid sizes was chosen to present and evaluate, and not show the apparent length, because of the variance in the number of evaluable molecules (N) on mica surfaces for each experimental condition. Figure 6 presents a typical topographic AFM image of plasmid on mica (see more in Figure 1 in Appendix A) and the relative frequency distribution of the lengths of 0 Gy (control) and 10 Gy. The 0 Gy distribution shows the detection of tight-binding DNA conformations of total length mostly of ~200–300 nm, underestimating the length of the supercoiled fraction due to the adsorption of the 3D molecules on the 2D mica surface. On the other hand, 10 Gy distribution reveals the segmentation of the initially supercoiled plasmid into one-stranded unfolded DNA pieces by recording molecules along the whole distribution range.

With increasing dose (Figure 7), there is a shift to smaller plasmid lengths revealed as increased DNA fragmentation due to multiple breaks. The same trend seems to follow the LET increase, since even in the case of small increment as in our experiment (Figure 7a corresponds to proton beam entrance and LET = 1 keV/μm, while Figure 7b to SOBP fall-off plasmid position with LET = 9 keV/μm) the fragment distribution shifts to smaller linear recorded DNA forms.

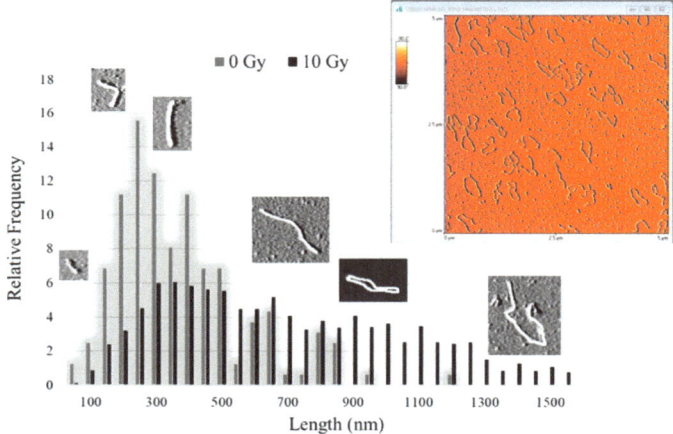

Figure 6. Atomic Force Microscopy (AFM) measurements: The relative frequency distribution of apparent molecule lengths for control sample (0 Gy) and irradiated with 10 Gy (proton beams) together with AFM images of DNA molecules of different forms. A representative AFM image (5 μm × 5 μm) of plasmid pBR322 on freshly cleaved mica surface, revealing the DNA macromolecule conformations. Such images are used as input for length evaluation and spread-out full-length circular molecules are utilized as calibration rulers for pixel-to-nm conversion. The length of the super-twisted supercoiled fraction is underestimated due to its adsorption on the mica surface. As a result, the apparent length of control plasmid is recorded smaller, while plasmid irradiated with plasmid is distributed along the whole range of lengths.

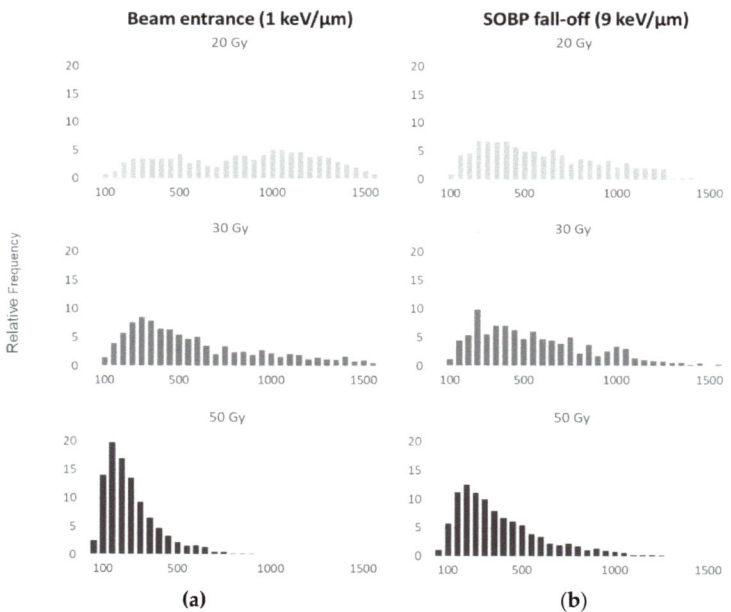

Figure 7. Relative frequency distributions of apparent molecule lengths measured using AFM for plasmid pBR322 irradiated with doses of 20, 30 and 50 Gy at (**a**) the entrance of proton beam (LET = 1 keV/μm) and (**b**) SOBP fall-off (LET = 9 keV/μm).

3. Materials and Methods

3.1. Sample Preparation

Plasmid pBR322, a vector of 4361 base pairs, dissolved in 10 mM Tris–Hcl, 1 mM EDTA (New England BioLabs Inc., Ipswich, MA, USA), was purified from salts via dialysis in ultrapure water (Pur-A-Lyzer dialysis kit from Sigma-Aldrich, St. Louis, MO, USA). Our study included two types of scavengers: coumarin-3-carboxylic acid (C3CA) (a water-soluble coumarin derivative) and 2-amino-2-(hydroxymethyl)propane-1,3-diol (Tris) with hydroxyl radicals (•OH) reaction rate constant $k_{C3CA} = 6.8 \times 10^9$ M^{-1} s^{-1} [41] and $k_{Tris} = 1.5 \times 10^9$ M^{-1} s^{-1} [42]. Three forms of plasmid samples were prepared: plasmid without scavenger, plasmid with C3CA and plasmid with Tris in total scavenging capacity of 10^6 s^{-1}, 10^7 s^{-1} and 10^8 s^{-1} for each compound. Scavenging capacity equals the product $k \times S$, where S is the scavenger concentration. Every sample contained 10 ng/μL of the plasmid in 20 mM potassium phosphate buffer, pH 7, ultrapure water and scavenger solution in a total volume of 160 μL irradiated in a polypropylene microtube (0.5 mL) with 0.85-mm-thick walls.

3.2. Irradiation and Dosimetry

Samples were irradiated at MedAustron Ion Beam Therapy Center in Wiener Neustadt, Austria, with doses up to 50 Gy at room temperature and kept on ice before and after irradiation.

3.2.1. Set-Up

The set-up that held all sample tubes consisted of a Teflon frame holder that allowed positioning of a removable plastic base at different heights. This frame was always placed vertically in the metal base of the solid water RW3 slab phantom, which was also used for a standard dosimetric quality assurance procedure by means of UNIDOSwebline with the ionization chamber ROOS (PTW, Freiburg, Germany).

3.2.2. Proton Irradiation

Treatment planning and dose calculations were performed with the RayStation TPS V5.99 (RaySearch, Stockholm, Sweden) for a hypothetical scenario of an existing tumor, 4 cm thick and 13 cm behind the skin. The set-up was placed on a robotic table (KUKA robot, Reutlingen BEC GmbH, Pfullingen, Germany), and then the table was placed in front of the beam, in a position that was calculated during the treatment planning. The proton beams were of energy range 137–198 MeV with the corresponding LET values 1–10 keV/μm along the clinical SOBP (Figure 3), a LET range that is important to cell killing [43]. The samples were irradiated in order of minutes under room temperature, and they were otherwise kept on ice. Doses of 0, 1, 2, 4, 8, 10, 15, 20, 30 and 50 Gy were delivered in different positions along the proton treatment plan, and an ionization chamber was used for dose monitoring. The chosen positions were achieved by interfering with polymethyl methacrylate (PMMA) plates of calculated thicknesses in front of the samples (Table 1).

3.2.3. X-rays

A YXLON X-ray unit (Yxlon International X-ray GmbH, Hamburg, Germany) was employed for plasmid irradiation. The X-ray tube was adjusted to 200 kV, 20 mA, and the dose rate was found to be constant at 1.25 Gy/min. Since the source tube was horizontal and the ROOS chamber set-up prerequisites 1 mm PMMA plate to position the plane parallel chamber vertically to the irradiation axis, all samples were exposed and taped on the back side of that PMMA plate and kept on ice before and after irradiation.

3.3. Post-Irradiation Treatment—DNA Damage Detection

3.3.1. Agarose Gel Electrophoresis in Tris-Acetate-EDTA (TAE) Buffer

Three subsamples of 5 μL, derived from each sample, were incubated at 37 °C for 1 h without or with enzymes: Formamidopyrimidine DNA glycosylase (Fpg) or Endonuclease III (Nth) in specific complementary reaction buffers (New England BioLabs Inc.).

Both enzymes are *E. coli* base excision repair enzymes and catalyze cleavage of oxidized nitrogenous bases. Fpg catalyzes lesions in purines, while Nth in pyrimidines and, due to associated lyase activity, they convert both existing and resulting abasic sites and oxidized bases into DNA strand breaks [44]. The optimal enzyme concentration was found by titration of each enzyme to succeed maximum specific along with minimum non-specific cutting activity and by comparing irradiated with non-irradiated samples treated with different enzyme concentrations. Enzymatic reactions were quenched by adding 2 µL of DNA loading dye (MassRuler, ThermoFisher, Waltham, MA, USA) containing bromophenol blue, 3.3 mM Tris–HCl and 11 mM EDTA. The different forms of plasmid DNA were separated and then visualized by employing agarose gel electrophoresis on 1% agarose gel stained with fluorescent dye SYBR Green I (Sigma-Aldrich) under electric field of 100 V in 0.5 × TAE.

At this stage and under the presence of single- and double-strand breaks, plasmid DNA is separated into bands-fractions of different conformations: supercoiled (SC), circular (C) and linear (L) and fragments (F), with the last one being non-detectable due to method limitations (Figure 8). These patterns were visualized with green filter on an MYECL Imager, and band analysis was performed with the image processing program MYImageAnalysis™ v2.0 Software (Thermo Scientific, Waltham, MA, USA). The full-length molecule bands of SC, R and L were identified and integrated. The attempt to include F in the analysis was not always possible, as shorter-than-linear plasmid lengths have greater mobility in the electric field, appearing as a smear under L and SC bands that were not always countable. Averaged SC, C and L relative fractions are quantified by gel luminosity and translated into DNA breaks using Cowan model [45,46] (Equations in Figure 8).

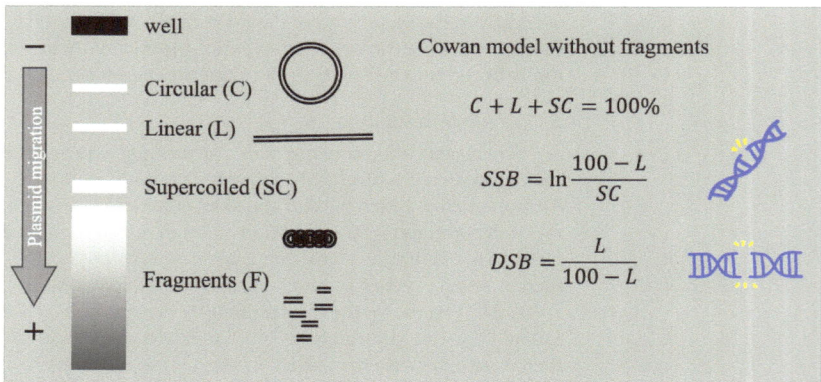

Figure 8. The electrophoresis concept: Each plasmid sample is added in a well (cathode side), electric field is applied at the gel edges and under the electric potential difference, the negatively charged DNA migrates to the anode side through the gel net. Due to the net-like agarose gel, different DNA forms are separated according to the size of each form that created three clearly distinguishable bands. Supercoiled (SC) plasmid (small-sized twisted DNA) is moving easier and faster, crossing a larger pathway inside the gel and appearing as a more distant band. The large circular (C) and linear (L) molecules have lower mobility than SC, and they are trapped in areas closer to the well. Therefore, the unfolded C appears as higher band in the gel, and L forms a band in between. Additionally, smaller DNA fragments (F) of higher mobility appear as a smear inside the gel. SC is the compact initial DNA with no break; C is caused by the cleavage of one DNA strand (SSB) and L by the cleavage of two strands (DSB). F results from further nicking cannot be safely measured via AGE and is excluded from present analysis. By defining the amount of SC, C and L and employing Cowan model [45] (equations above), we translate it into number of SSB and DSB.

The slope of SSB and DSB vs. dose plots converts results into the useful quantity of G-values (breaks per Gy per Mbp). To improve the statistics, AGE was performed twice for each irradiation condition, and image analysis was performed twice for each gel. The irradiation was only repeated for the middle of SOBP. Results are the mean values accompanied by the error of the mean.

Base lesions and non-DSB clustered damage are calculated via the difference between enzymatic cleavage and strand breaks. Base lesions correspond to the excessive SSB, and non-DSB clustered damage is the excessive DSB that is produced by Nth and Fpg enzymes.

3.3.2. AFM Analysis

Samples were also analyzed with an atomic force microscope. A part of the dialyzed (or/and also irradiated) plasmid sample was diluted to 1 ng/µL pBR322 in 1 mM $MgCl_2$. Mg^{2+} cations of such a concentration stabilize double-stranded DNA, prevents complete denaturation of the DNA and enhances adsorption (via a weak electrostatic attachment) of the molecule onto mica substrate [28,47]. AFM images (Figure 1) were acquired with Nanoscope diInnova device (Veeco Metrology, Santa Barbara, CA, USA) with an Innova scanner possessing a maximum range of 100 µm × 100 µm in tapping mode. Antimony (n) doped silicon tips with a nominal constant 3 N/m and 42 N/m (Bruker, Billerica, MA, USA) were used to acquire several high-resolution DNA topographies of 5 × 5 µm^2 at a scanning speed 1 Hz and with lateral resolution 512 × 512 pixels. The images were processed with the AFM apparatus software (SPMLab 5.01, Sunnyvale, CA, USA), they were flattened, and a histogram equalization was applied for the background noise subtraction and image contrast increase.

Images were input into the semi-automatic algorithm "lemeDNA" (Length Measurement of DNA) [48]. This algorithm uses 8-connected Freeman chain code to compute the pixel lengths and estimate the length of each molecule in pixels. Since the length of an intact plasmid pBR322 molecule is known to be 4361 base pairs, with each base pair 0.34 nm long (X-ray crystallography studies), calibration from pixels to nm is feasible and arbitrary fragments of DNA can be organized in length distributions.

4. Conclusions

The damage induction rate that follows the increasing capacity was found to decrease, underlining dominant indirect effects and the leading role of ROS in proton irradiation treatment. Enzyme analysis reveals that base lesions and non-DSB clusters are increased compared to SSB and DSB, respectively, with base lesions being the leading type of damage. Different positioning along the proton treatment plan shows no remarkable difference between DNA damage recorded at the beam entrance and at the middle of the SOBP position, probably due to very similar LET values. The fact that there is no higher damage induction rate at the distal fall-off of SOBP, as hypothesized for increasing LET, is raising the question about possible underestimation of highly complex damage and if there is multifragmented DNA that is not detectable with AGE and/or other types of interactions between DNA and protons that we do not fully comprehend.

Comparison with the literature suggests a great variety of results since one finds experiments with different beam energy, irradiation conditions and set-ups Furthermore, although there are studies that invoke the plasmid model, the systems are finally different because there is strong dependence on plasmid type and geometry, scavenging capacity and plasmid hydration level. All these parameters blend together, complicating result interpretation.

AFM provides impressive images of DNA conformations and visualizes fragments as short as 42 bp (equal to 14 nm). The present analysis with the LemeDNA algorithm qualitatively records the shift of the relative frequency distribution of the apparent DNA length towards shorter lengths following the dose increment. On the other hand, quantitatively there is not enough to contribute since there is no discrimination between different DNA forms, and only the apparent size is recorded. In order to reproduce results comparable to that of AGE, there is a need for an algorithm that also distinguishes and counts the SC and C and separates the L conformations into categories according to their measured length. This way, users will have the option to perform a similar but stronger analysis than this of traditional AGE.

Proton therapy-induced DNA damage in vitro studies employing biological models like plasmid DNA or cells using real therapeutic beams and exposure conditions are always challenging and quite limited. The cost of proton irradiations is high, and irradiation time is distributed on a priority basis, with patients being the first concern, with clinical research and applied and basic research activities following. At the same time, each ion facility is developed using different technologies (beam physical characteristics, dose delivery system, irradiation set-up, etc.), producing results that are not always repeatable from another beam facility. Therefore, non-clinical studies are difficult to perform and repeat in ion therapy facilities, with the available proton DNA damage data sourcing from the not plentiful literature of different parameters.

Consequently, the present study provides results from experiments performed in a cutting-edge ion therapy facility and analyzed with updated methods. The current results constitute a fresh input for early physical-chemical events of DNA damage induction. At the same time, this work strengthens the challenging attempt toward the modeling and deeper understanding of IR therapeutic modalities' effects on biological systems that may discharge research from demanding experiments in the future. Last but not least, DNA-based systems have been recently used as reliable dosimeters in therapy beam set-up. More specifically, recent independent studies on DNA double-strand breaks measurement were performed using a DNA dosimeter, consisting of magnetic streptavidin beads attached to a properly labeled four kbp DNA molecule suspended in phosphate-buffered saline (PBS) and utilized as a method of radiation measurements for therapeutic beams and high doses > 25 Gy where cellular systems are very difficult to be utilized [49]. Based on all the above, our results may also prove useful in the development of more accurate bio-dosimetry in proton or carbon-therapy treatment planning incorporating the biological signature of radiation and aid reduce damage to normal tissues and toxicity.

Author Contributions: Conceptualization, L.S. and A.G.G.; methodology, M.P.S., Z.N., M.P., K.P.B., and E.S.; formal analysis, M.P.S., Z.N., and E.S.; investigation, M.P.S., A.G.G., and L.S.; writing—original draft preparation, M.P.S. and A.G.G.; writing—review and editing, M.P.S., M.P., K.P.B., E.S., P.K., E.P.E., M.H., A.G.G., and L.S.; supervision, L.S. and A.G.G.; project administration, L.S; funding acquisition, L.S. All authors have read and agreed to the published version of the manuscript.

Funding: This research was funded by TU Wien, Austria and MedAustron, Wiener Neustadt, Austria and the project '21GRD02 BIOSPHERE', which has received funding from the European Partnership on Metrology, co-financed by the European Union's Horizon Europe Research and Innovation Programme and by the Participating States.

Institutional Review Board Statement: Not applicable.

Informed Consent Statement: Not applicable.

Data Availability Statement: All data will be provided by corresponding authors upon logical request.

Conflicts of Interest: The authors declare no conflict of interest.

Appendix A

Table 1. IR (protons, ions and electromagnetic radiation) damage induction rate on plasmid systems: results from the present study and reported in the literature.

	Type Rad/Proton Energy (MeV)	LET (keV/μm)	Plasmid	Scavenger	Plasmid Concentration (ng/μL)	Scav. Capacity (s^{-1})	SSB Mbp^{-1}Gy^{-1}	Error	DSB Mbp^{-1}Gy^{-1}	Error	Base Lesions Mbp^{-1}Gy^{-1}	Error	Non−DSB Clusters Mbp^{-1}Gy^{-1}	Error
this study	X-rays		pBR322 in solution	no scav (residual TRIS)	10	10^5	89.559	4.490	3.147	0.141	191.102	10.867	14.723	0.856
				TRIS		10^6	30.232	1.094	0.532	0.215	65.596	3.163	3.919	0.836
						10^7	4.551	0.746	0.103	0.010	18.656	3.415	0.631	0.036
						10^8	1.135	0.300	0.108	0.077	4.654	1.005	0.263	0.026
				C3CA		10^6	24.306	1.194	0.606	0.109	61.223	6.884	3.991	−0.054
						10^7	4.921	0.108	0.117	0.011	9.562	0.111	0.726	0.037
						10^8	1.370	0.054	0.121	0.077	2.139	0.133	0.137	0.032
this study	p 198 MeV	1	pBR322 in solution	no scav (residual TRIS)	10	10^5	101.101	16.868	1.914	0.247	275.852	114.295	10.908	1.778
		1		TRIS		10^6	45.848	5.031	1.534	0.247	130.510	40.667	13.270	1.411
		1				10^7	11.609	4.668	0.092	0.047	30.405	−0.222	0.426	−0.015
		1				10^8	2.083	1.355	0.025	0.015	5.103	0.227	0.078	−0.011
		1		C3CA		10^6	34.349	4.683	0.458	0.044	75.715	16.431	3.175	−0.042
		1				10^7	9.434	1.499	0.163	0.022	32.678	8.270	0.658	0.023
		1				10^8	4.141	0.861	0.041	0.014	10.709	3.961	0.052	−0.013
	p 167–137 MeV	4	pBR322 in solution	no scav (residual TRIS)	10	10^5	96.012	27.211	1.529	0.169	52.085	2.365	10.415	1.666
		4		TRIS		10^6	39.171	0.754	0.473	0.048	74.808	5.202	2.912	0.305
		4				10^7	12.888	2.234	0.096	0.035	25.294	4.359	0.509	0.039
		4				10^8	2.727	1.152	0.028	0.005	37.634	25.479	1.727	1.516
		4		C3CA		10^6	37.170	3.826	0.490	0.107	63.820	−1.111	4.053	0.178
		4				10^7	9.928	2.765	0.125	0.009	18.926	0.070	0.642	0.003
		4				10^8	2.220	0.786	0.039	0.006	4.596	0.446	0.081	0.005
	p 167–137 MeV	9	pBR322 in solution	no scav (residual TRIS)	10	10^5	51.069	6.923	0.579	0.060	54.453	6.350	3.255	0.092
		9		TRIS		10^6	9.581	0.945	0.138	0.052	17.400	8.311	0.671	0.338
		9				10^7	2.274	0.235	0.032	0.001	3.745	1.864	0.106	0.085
		9				10^8	0.299	0.089	0.005	0.009	1.269	0.619	0.115	0.121
		9		C3CA		10^6	11.545	2.456	0.172	0.036	12.770	5.628	0.716	0.481
		9				10^7	3.085	0.691	0.055	0.004	4.010	1.940	0.157	1.495
		9				10^8	0.717	0.237	0.032	0.016	0.867	0.253	0.009	0.018
Pachnerová 2015 [32]	p 30 MeV	1.9	pBR322 in solution	TE buffer		1.5×10^3	113.760	17.064	3.990		113.090		14.580	
				C3CA		6.8×10^5	24.790	3.718	1.930		18.020		1.540	
				C3CA		6.8×10^6	9.170	1.376	0.890		13.320		0.410	
				C3CA		6.8×10^7	1.220	0.182	0.760		3.390		0.000	
Sui 2013 [33]	p 15 MeV	3.6	pUC19 in solution	TRIS−HCl	100	3×10^8	9.950	0.790	0.064	0.009	16.560	1.400	0.100	0.016

Table 1. *Cont.*

	Type Rad/Proton Energy (MeV)	LET (keV/μm)	Scavenger	Plasmid	Plasmid Concentration (ng/μL)	Scav. Capacity (s^{-1})	SSB Mbp^{-1} Gy^{-1}	Error	DSB Mbp^{-1} Gy^{-1}	Error	Base Lesions Mbp^{-1} Gy^{-1}	Error	Non–DSB Clusters Mbp^{-1} Gy^{-1}	Error
Leloup 2005 [34]	p 249 MeV	0.39	glycerol	pHAZE liquid film		3.8×10^6	18.850	3.900	0.338	0.039			1.495	0.260
	p 19.3 MeV	2.7				3.8×10^6	5.005	1.950	0.104	0.026			0.377	0.163
	p 1.03 MeV	25.5				3.8×10^6	1.690	0.260	0.163	0.020			0.533	0.130
	p 249 MeV	0.39	glycerol			3.8×10^8	0.917	0.195	0.029	0.006			0.176	0.026
	p 19.3 MeV	2.7				3.8×10^8	0.397	0.091	0.011	0.004			0.037	0.020
	p 1.03 MeV	25.5				3.8×10^8	0.384	0.059	0.018	0.002			0.085	0.020
Vyšín 2015 [50]	p 10 MeV	6.39	TE buffer	pBR322 dry	30		0.009	0.007	0.003	0.001	0.082		0.001	
	p 20 MeV	3.64					0.053	0.000	0.001	0.001	0.088		0.006	
	p 30 MeV	2.61					0.044	0.006	0.001	0.000	0.088		0.004	
	p 20 MeV	3.1–6.95	TE buffer	pBR322 liquid			58.900	2.600	2.000	0.200	45.800		4.500	
	p 30 MeV	1.96–2.34					39.700	8.200	1.500	0.800	45.900		3.900	
Ohsawa 2021 [51]	p 27.5 MeV	2.3	TE buffer	pBR322 in solution	50		2.476	0.032	0.027	0.005				
	p 27.5 MeV FLASH	2.3					2.016	0.156	0.025	0.004				
Small 2021 [52]	e 100 MeV		no scav	pBR322 in solution			15.420	0.860	0.350	0.020				
	e 100 MeV FLASH						20.310	0.200	0.370	0.030				
	e 150 MeV						17.630	0.570	0.350	0.030				
	e 150 MeV FLASH						18.740	0.520	0.370	0.040				
	e 200 MeV						20.190	0.560	0.380	0.020				
	e 200 MeV FLASH						21.220	0.380	0.380	0.020				
	e 100 MeV	0.22		pBR322 dry			69.810	8.720	3.660	0.430				
	e 150 MeV	0.22					80.300	3.060	3.710	0.110				
	e 200 MeV	0.23					50.270	4.190	3.830	0.450				
Small 2019 [53]	60–Co – 6 MeV	0.19	no scav	pBR322			7.940	0.140	0.970	0.100				
	60–Co – 10 MeV	0.20					11.000	0.660	1.130	0.080				
	60–Co – 15 MeV	0.20					7.710	0.030	1.220	0.010				
Pachnerová 2019 [28]	Carbon ions 400 MeV/u	11	TE buffer	pBR322	10	1.5×10^3	128.600	1.900	4.800	0.400				
Souici 2016 [54]	Ultra Soft X-rays 1.5 keV		TRIS	pBR322	5	1.5×10^6	2.477	0.130	0.228	0.026				
						1.5×10^7	0.780	0.059						
						1.5×10^8	0.163	0.072						
					10	1.5×10^6	2.386	0.052	0.208	0.020				
						1.5×10^7	0.845	0.013						
						1.5×10^8	0.182	0.020						
					50	1.5×10^6	2.106	0.091	0.137	0.013				
						1.5×10^7	0.800	0.039						
						1.5×10^8	0.228	0.026						

Table 1. Cont.

	Type Rad/Proton Energy (MeV)	LET (keV/μm)	Scavenger	Plasmid	Plasmid Concentration (ng/μL)	Scav. Capacity (s^{-1})	SSB Mbp^{-1}Gy^{-1}	Error	DSB Mbp^{-1}Gy^{-1}	Error	Base Lesions Mbp^{-1}Gy^{-1}	Error	Non-DSB Clusters Mbp^{-1}Gy^{-1}	Error
Shiina 2013 [55]	X-rays		TRIS	pUC18 in solution	50	1×10^6	5.720		0.111		9.035		0.481	
						1.5×10^7	1.105		0.029		1.430		0.092	
						3×10^8	0.163		0.008		0.650		0.020	
						1×10^{10}	0.124		0.010					
	C6+ 290 MeV	13	TRIS	pUC18 in solution	50	1×10^6	5.590		0.228		4.290		0.481	
						1.5×10^7	1.300		0.008		2.795		0.182	
						3×10^8	0.325		0.013		1.300		0.059	
Ushigome 2012 [56]	He2+	2.2		pUC18 hydrated films			0.058	0.013	0.005	0.001	0.141		0.004	
		6					0.064	0.012	0.004	0.001	0.169		0.007	
	C5+, C6+	13		pUC18 hydrated films			0.107	0.026	0.008	0.004	0.255		0.009	
		87					0.040	0.003	0.003	0.000	0.057		0.003	
		122					0.037	0.003	0.004	0.000	0.074		0.004	
		342					0.030	0.004	0.005	0.000	0.047		0.001	
		507					0.033	0.003	0.005	0.001	0.061		0.000	
	Ne10+	31		pUC18 hydrated films			0.092	0.023	0.005	0.001	0.180		0.006	
		361					0.038	0.003	0.007	0.001	0.066		0.002	
		491					0.031	0.001	0.007	0.001	0.067		0.002	
		842					0.031	0.005	0.008	0.001	0.038		0.002	
Urushibara 2008 [57]	gamma 60–Co			pUC18			0.047	0.003	0.005	0.000	0.138		0.014	
	α He	19		pUC18			0.045	0.007	0.002	0.001	0.166		0.006	
	α He	63					0.047	0.001	0.005	0.001	0.085		0.006	
	α He	95					0.044	0.002	0.007	0.000	0.047		0.004	
	α He	121					0.031	0.003	0.003	0.001	0.040		0.003	
	α He	148					0.025	0.002	0.006	0.000	0.012		0.002	
Yokoya 2003 [57]	α Pu						0.039	0.006	0.011	0.001	0.016		0.003	
Klimczak 1993 [58]	gamma 60–Co			pBR322	100	1.5×10^6	26.00		0.26					
						1.5×10^7	5.85		0.07					
						1.5×10^8	1.30		0.02					

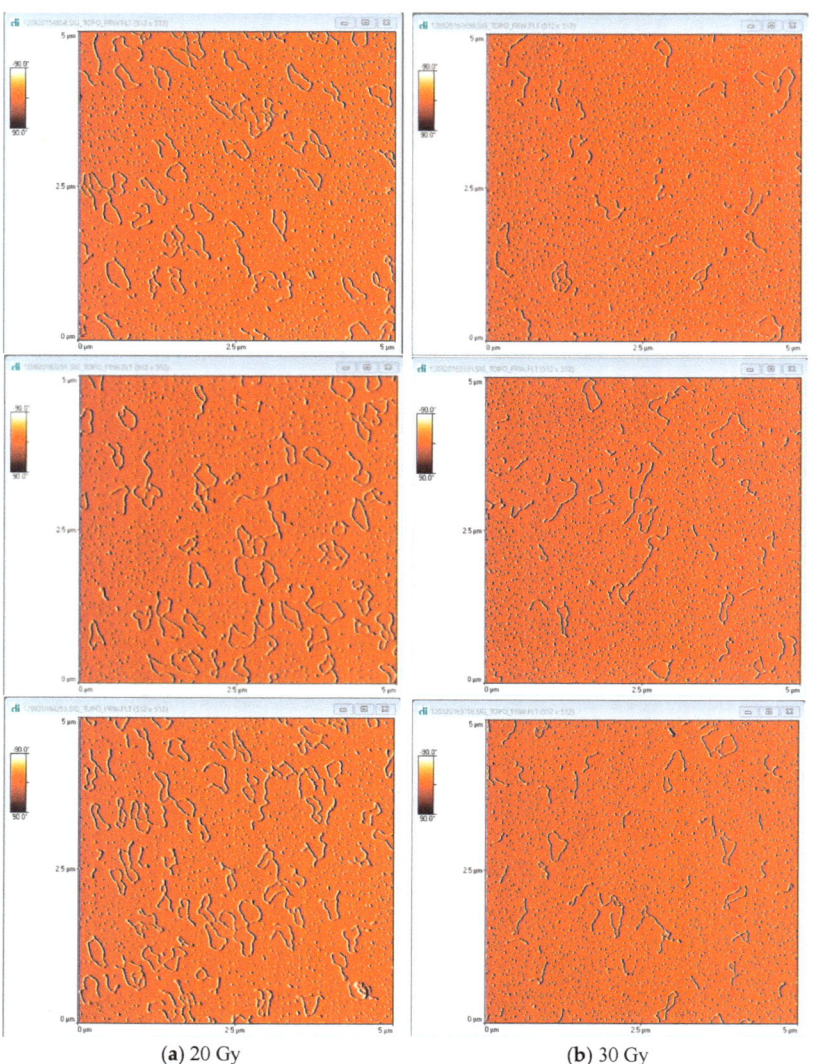

(a) 20 Gy (b) 30 Gy

Figure 1. AFM topographic images of plasmid pBR322 on mica substrate irradiated with protons: (**a**) 20 Gy and (**b**) 30 Gy. AFM reveals the different conformations of DNA from simple linear to complex twisted loops. The difference in plasmid concentration between the two doses is incidental.

References

1. Nikitaki, Z.; Velalopoulou, A.; Zanni, V.; Tremi, I.; Havaki, S.; Kokkoris, M.; Gorgoulis, V.G.; Koumenis, C.; Georgakilas, A.G. Key biological mechanisms involved in high-LET radiation therapies with a focus on DNA damage and repair. *Expert Rev. Mol. Med.* **2022**, *24*, e15. [CrossRef] [PubMed]
2. Ward, J.F. DNA Damage Produced by Ionizing Radiation in Mammalian Cells: Identities, Mechanisms of Formation, and Reparability. In *Progress in Nucleic Acid Research and Molecular Biology*; Cohn, W.E., Moldave, K., Eds.; Academic Press: New York, NY, USA, 1988; Volume 35, pp. 95–125.
3. Ward, J.F. The complexity of DNA damage: Relevance to biological consequences. *Int. J. Radiat. Biol.* **1994**, *66*, 427–432. [CrossRef] [PubMed]

4. Sage, E.; Harrison, L. Clustered DNA lesion repair in eukaryotes: Relevance to mutagenesis and cell survival. *Mutat. Res.* **2011**, *711*, 123–133. [CrossRef] [PubMed]
5. Asaithamby, A.; Hu, B.; Chen, D.J. Unrepaired clustered DNA lesions induce chromosome breakage in human cells. *Proc. Natl. Acad. Sci. USA* **2011**, *108*, 8293–8298. [CrossRef]
6. Mavragani, I.V.; Nikitaki, Z.; Kalospyros, S.A.; Georgakilas, A.G. Ionizing Radiation and Complex DNA Damage: From Prediction to Detection Challenges and Biological Significance. *Cancers* **2019**, *11*, 1789. [CrossRef]
7. Schipler, A.; Mladenova, V.; Soni, A.; Nikolov, V.; Saha, J.; Mladenov, E.; Iliakis, G. Chromosome thripsis by DNA double strand break clusters causes enhanced cell lethality, chromosomal translocations and 53BP1-recruitment. *Nucleic Acids Res.* **2016**, *44*, 7673–7690. [CrossRef]
8. Sutherland, B.M.; Bennett, P.V.; Sidorkina, O.; Laval, J. Clustered Damages and Total Lesions Induced in DNA by Ionizing Radiation: Oxidized Bases and Strand Breaks. *Biochemistry* **2000**, *39*, 8026–8031. [CrossRef]
9. Hada, M.; Georgakilas, A.G. Formation of clustered DNA damage after high-LET irradiation: A review. *J. Radiat. Res.* **2008**, *49*, 203–210. [CrossRef]
10. Fakir, H.; Sachs, R.K.; Stenerlöw, B.; Hofmann, W. Clusters of DNA double-strand breaks induced by different doses of nitrogen ions for various LETs: Experimental measurements and theoretical analyses. *Radiat. Res.* **2006**, *166*, 917–927. [CrossRef]
11. Asaithamby, A.; Chen, D.J. Mechanism of cluster DNA damage repair in response to high-atomic number and energy particles radiation. *Mutat. Res.* **2011**, *711*, 87–99. [CrossRef]
12. Lorat, Y.; Brunner, C.U.; Schanz, S.; Jakob, B.; Taucher-Scholz, G.; Rübe, C.E. Nanoscale analysis of clustered DNA damage after high-LET irradiation by quantitative electron microscopy—The heavy burden to repair. *DNA Repair* **2015**, *28*, 93–106. [CrossRef] [PubMed]
13. Nikitaki, Z.; Nikolov, V.; Mavragani, I.V.; Mladenov, E.; Mangelis, A.; Laskaratou, D.A.; Fragkoulis, G.I.; Hellweg, C.E.; Martin, O.A.; Emfietzoglou, D.; et al. Measurement of complex DNA damage induction and repair in human cellular systems after exposure to ionizing radiations of varying linear energy transfer (LET). *Free Radic. Res.* **2016**, *50*, S64–S78. [CrossRef] [PubMed]
14. Kalospyros, S.A.; Gika, V.; Nikitaki, Z.; Kalamara, A.; Kyriakou, I.; Emfietzoglou, D.; Kokkoris, M.; Georgakilas, A.G. Monte Carlo Simulation-Based Calculations of Complex DNA Damage for Incidents of Environmental Ionizing Radiation Exposure. *Appl. Sci.* **2021**, *11*, 8985. [CrossRef]
15. Surdutovich, E.; Solov'yov, A.V. Multiscale approach to the physics of radiation damage with ions. *Eur. Phys. J. D* **2014**, *68*, 353. [CrossRef]
16. Surdutovich, E.; Gallagher, D.C.; Solov'yov, A.V. Calculation of complex DNA damage induced by ions. *Phys. Rev. E Stat. Nonlinear Soft Matter Phys.* **2011**, *84*, 051918. [CrossRef] [PubMed]
17. Ray, S.; Cekanaviciute, E.; Lima, I.P.; Sørensen, B.S.; Costes, S.V. Comparing Photon and Charged Particle Therapy Using DNA Damage Biomarkers. *Int. J. Part. Ther.* **2018**, *5*, 15–24. [CrossRef]
18. Carter, R.J.; Nickson, C.M.; Thompson, J.M.; Kacperek, A.; Hill, M.A.; Parsons, J.L. Complex DNA Damage Induced by High Linear Energy Transfer Alpha-Particles and Protons Triggers a Specific Cellular DNA Damage Response. *Int. J. Radiat. Oncol. Biol. Phys.* **2018**, *100*, 776–784. [CrossRef]
19. Chaudhary, P.; Marshall, T.I.; Currell, F.J.; Kacperek, A.; Schettino, G.; Prise, K.M. Variations in the Processing of DNA Double-Strand Breaks Along 60-MeV Therapeutic Proton Beams. *Int. J. Radiat. Oncol. Biol. Phys.* **2016**, *95*, 86–94. [CrossRef]
20. Dizdaroglu, M.; Jaruga, P. Mechanisms of free radical-induced damage to DNA. *Free Radic. Res.* **2012**, *46*, 382–419. [CrossRef]
21. Le Caër, S. Water Radiolysis: Influence of Oxide Surfaces on H2 Production under Ionizing Radiation. *Water* **2011**, *3*, 235–253. [CrossRef]
22. Peddi, P.; Loftin, C.W.; Dickey, J.S.; Hair, J.M.; Burns, K.J.; Aziz, K.; Francisco, D.C.; Panayiotidis, M.I.; Sedelnikova, O.A.; Bonner, W.M.; et al. DNA-PKcs deficiency leads to persistence of oxidatively induced clustered DNA lesions in human tumor cells. *Free Radic. Biol. Med.* **2010**, *48*, 1435–1443. [CrossRef] [PubMed]
23. LaVerne, J.A.; Pimblott, S.M. Yields of hydroxyl radical and hydrated electron scavenging reactions in aqueous solutions of biological interest. *Radiat. Res.* **1993**, *135*, 16–23. [CrossRef] [PubMed]
24. Pang, D.; Thierry, A.R.; Dritschilo, A. DNA studies using atomic force microscopy: Capabilities for measurement of short DNA fragments. *Front. Mol. Biosci.* **2015**, *2*, 1. [CrossRef] [PubMed]
25. Pyne, A.L.B.; Noy, A.; Main, K.H.S.; Velasco-Berrelleza, V.; Piperakis, M.M.; Mitchenall, L.A.; Cugliandolo, F.M.; Beton, J.G.; Stevenson, C.E.M.; Hoogenboom, B.W.; et al. Base-pair resolution analysis of the effect of supercoiling on DNA flexibility and major groove recognition by triplex-forming oligonucleotides. *Nat. Commun.* **2021**, *12*, 1053. [CrossRef] [PubMed]
26. Melters, D.P.; Dalal, Y. Nano-Surveillance: Tracking Individual Molecules in a Sea of Chromatin. *J. Mol. Biol.* **2021**, *433*, 166720. [CrossRef]
27. Küpeli Akkol, E.; Genç, Y.; Karpuz, B.; Sobarzo-Sánchez, E.; Capasso, R. Coumarins and Coumarin-Related Compounds in Pharmacotherapy of Cancer. *Cancers* **2020**, *12*, 1959. [CrossRef]
28. Pachnerová Brabcová, K.; Sihver, L.; Ukraintsev, E.; Štěpán, V.; Davídková, M. HOW DETECTION OF PLASMID DNA FRAGMENTATION AFFECTS RADIATION STRAND BREAK YIELDS. *Radiat. Prot. Dosim.* **2019**, *183*, 89–92. [CrossRef]
29. Pouget, J.P.; Frelon, S.; Ravanat, J.L.; Testard, I.; Odin, F.; Cadet, J. Formation of modified DNA bases in cells exposed either to gamma radiation or to high-LET particles. *Radiat. Res.* **2002**, *157*, 589–595. [CrossRef]

30. Nikitaki, Z.; Hellweg, C.E.; Georgakilas, A.G.; Ravanat, J.-L. Stress-induced DNA damage biomarkers: Applications and limitations. *Front. Chem.* **2015**, *3*, 35. [CrossRef]
31. Ravanat, J.L.; Breton, J.; Douki, T.; Gasparutto, D.; Grand, A.; Rachidi, W.; Sauvaigo, S. Radiation-mediated formation of complex damage to DNA: A chemical aspect overview. *Br. J. Radiol.* **2014**, *87*, 20130715. [CrossRef]
32. Pachnerová Brabcová, K.; Štěpán, V.; Karamitros, M.; Karabín, M.; Dostálek, P.; Incerti, S.; Davídková, M.; Sihver, L. Contribution of indirect effects to clustered damage in DNA irradiated with protons. *Radiat. Prot. Dosim.* **2015**, *166*, 44–48. [CrossRef]
33. Sui, L.; Wang, Y.; Wang, X.; Kong, F.; Liu, J.; Zhou, P. Clustered DNA damage induced by protons radiation in plasmid DNA. *Chin. Sci. Bull.* **2013**, *58*, 3217–3223. [CrossRef]
34. Leloup, C.; Garty, G.; Assaf, G.; Cristovão, A.; Breskin, A.; Chechik, R.; Shchemelinin, S.; Paz-Elizur, T.; Livneh, Z.; Schulte, R.W.; et al. Evaluation of lesion clustering in irradiated plasmid DNA. *Int. J. Radiat. Biol.* **2005**, *81*, 41–54. [CrossRef] [PubMed]
35. Chapman, J.D.; Reuvers, A.P.; Borsa, J.; Greenstock, C.L. Chemical Radioprotection and Radiosensitization of Mammalian Cells Growing in Vitro. *Radiat. Res.* **1973**, *56*, 291–306. [CrossRef]
36. Roots, R.; Okada, S. Estimation of Life Times and Diffusion Distances of Radicals Involved in X-Ray-Induced DNA Strand Breaks or Killing of Mammalian Cells. *Radiat. Res.* **1975**, *64*, 306–320. [CrossRef]
37. Dang, H.M.; van Goethem, M.J.; van der Graaf, E.R.; Brandenburg, S.; Hoekstra, R.; Schlathölter, T. Heavy ion induced damage to plasmid DNA: Plateau region vs. spread out Bragg-peak. *Eur. Phys. J. D* **2011**, *63*, 359–367. [CrossRef]
38. Dang, H.M.; van Goethem, M.J.; van der Graaf, E.R.; Brandenburg, S.; Hoekstra, R.; Schlathölter, T. Plasmid DNA damage by heavy ions at spread-out Bragg peak energies. *Eur. Phys. J. D* **2010**, *60*, 51–58. [CrossRef]
39. Vanderwaeren, L.; Dok, R.; Verstrepen, K.; Nuyts, S. Clinical Progress in Proton Radiotherapy: Biological Unknowns. *Cancers* **2021**, *13*, 604. [CrossRef]
40. Paganetti, H. Relative biological effectiveness (RBE) values for proton beam therapy. Variations as a function of biological endpoint, dose, and linear energy transfer. *Phys. Med. Biol.* **2014**, *59*, R419–R472. [CrossRef]
41. Yamashita, S.; Baldacchino, G.; Maeyama, T.; Taguchi, M.; Muroya, Y.; Lin, M.; Kimura, A.; Murakami, T.; Katsumura, Y. Mechanism of radiation-induced reactions in aqueous solution of coumarin-3-carboxylic acid: Effects of concentration, gas and additive on fluorescent product yield. *Free Radic. Res.* **2012**, *46*, 861–871. [CrossRef]
42. Hicks, M.; Gebicki, J.M. Rate constants for reaction of hydroxyl radicals with Tris, Tricine and Hepes buffers. *FEBS Lett.* **1986**, *199*, 92–94. [CrossRef]
43. Wéra, A.C.; Heuskin, A.C.; Riquier, H.; Michiels, C.; Lucas, S. Low-LET proton irradiation of A549 non-small cell lung adenocarcinoma cells: Dose response and RBE determination. *Radiat. Res.* **2013**, *179*, 273–281. [CrossRef] [PubMed]
44. Sutherland, B.M.; Bennett, P.V.; Sidorkina, O.; Laval, J. Clustered DNA damages induced in isolated DNA and in human cells by low doses of ionizing radiation. *Proc. Natl. Acad. Sci. USA* **2000**, *97*, 103. [CrossRef] [PubMed]
45. Cowan, R.; Collis, C.M.; Grigg, G.W. Breakage of double-stranded DNA due to single-stranded nicking. *J. Theor. Biol.* **1987**, *127*, 229–245. [CrossRef]
46. Śmiałek, M.A. Early models of DNA damage formation. *J. Phys. Conf. Ser.* **2012**, *373*, 012013. [CrossRef]
47. Bezanilla, M.; Manne, S.; Laney, D.E.; Lyubchenko, Y.L.; Hansma, H.G. Adsorption of DNA to Mica, Silylated Mica, and Minerals: Characterization by Atomic Force Microscopy. *Langmuir* **1995**, *11*, 655–659. [CrossRef]
48. Pachnerová Brabcová, K.; Sihver, L.; Ukraintsev, E.; Štěpán, V.; Davídková, M. Length computation of irradiated plasmid DNA molecules. *Biointerphases* **2018**, *13*, 061005. [CrossRef]
49. Obeidat, M.; McConnell, K.A.; Li, X.; Bui, B.; Stathakis, S.; Papanikolaou, N.; Rasmussen, K.; Ha, C.S.; Lee, S.E.; Shim, E.Y.; et al. DNA double-strand breaks as a method of radiation measurements for therapeutic beams. *Med. Phys.* **2018**, *45*, 3460–3465. [CrossRef]
50. Vyšín, L.; Pachnerová Brabcová, K.; Štěpán, V.; Moretto-Capelle, P.; Bugler, B.; Legube, G.; Cafarelli, P.; Casta, R.; Champeaux, J.P.; Sence, M.; et al. Proton-induced direct and indirect damage of plasmid DNA. *Radiat. Environ. Biophys.* **2015**, *54*, 343–352. [CrossRef]
51. Ohsawa, D.; Hiroyama, Y.; Kobayashi, A.; Kusumoto, T.; Kitamura, H.; Hojo, S.; Kodaira, S.; Konishi, T. DNA strand break induction of aqueous plasmid DNA exposed to 30 MeV protons at ultra-high dose rate. *J. Radiat. Res.* **2021**, *63*, 255–260. [CrossRef]
52. Small, K.L.; Henthorn, N.T.; Angal-Kalinin, D.; Chadwick, A.L.; Santina, E.; Aitkenhead, A.; Kirkby, K.J.; Smith, R.J.; Surman, M.; Jones, J.; et al. Evaluating very high energy electron RBE from nanodosimetric pBR322 plasmid DNA damage. *Sci. Rep.* **2021**, *11*, 1–12. [CrossRef] [PubMed]
53. Small, K.L.; Henthorn, N.T.; Angal-Kalinin, D.; Chadwick, A.L.; Edge, R.; Henthorn, N.T.; Jones, R.M.; Kirkby, K.; Merchant, M.J.; Morris, R.; et al. A Comparative Study of Biological Effects of Electrons and Co-60 Gamma Rays on pBR322 Plasmid DNA. In Proceedings of the IPAC2019, Melbourne, Australia, 19–24 May 2019; pp. 3533–3536.
54. Souici, M.; Khalil, T.T.; Boulanouar, O.; Belafrites, A.; Mavon, C.; Fromm, M. DNA strand break dependence on Tris and arginine scavenger concentrations under ultra-soft X-ray irradiation: The contribution of secondary arginine radicals. *Radiat. Environ. Biophys.* **2016**, *55*, 215–228. [CrossRef] [PubMed]
55. Shiina, T.; Watanabe, R.; Shiraishi, I.; Suzuki, M.; Sugaya, Y.; Fujii, K.; Yokoya, A. Induction of DNA damage, including abasic sites, in plasmid DNA by carbon ion and X-ray irradiation. *Radiat. Environ. Biophys.* **2013**, *52*, 99–112. [CrossRef] [PubMed]

56. Ushigome, T.; Shikazono, N.; Fujii, K.; Watanabe, R.; Suzuki, M.; Tsuruoka, C.; Tauchi, H.; Yokoya, A. Yield of single- and double-strand breaks and nucleobase lesions in fully hydrated plasmid DNA films irradiated with high-LET charged particles. *Radiat. Res.* **2012**, *177*, 614–627. [CrossRef]
57. Urushibara, A.; Shikazono, N.; O'Neill, P.; Fujii, K.; Wada, S.; Yokoya, A. LET dependence of the yield of single-, double-strand breaks and base lesions in fully hydrated plasmid DNA films by 4He(2+) ion irradiation. *Int. J. Radiat. Biol.* **2008**, *84*, 23–33. [CrossRef]
58. Klimczak, U.; Ludwig, D.C.; Mark, F.; Rettberg, P.; Schulte-Frohlinde, D. Irradiation of plasmid and phage DNA in water-alcohol mixtures: Strand breaks and lethal damage as a function of scavenger concentration. *Int. J. Radiat. Biol.* **1993**, *64*, 497–510. [CrossRef]

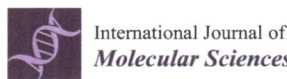

Review

The Molecular and Cellular Strategies of Glioblastoma and Non-Small-Cell Lung Cancer Cells Conferring Radioresistance

Lina Alhaddad [1,2], Andreyan N. Osipov [1,3,4,*] and Sergey Leonov [1,5]

1. School of Biological and Medical Physics, Moscow Institute of Physics and Technology, 141700 Dolgoprudny, Russia
2. Department of Environmental Sciences, Faculty of Science, Damascus University, Damascus P.O. Box 30621, Syria
3. State Research Center-Burnasyan Federal Medical Biophysical Center of Federal Medical Biological Agency (SRC-FMBC), 123098 Moscow, Russia
4. N.N. Semenov Research Center of Chemical Physics, Russian Academy of Sciences, 119991 Moscow, Russia
5. Institute of Cell Biophysics, Russian Academy of Sciences, 142290 Pushchino, Russia
* Correspondence: aosipov@fmbcfmba.ru

Abstract: Ionizing radiation (IR) has been shown to play a crucial role in the treatment of glioblastoma (GBM; grade IV) and non-small-cell lung cancer (NSCLC). Nevertheless, recent studies have indicated that radiotherapy can offer only palliation owing to the radioresistance of GBM and NSCLC. Therefore, delineating the major radioresistance mechanisms may provide novel therapeutic approaches to sensitize these diseases to IR and improve patient outcomes. This review provides insights into the molecular and cellular mechanisms underlying GBM and NSCLC radioresistance, where it sheds light on the role played by cancer stem cells (CSCs), as well as discusses comprehensively how the cellular dormancy/non-proliferating state and polyploidy impact on their survival and relapse post-IR exposure.

Keywords: ionizing radiation; radioresistance; radiosensitivity; cancer stem cells; epithelial mesenchymal transition; polyploid/multinucleated giant cancer cells

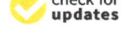

Citation: Alhaddad, L.; Osipov, A.N.; Leonov, S. The Molecular and Cellular Strategies of Glioblastoma and Non-Small-Cell Lung Cancer Cells Conferring Radioresistance. *Int. J. Mol. Sci.* **2022**, *23*, 13577. https://doi.org/10.3390/ijms232113577

Academic Editor: François Chevalier

Received: 12 October 2022
Accepted: 3 November 2022
Published: 5 November 2022

Publisher's Note: MDPI stays neutral with regard to jurisdictional claims in published maps and institutional affiliations.

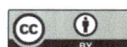

Copyright: © 2022 by the authors. Licensee MDPI, Basel, Switzerland. This article is an open access article distributed under the terms and conditions of the Creative Commons Attribution (CC BY) license (https://creativecommons.org/licenses/by/4.0/).

1. Introduction

Glioblastoma (GBM; grade IV) is classified as the most aggressive, heterogeneous, and invasive primary brain tumor [1] in adults and often occurs in patients over 65 years of age [2]. GBM accounts for 15% of all brain tumors [3–5]. Non-small-cell lung cancer (NSCLC), a heterogeneous class of tumors, represents approximately 85% of all lung cancer diagnoses [6]. Radiotherapy represents the mainstay of therapy in patients with inoperable early-stage NSCLC [7] and GBM [8], yet the prognosis of GBM and NSCLC patients still remains poor due to a refractory response to ionizing radiation (IR) [9,10]. Therefore, a high radioresistance of these tumors still limits therapeutic success. The median survival for elderly patients with GBM remains approximately 8 months with RT alone [11], whereas the observed improvement in median survival of NSCLC time is only 5 to 7 months, and radiotherapy does not offer the possibility of a cure [12]. Tumor heterogeneity accounts for therapeutic failure [13]. Tumor recurrence occurs when therapy-surviving residual tumor cells tenaciously propagate and re-establish the tumor. Many studies have suggested that the heterogeneity of tumors can be explained not only with the characteristic of genetic instability and epigenetic changes but also with the help of cancer stem cells (CSCs) supported by antiapoptotic signaling [14–16]. CSCs thwart harmful insults resulting from radiotherapy due to their distinctive inherent properties of self-renewal for unlimited time, increased aggressiveness, resistance to stress, and preferential activation of the DNA damage checkpoint [10,14,17–21] (Figure 1). CSCs are capable of evading cell death, albeit they can become dormant for extended periods of time [22]. Plasticity of CSCs, therapy resistance, and dormancy are substantially interrelated processes [23,24]. It has been suggested that tumor progression depends profoundly on the CSC niche within it [23]. Invasion and metastasis have been known to be the main obstacles to successful therapy and are closely linked to the mortality rate of GBM [25] and NSCLC [26]. Epithelial-to-mesenchymal transition (EMT) is a very complex process regulated by several families of transcriptional factors through many signaling pathways that form a network that allows tumor cells to acquire invasive properties and penetrate the neighboring stroma, leading to the formation of a privileged microenvironment for tumor progression and metastasis [27]. EMT is hallmarked by the combined loss of epithelial cell junction proteins, such as E-cadherin, and the gain of mesenchymal markers, such as vimentin and N-cadherin [28,29]. EMT is an important inducer of the CSCs' plasticity [30]. IR is one of the exogenous genotoxic agents that are capable of eliciting DNA damage [31]. GBM and NSCLC cells have network mechanisms in response to DNA damage, including initiation of DNA repair and, in certain cases, induction of apoptosis to annihilate dysregulated and damaged cells [32,33]. It has been reported that IR can induce proliferation arrest of tumor cells [34], which is often accompanied by senescence and/or quiescence [35,36]. The mechanisms dictating the exit from cycle arrest have considerable implications on cell fate and can thus affect the outcome of DNA damage-based tumor therapies [36]. Rarely dividing/non-proliferating tumor cells are regarded as deeply resistant to these agents, thereby causing therapeutic failure and tumor recurrence [37]. It has been suggested that tumor cells can recuperate from temporary arrest after DNA damage is repaired [36]. It has been demonstrated that IR can result in the development of polyploid tumor cells [38]. These giant cells have been reported to be adequately pliable to meet developmental tumor needs by facilitating the rapid evolution of tumors and the acquisition of therapy resistance in multiple incurable tumors [39]. Moreover, they have been shown to undergo depolyploidization [40] and produce a limited number of para-diploid clones [41,42]. It should also be noted that the radioresistance of GBM and NSCLC may be attributable to the interlink between the tumor cells and their tumor microenvironment (TME) [43,44].

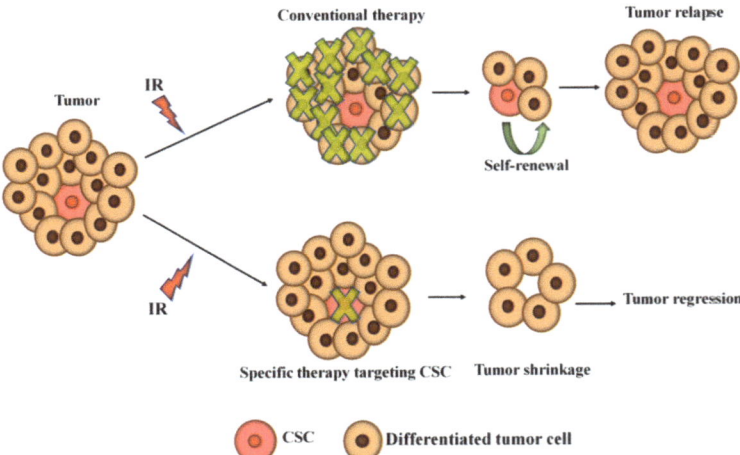

Figure 1. Targeting of CSCs. CSCs remaining after radiotherapy can then emerge and repopulate.

2. Tumor Heterogeneity

One of the most important hallmarks of GBM [45] and NSCLC [46] is cellular heterogeneity. The heterogeneity of tumor cells is a continuous cause of incomplete molecular response to radiotherapy [13,47,48] due to the diversity of tumor cells within the same tumor, leading to different responses to radiotherapy and inevitable repopulation post-IR [49,50]. Tumor heterogeneity arises from subpopulations of cells with marked genomic and/or epigenetic change and molecular signatures, a phenomenon termed intra-tumor heterogeneity [51]. Intra-tumoral heterogeneity results in the ability of a tumor to harbor anomalies in a variety of signaling pathways and cells with different levels of sensitivity to established antitumor agents [48]. Three models of tumor progression and metastasis have been postulated to explain this phenomenon—the clonal evolution, the classical CSC, and the plastic CSC models [52] (Figure 2).

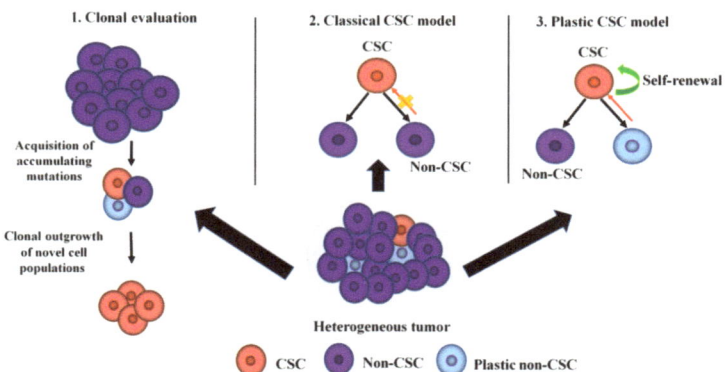

Figure 2. Models of tumor heterogeneity and progression of metastatic disease.

The clonal evolution theory was the first model to describe a way in which tumor cells evolve progressively due to genomic instability resulting from an accumulation of successive mutations. These stochastic events generate the raw material for the clonal outgrowth of novel cell populations that can thrive under selective pressures imposed by the TME, dictating more malignant phenotypes [52,53]. Moreover, heritable changes in the epigenome permit the cells to acquire advantageous traits and to be selected in a neo-Darwinian-like evolutionary paradigm [54]. The classical CSC theory hypothesizes that tumors are immortalized by CSCs identified by their ability to initiate tumor growth, sustain self-renewal, and re-establish a heterogeneous tumor cell population [21,55–57]. This model focuses on the internal heterogeneity within individual clonal subsets. According to this theory, most tumorigenic cells within such a clonal population reside at the peak of the hierarchy [52]. A defining feature of this model is its unidirectional nature, whereby CSCs undergo symmetric division to replenish the CSC pool within a tumor or irreversible asymmetric division to generate more differentiated progeny with low metastatic potential. In this case, the divergent cell phenotypes are regulated by endogenous and exogenous stimuli arising in the TME. These stimuli can lead to the induction of specific growth factor and cytokine pathways that, in turn, affect subtle epigenetic changes in CSCs and their non-CSC progeny. The CSC hierarchical model has been extended to many solid human tumors, including GBM and NSCLC [58,59]. The plastic CSCs theory portrays the phenotypic conversion between the CSC and non-CSC compartments as a bidirectional process [52], highlighting an evolving mechanism by which non-CSCs can dynamically move back up the hierarchy and re-enter the CSC state due to dedifferentiation process [52]. Moreover, this model describes the basic aspects of non-CSC-to-CSC bidirectional interconversions. According to this theory, CSCs may be derived by the oncogenic transformation of normal tissue stem cells, by EMT, by mutations in key regulators of differentiation, or by a spontaneous conversion process [52]. Numerous studies have reported that IR can promote non-CSCs to obtain the phenotype and function of CSCs, so-called "awakened" CSCs [60,61].

3. Cancer Stem Cells Concept, History, and Properties

Cancer stem (-like) cells (CSCs) or (CSLCs), also referred to as cancer-initiating cells (CICs), are a small subgroup of cancer cells with the capability of self-renewal and differentiation into heterogeneous tumor cells, and they have been believed to be accountable for tumor initiation, growth, and recurrence [62]. Other terms used for these cells are tumor or rescuing units, tumor-progenitor cells, and functional tumor stem cells [63]. Large-scale studies have indicated that the biological characteristics of tumors, including radioresistance, are determined by CSCs [64,65]. It has been demonstrated that CSCs can be enriched both in vitro and in vivo by IR, indicating the possibility of IR-induced generation of CSCs [66,67]. CSCs are considered to have innately higher radioresistance, invasion capability, and metastatic capacity than their differentiated counterparts [61]. Targeting CSCs in tumors may represent an effective antitumor therapeutic strategy and improve the efficacy of radiotherapy. CSCs share some, or all, properties of SCs, that endow these cells with key traits in tumorigenesis, relative quiescence, activation of survival responses, promotion of blood vessel formation, and enhanced motility [10,68]. For example, miR-200 regulates both normal stem/progenitor cells and CSCs by targeting BMI,1 which is necessitated for SC self-renewal [69,70]. Among the early investigators of the 1800s, Virchow and Cohnheim postulated the existence of CSCs that arise from what they believed to be the "activation of dormant embryonic tissue remnants" [71]. CSCs were first proposed by Fiala in 1968 [72]. Although the modern concept of SC biology was absent, a CIC was clearly hypothesized to be an SC unable to differentiate. Researchers in the 1970s advanced the theory that tissue-specific SCs might be the cells of origin for specific tumors [71]. Bayard Clarkson and coworkers identified a small subpopulation of slow-cycling cells, which they termed "dormant cells". These cells were able to escape anti-proliferative chemotherapy and were supposed to be responsible for the relapse of lymphoblastic leukemia in adults [73,74]. The tumor colony assay in soft agar medium proposed by Hamburger and Salmon in the late 1970s introduced the concept that only a small proportion of tumor cells, yielding a plating efficiency of 0.001 to 0.1%, are tumorigenic, and the authors identified these cells as the essential target of therapy [75]. Eventually, compelling evidence for the role of CSCs in the metastatic progression of the tumors was first validated in 1997 when Dick and Bonnet isolated a set of stem cells from human acute myeloid leukemia, and the samples were capable of transferring human acute myeloid leukemia to nonobese diabetic/severe combined immunodeficient mice [56]. In this case, it was observed only that CD34+ CD38− subpopulation [56] was able to reconstitute human acute myeloid leukemia that resembled the human disease in nonobese diabetic/severe combined immunodeficient mice [56,76–78]. CD34+ CD38− cell fraction was shown to represent 0.1–1% of the total cells and possess the proliferative, differentiation, and self-renewal capacities expected of normal stem cells [56,76]. The first time the CSCs concept was applied to solid tumors was in 2003 by Al-Hajj and colleagues [78], when they identified that only a small subset of breast cancer cells expressing markers CD44+/CD24− possessed a marked proliferative capacity, differentiation, self-renewal, and in vivo tumor-forming ability, while the remaining bulk of cells from this tumor had none, even when injected at many-fold higher cell doses [79]. Within the same year, Singh et al. purified CD133+ CSCs from human brain tumors of different phenotypes [80]. In 2004, it was also shown that multiple myeloma contains a rare subset of cells, defined by their lack of expression of the plasma cell marker CD138, that are clonogenic in vitro and tumorigenic in vivo [81]. In 2006, a workshop of the American Association for Cancer Research discussed the rapidly emerging CSC model for tumor progression and established the definition of a CSCs as "a small subset of cells within a tumor that possesses the capacity to self-renewal and to generate the heterogeneous lineages of cancer cells that comprise the tumor" [82]. During the last decade, CSCs have been identified in many solid tumors, including lung [83], pancreas [84], prostate [85], colon [86], liver [87], blood [88], skin [89], thyroid [90], cervix [91], ovary [92], and stomach [93], as well as their functional and phenotypic features have been investigated. CSCs have been previously identified through different criteria, including increased glycolysis and glycine/serine metabolism or low concentrations of reactive oxygen species (ROS) and ATP [94]. The vast majority of studies, such as colony forming unit and marker expression, have been performed to check CSCs' radioresistance [82,95]. CSCs have been found to display enhanced chromosomal instability, possibly highlighting a role in clonal evolution in their propagation [96]. One of the intrinsic properties of CSCs is their ability to grow in a serum-free medium supplemented with growth factors in non-adherent culture plates [97]. In general, CSCs are considered quiescent or at least slow-cycling [98–101]. These cells can stay dormant for extended periods after treatment but eventually re-enter the cell cycle, leading to tumor regrowth [102]. Furthermore, CSCs exhibit certain properties, such as long-term survival, high expression of drug efflux transporters, abnormal cellular metabolism, deregulated self-renewal pathways, acquisition of EMT phenotype [103], more efficient DNA damage repair than bulk tumor cells after IR [104] (Figure 3).

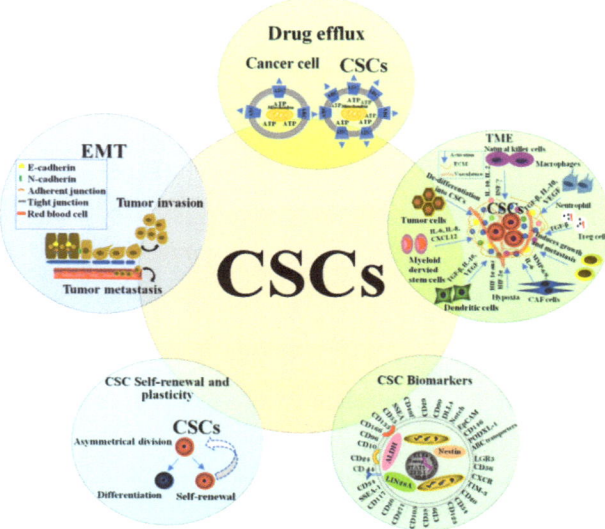

Figure 3. The defining properties CSCs.

It has been reported that CSCs withstand anoikis and display immune evasion, which may result in tumor metastasis and relapse [105,106]. Complicated cellular and molecular mechanisms, such as stemness maintenance, EMT, and ROS production, are intimately involved in the process of CSC initiation and facilitation of tumor recurrence and metastasis after treatment [107–110]. Metabolic stressors, which result in numerous enlarged, elongated, and interconnected mitochondria and increase oxidative capacity and ATP production in CSCs [111]. CSCs have been reported to overexpress ROS free-radical scavengers in order to reinforce their defense against ROS-induced damage [18,112–114], leading to tumor radioresistance. Compared to regular stem cells, CSCs are believed to reside predominantly in niches within the TME, including stromal cells, cancer-associated fibroblasts, infiltrating immune/inflammatory cells, and vascular endothelial cells [67,115,116], to retain their unique properties [117,118]. CSCs niche facilitates their metastatic potential and preserves their plasticity [22,23]. Furthermore, a variety of conditions, such as EMT [30], hypoxia [119], inflammatory cytokines, such as IL-1 β, IL-6, C-X-C motif chemokine ligand 12 (CXCL12), and IL-8 generate cells harboring CSCs properties [120]. The acidic TME has been reported to enhance CSCs radioresistance and angiogenesis through the induction of vascular endothelial growth factor (VEGF) [121,122]. Experimental and clinical studies have indicated that CSCs also possess the ability to initiate tumor formation in the host's body [123]. Interestingly, as few as 100 CSCs have been shown to be able to recreate tumors in nonobese diabetic/severe combined immunodeficient mice [124]. The frequency of CSC varies broadly between different tumor types, spanning from small populations of <1% in human acute myeloid leukemia and liver cancer up to 82% in acute lymphoblastic leukemia [110]. When leukemic cells were transplanted in vivo, only 1–4% of cells could form spleen colonies [67,125]. In vitro data have shown that only 1 in 1000 to 5000 lung cancer cells generates colonies in soft agar assay, indicating that not every lung cancer cell is capable of clonal tumor initiation [126].

3.1. Cancer Stem Cells Related Markers

A large panel of highly specific CSCs markers provides molecular targeted therapies for various tumors, using therapeutic antibodies specific to these markers [127]. These markers are categorized according to cellular localization [128–131]. Many CSCs surface membrane markers have been identified, including podocalyxin, stage-specific mouse embryonic antigen, trophoblast cell-surface antigen 2, epithelial cell adhesion molecule (EpCAM), leucine-rich repeat-containing G-protein coupled receptor 5, aldehyde dehydrogenase 1 family member A1 (ALDH1A1), CD13, CD14, CD19, CD20, CD24, CD26, CD27, CD34, CD38, CD44, CD45, CD47, CD66c, CD90, CD166, CD105, CD133, CD138, CD117/c-kit, CD151, CD166 [129], CD 29 [132], CD271 [133], CD 114 [127], CD 73 [134], integrin α6 (CD49), integrin β1(CD29), integrin β3 (CD61) [135,136], Jagged 1–2 [137], ATP-binding cassette sub-family G member (ABC) transporter family [138], neural cell adhesion molecule (NCAM) [139], and to name a few. Cell surface molecules mediate interactions between cells and their microenvironment [129]. Of note, CD44 and CD133 have been published to be the most widely used markers for isolating CSCs [129,140]. CSCs can be phenotyped by certain stemness-related transcription factors, such as (Yamanaka factors; octamer-binding transcription factor 3/4 (Oct3/4), cellular myelocytomatosis oncogene (c-Myc), SRY (sex determining region Y)-box 2 (SOX2), kruppel-like factor 4 (KLF4), Nanog, Spalt like transcription factor 4 [129], special AT-rich sequence-binding protein 2 (SATB2) [141], forkhead box M1 (FOXM1) [142], mouse nucleoside diphosphate kinase B (NME2) [143], and hypoxia-inducible factor 1-alpha (HIF-1) [144]. These transcription factors contribute to the pathologic self-renewal characteristics of CSCs [145]. Additionally, there is a number of stemness-related markers that are neither cell surface proteins nor transcription factors, including B lymphoma Mo-MLV insertion region 1 homolog (BMI1), Nestin, β-catenin, T-cell immunoglobulin and mucin-domain containing-3 (TIM-3), Musashi-1, ALDH, CXC chemokine receptors (CXCRs) [129,146], transcriptional co-activators (e.g., transformation/transcription domain associated protein TRRAP [147], yes-associated protein 1 (YAP), and transcriptional co-activator with PDZ-binding motif (TAZ) [148], and antiapoptotic genes (e.g., B-Cell Leukemia/Lymphoma 2 (BCL -2), Bcl-2-associated X protein (BAX), cellular FLICE-inhibitory protein (c-FLIP) [149,150]), Survivin [151], B-cell lymphoma-extra-large (Bcl-XL), and myeloid leukemia 1 (MCL-1) [152]. The CSCs phenotype can differ essentially between patients [153]. For example, a small subpopulation of cancer cells is present within some human breast cancers that exhibit a CD44 +/CD24 (−/low) phenotype; these tumorigenic cells have been shown to be highly enriched for CICs in xenografts compared to their counterparts [154], and display a mesenchymal phenotype in the invasive front of the tumor [155]. High CD133 expression is linked to multiple tumor recurrence, increased metastatic potential, and radioresistance [156–158]. It has been reported that CD44 overexpression, in particular CD44v, contributes to tumor radioresistance through the protection against ROS by stimulating the synthesis of reduced glutathione (GSH) level, a primary intracellular antioxidant [159,160]. It has been confirmed that HIF-1 α inactivates the T-cell factor-4 (Tcf-4) for direct binding to β-catenin [161], indicating a role of β-catenin–HIF-1α interaction in promoting CSCs adaptation to hypoxia after IR [161,162]. BMI1 upregulation has been found to confer radioresistance in tumors through stimulating telomerase activity and enhancing ATM recruitment to the chromatin, leading, in turn to tumor perpetuation [163]. Recent studies have confirmed that SATB2 acts as a regulator of stemness and self-renewal by augmenting the expression of pluripotency maintenance-associated transcription factors, such as SOX2, Oct4, c-Myc, KLF4, and Nanog [141,164]. ABC transporters overexpression has been reported in several tumors [165,166] and more predominantly in CSCs [137]. Multi-drug resistant proteins (MDR) have been known to mediate the transport of a variety of cytotoxic compounds out of the cells [137]. It has been shown that members of the ABC transporter superfamily have a wide range of physiological activity: (a) detoxification, permeability glycoprotein (P-gp, also known as MDR1 or ABCB1), and multi-drug resistance-associated protein 1 (MRP1, also known as ABCC1); (b) xenobiotic oxidative stress alleviation (MRPs and ABCCs); (c) cellular lipid metabolism (MDR3, ABCG, and ABCA families), and antigen presentation ATP-binding cassette subfamily-B member 2 and 3, antigen peptide transporter 1 and 2 (ABCB2/transporter associated with antigen processing 1 (TAP1) and ABCB3/TAP2) [167]. A drug-resistance characteristic of CSCs has been identified as a side population [168]. The activity of ABC transporters can be gauged by pumping out fluorescent dyes, such as rhodamine 123 and Hoechst 33342, which can be extruded by ATP-binding cassette subfamily-G member 2 (ABCG2, also known as CDw338/ breast cancer resistance protein (BCRP)) and ATP-binding cassette subfamily-B member 1 (ABCB1), respectively [169,170]. YAP/TAZ activation leads to the induction and maintenance of CSC properties in a wide range of human tumors, including GBM [171,172] and NSCLC [173]. YAP/ TAZ activation in response to IR has been shown to drive tumor growth, transformation, and metastasis [174]. Nestin overexpressing after IR has been demonstrated to correlate with the transformation of various human malignancies [175].

3.2. Cancer Stem Cells Signaling Pathways

CSCs exhibit deregulated activation of self-renewal pathways [103], a process that can lead to extensive cell proliferation and malignant transformation [176].

Furthermore, IR is an antitumor treatment modality that triggers multiple signal transduction networks [177]. Exploring CSC-specific signaling mechanisms and characteristics is clinically important for better-targeted radiotherapy strategies. Regulatory networks consisting of the Notch, Hedgehog (Hh), Janus kinase/signal transducer and activator of transcription (JAK-STAT), canonical and non-canonical Wingless and Int-1 (WNT/β- catenin), nuclear factor kappa-light-chain-enhancer of activated B cells (NF-κB), phosphatase and tensin homolog (PTEN) [129], transforming growth factor and mothers against decapentaplegic (TGF/SMAD), phosphatidylinositol-3-kinase (PI3K)/Akt and the mammalian target of rapamycin (mTOR), peroxisome proliferator-activated receptors (PPAR) [178,179], Hippo-YAP/TAZ [148], mitogen-activated protein kinase and extracellular signal-regulated kinase (MAPK/ERK) [180,181], and miRNAs [179] pathways have all been shown experimentally to play an essential role in regulating CSCs functions [129], controlling their properties [67], and causing radioresistance by expediting tumor recurrence [182,183]. Many of these pathways are inextricably interwoven networks of signaling mediators that feed one another, facilitating inter-pathway crosstalk [184]. For example, Notch signaling inhibition in GBM has been shown to downregulate its target Hes1, a transcriptional repressor, which in turn upregulates GLI transcription in the Hh pathway [185]. NF-κB and TGF proinflammatory signaling pathways have been shown to be activated in tumor cells in response to IR [186]. Recent studies have reported that the canonical WNT/β-catenin signaling cascade participates in the formation of tumor radioresistance by affecting the cell cycle, proliferation, apoptosis, invasion, and DNA damage repair (DDR) [187]. Hh signaling has been reported to play a fundamental role in growth, recurrence, metastasis, radioresistance, and acquisition of a CSC-like phenotype via the EMT process in various tumors [62,188]. It has been confirmed that Notch signaling is an important mediator of IR-induced EMT and responsible for IR-enhanced tumor malignancy [182,189–191]. Many studies have supported the role of the Hippo-YAP/TAZ signaling pathway in the induction of EMT, tumorigenesis, and chromatin remodeling. Moreover, this pathway has been shown to promote tumor radioresistance via escalating DDR [192–194].

3.3. DNA Damage Repair in Response to Ionizing Radiation

The biological consequences of IR are highly influenced by the activation of the DNA damage response mechanisms [195]. A high DDR capacity after IR has been described for CSCs in different tumor entities, including GBM and NSCLC [18,157,196]. Among the various types of DNA damages produced directly and indirectly by IR, such as single-strand breaks (SSBs), double-strand breaks (DSBs), and damaged nucleotide bases or abasic sites, DSBs represent the principal lesions that might lead to cell death or loss of reproductive capacity via activation of different pathways, such as mitotic catastrophe, apoptosis or senescence, if not adequately corrected [197–200]. It has been reported that about 1000 SSBs and 40 DSBs are produced per Gy/cell [201]. Two major mechanisms of DSBs repair have been extensively studied: error-prone non-homologous end joining (NHEJ) and error-free homology-directed recombination (HR) [202,203]. DSBs have been reported to activate three key phosphatidylinositol 3-kinase-related kinase (PIKK) family kinases: ataxia telangiectasia mutated kinase (ATM), ATM-related kinase (ATR), and DNA-dependent protein kinase (DNA-PK) [204,205]. NHEJ is initiated by the binding of the Ku70/Ku80 heterodimer to the end of the DSB [206], allowing the recruitment of catalytic subunit DNA-PKcs forming the protein complex DNA-PK [206]. DNA-bound DNA-PK is activated and phosphorylates numerous proteins, including histone H2AX (γ-H2AX) [207], Artemis [208], X-ray repair cross-complementing 4 (XRCC4), ligase IV complex [209], and XRCC4-like factor [210] that are aggregated on the site of IR-induced foci (IRIF) [211,212]. Inversely, HR uses undamaged homologous chromosome or sister chromatid as a template [213]. Consequently, this mechanism only functions in late S/G2 cell cycle phases [202] and requires the presence of breast cancer proteins [202]. NHEJ has been known to be an efficient and rapid process due to the avid end-binding ability of Ku and its high abundance [214], whereas HR is the least error-prone repair mechanism [202].

3.4. Cancer Stem Cells in Glioblastoma

It has been reported that a single GBM can contain heterogeneous clones of GBM stem-like cells (referred to as GSCs) with different morphologies, self-renewal, aggressive phenotype, and proliferative capacities [49,215–219]. The similarity of the gene-expression profiles of GSCs and normal neural stem cells (NSCs) provides support to the idea that CSCs are malignant variants of normal neural stem cells [220,221]. It has been shown that GSCs are able to grow under serum-free culture conditions identical to normal neural stem cells [222], efflux fluorescent dyes [223], and generate progeny comprised of a mixture of stem cells and more restricted non-stem cells descendants through symmetrically dividing [1,49,224]. GSCs tend to be more tumorigenic, pro-angiogenic, and radioresistant than the majority of GBM cells [10,131,225]. Recent accumulating evidence has revealed that GSCs can enhance radioresistance in GBM through activation of DNA damage checkpoint proteins, including checkpoint kinase 1 (Chk1), checkpoint kinase 2 (Chk2), ATM, structural maintenance of chromosomes (SMC1), and p53 [226]. GSCs have been reported to express cell surface CSCs markers, such as stage-specific mouse embryonic antigen, CD34, CD44, α6-integrin, CD133, L1CAM (L1 Cell Adhesion Molecule), CD54, and A2B5 [97,217,227–235]; cytoskeleton proteins (also referred as; intermediate filaments or nanofilaments), such as glial fibrillary acidic protein (GFAP) [236], vimentin [237–239], and Nestin; transcription factors, such as SOX2, Nanog, Oct3/4 [240,241], nuclear factor erythroid 2-related factor 2 (Nrf2) [241,242], oligodendrocyte transcription factor (Olig2) [243], FoxM1 [244], and zinc finger protein 281 (ZNF281) [245], POU class 3 Homeobox 2 [246], and melanocyte inducing transcription factor (MITF) [247]; posttranscriptional factors, such as Musashi 1 [248] and microRNAs [249]; polycomb (Pc) transcriptional suppressors, such as enhancer of zeste homolog 2 and BMI 1 [248]; transcriptional co-activators, such as YAP/TAZ [171] and TRRAP [250], yet no single marker is able to define a general GSC population. It has been reported that GSCs metabolism undergoes different changes than that of traditional GBM tumor cells following IR [251]. Gene expression analyses of GBM cells treated by IR have revealed that many genes are modulated after treatment [252–254]. These genes are closely involved in a variety of cellular processes, such as cell cycle, apoptosis, DNA replication/damage repair, cytoskeleton organization, and metabolism [255]. There is a growing body of evidence that the fraction of GSCs expressing CD133 increases after IR [80]. CD133+ GSCs have been reported to represent the cellular subpopulation that confers radioresistance and drives GBM recurrence [225,229,256]. It has been observed that injection of 10^2 CD133+ cells forms a tumor that regenerates a phenocopy of the patient's original tumor upon transplantation, whereas transplantation of 10^4 CD133− cells does not lead to producing a tumor [225,229]. CD133+ GSCs radioresistance is attributed to preferential activation of the DNA damage checkpoint proteins (e.g., Chk1 and Chk2 kinases) [225,257]. It has been found that the CD133+ subpopulation is able to repair IR-induced DNA damage more efficiently and undergo less apoptosis compared to CD133− counterparts [225,258]. The CD133+ fraction among highly aggressive GBMs ranges from 0.1 to 50% [229]. It should be emphasized that some GBM tumors do not contain any CD133+ cells [259–261]. For example, GBM xenografts irradiated in vivo have been reported to be enriched 3–5-fold for CD133+ cells compared to untreated xenografts [225]. Bao et al. observed using a colony-forming unit assay that CD133− non-GSCs cultures irradiated at a dose of 5 Gy form fewer colonies compared to CD133+ GSC cultures [225]. Overexpression of Olig2 and CD44 after exposure to 6 Gy of cobalt-60 has been found to be related to the proliferative and invasive state of GBM [262]. Many authors have pointed out the role of α6-integrin in GBM radioresistance by increasing the efficiency of DDR [263]. IR-treated GBM cells have been reported to produce sICAM-1, resulting in a mesenchymal shift of GBM only in vivo [235,264]. Side population cells have been identified in GBM cells [168]. In 2003, Trog et al. first reported on the upregulation of the ABC-1 transporter in human GBM in response to DNA-damaging agents in an IR-dose-dependent manner. They also found that IR has a higher inducible effect on the ABC-1 expression rates depending on GBM cell density [265]. A high expression of KLF4 has been shown to promote the proliferation of the GSC population and the regrowth of GBM, even after aggressive radiotherapy [266]. An increased expression of Nrf2 post-IR has been reported to protect GBM against IR-induced oxidative stress by activating several downstream genes related to detoxification and antioxidant response, such as glutathione peroxidase and superoxide dismutase [241,267–271]. It has been documented that a pronounced enrichment of BMI1 after IR at the chromatin confers radioresistance in GBM through copurifying with NHEJ repair proteins, such as DNA-PK, poly [ADP-ribose] polymerase 1 (PARP-1), hnRNP U, and histone H1 in CD133+ GSCs [272]. Epidermal growth factor receptor (EGFR) and epidermal growth factor receptor variant III (EGFR^{VIII}) have been shown to mediate radioresistance in GBM by maintaining EMT and activating both NHEJ and HR [273,274]. IR-induced VEGF secretion enhances the angiogenic potential of GBM [275]. Compelling preclinical proof has shown that anti-VEGF growth therapy stimulates IR-induced cell death in U-87 under normoxic and hypoxic conditions [276]. Maachani U. B. et al. demonstrated that both FOXM1 and STAT3 proteins interact together and co-localize in the nucleus under radiotherapy, facilitating the DDR processes [277]. It has been shown that GBM become more radioresistant through the overexpression of proliferating cell nuclear antigen (PCNA)-associated factor, which facilitates DNA damage bypass [278]. Accumulating evidence has pointed out the potential role of antioxidant enzymes, such as superoxide dismutase, catalase, glutathione peroxidase, glutathione reductase, in GBM radioresistance [279]. These enzymes have been reported to be activated up to 5-fold in a radioresistant variant clone isolated from a human U251 cell line compared to the parent cells after IR [279,280]. Enhanced expression of cyclooxygenase-2, also known as prostaglandin endoperoxide/H synthase 2, in GSCs has been reported to be potently involved in progressive GBM growth, as well as radioresistance [281,282]. It has been evinced that overexpression of cathepsin L, a lysosomal endopeptidase enzyme, enhances GSCs' radioresistance through inducing expression of CD133 and phosphorylation of DNA damage checkpoint proteins [283]. Cyclin-dependent kinase 2 (CDK2) expression has been shown to be significantly enriched in GBM and is functionally required for their proliferation and growth both in vitro and in vivo [284]. CDK2 has also been to induce radioresistance in GBM cells, and its knockdown enhances cell apoptosis when combined with radiotherapy [284]. Histone deacetylase 4 and -6 have been shown to induce radioresistance in GBM by maintaining the GSC phenotype [285]. Many studies have reported that the radiosensitivity of GBM can be altered by targeting microRNAs. The expression of miR-1, miR-221/222, and miR-124 has been shown to effectively regulate IR-related signal transduction pathways in GBM [286]. Another study has revealed that miR-1, miR-125a, miR-150, and miR-425 induce radioresistance in GBM through upregulation of the cell cycle checkpoint response [287]. Many reports have stated that high Ki-67 is rigorously proportional to the high proliferative state of GBM cells [288,289]. It has been shown that the Ki-67 labeling index is significantly expressed in post-irradiated GBM cells compared to their respective pre-irradiated counterparts [290]. GSCs isolated from human LN18 cells with cell surface vimentin overexpression have been found to present 95% CD133 expression and 98% CD44 expression, suggesting that GSCs that express surface vimentin possess tumor-initiating properties [291]. Many studies have shown that vimentin regulates IR-induced migration of GBM cells [292]. Survivin has been reported to enhance GBM cell survival, regulate DSB repair capabilities, and contribute to a hypermetabolic state upon IR exposure [9,293]. Increased GFAP and insulin-like growth factor binding protein-2 (IGFBP-2) serum levels in GBM patients after radiotherapy have been shown to be correlated with the malignant degree and prognosis of GBM (wpr-669323). It has been indicated that overexpression of RCC2, a regulator of chromosome condensation 2, enhances proliferation and tumorigenesis, as well as confers radioresistance in GBM cells [294]. Alterations in several molecular and signaling pathways following IR have been shown to be closely involved in inducing radioresistance in GBM [295]. GSC functions are largely mediated by several deregulated signaling pathways, such as MEK/ERK [296], Notch [297], NF-κB [298], Hh [299], WNT/β-catenin [300], PI3K/AKT/mTOR [301], JAK-STAT [302,303], retinoblastoma protein (Rb), receptor tyrosine kinase (RTK) [304], transforming growth factor-β (TGF-β), platelet-derived growth factor [305,306], and PTEN [307], resulting in an aberrant expression of downstream signature molecules that drive radioresistance and recurrence of GBM. Marampon et al. showed that MEK/ERK pathway positively regulates HIF-1α protein activity through the sustained expression of DNA-PKcs, preserving GBM radioresistance in hypoxic conditions [296]. CD133 has been shown to promote the tumorigenic capacity of GCS by activation of the PI3K/Akt pathway by interacting with the p85 regulatory domain of PI3K [308]. It has been shown that Notch1 inhibition in GBM xenografts reduces the hypoxic fraction and delays tumor progression, suggesting a potential mechanism whereby Notch1 downregulation radiosensitizes GBM cells [309]. NF-κB signaling pathway has been found to be aberrantly activated in response to IR in GBM, where its IR-induced upregulation has been involved in GSCs maintenance, invasion, mesenchymal identity promotion, and DNA damage repair through NHEJ and HR processes [49,310–316]. In GBM, the most common genetic lesions, including p53, PTEN, and P16 (also known as p16^{INK4A}, cyclin-dependent kinase inhibitor 2A), have been reported to regulate the DNA damage response [10]. Around 40–50% of GBM has p53 mutations [317,318]. Indeed, it has been reported that the failure of p53 to induce p21^{BAX} expression causes radioresistance in GBM [319]. Moreover, loss of PTEN contributes to an increase in the cellular motility of neural precursor cells, alteration in Chk1 localization, and genetic instability, conferring radioresistance in GBM cells [320,321]. It has been established that the radiosensitivity of GSCs can be increased by inhibiting Becline-1 and ATG5, autophagy-related proteins, indicating that the induction of autophagy contributes to radioresistance in GSC [322]. The PI3K/Akt/mTOR pathway has been suggested to play an important role in IR-induced autophagy in GBM cells [323].

3.5. Cancer Stem Cells in Non-Small-Cell Lung Cancer

It has been demonstrated that IR-Surviving NSCLC cells display CSCs [324]. The expression of CSC-related markers after radiotherapy is significantly correlated with a poor prognosis in patients with NSCLC [325]. There is a huge number of lung CSC

(LCSC) markers, including cell surface markers, such as EpCAM [326], CD 24 [327,328], CD34 [329], CD44, CD90 [57,330], CD133 [94], CD166 [83], ALDH1 [331,332], sICAM-1 [333], ABCG2 [334], and NCAM [335]; stemness related-TFs, such as Yamanaka factors (Oct-3/4) [336], SOX-2 [337], KLF4 [338], c-Myc [339], Stabilin 2 [340], MITF [341], STAT3 [342], and HIF-1α [343]; other stemness-related markers, such as miRNAs [344], Nestin [345], BMI1 [346], Musashi-1 [347], PARP-1 [348], matrix metalloproteinases (MMPs) [349,350], VEGF, epidermal Growth Factor (EGF) [351], and chemokines (e.g., CXCL12/CXCR-4) [352]. CD24 expression in NSCLC cells has been reported to be associated with disease progression and aggressive tumor behavior [327,353]. It has been observed that CD24 is upregulated only in IR-surviving NSCLC cells [324]. It has been reported that CD44 is dramatically upregulated in IR-surviving NSCLC cells [324]. Knockdown of CD44 expression in NSCLC cells has been shown to suppress cell proliferation and colony formation in vitro [354]. Tirino et al. proposed that CD133+ cells isolated from NSCLC cells can form tumors and act as CICs [355,356]. The injection of 10^4 lung cancer CD133+ cells in immunocompromised mice has been reported to readily generate unlimited progeny phenotypically identical to the original tumor [94]. It has been observed that A549 but not H1299 cells expand their CD133+ population after exposure to 4 Gy IR, and isolated A549 CD133+ cells have been found to be radioresistant, and this resistance has been noted to correspond with upregulated expression of DSB repair genes in A549 cells [157]. Clinically relevant IR doses (1 or 3 Gy) have been reported to induce markedly HIF-1α expression in a subset of normoxic NSCLC lines in vitro, leading to modulating the cell viability and angiogenic activity [357] through the activation of anaerobic metabolism [358]. CXCR-4 has been found to use STAT3-mediated slug expression to maintain NSCLC radioresistance [359]. Many articles have proved that angiogenic factors, such as VEGF and EGF, are correlated with tumor growth, aggressiveness, survival, disease relapse, and radioresistance in NSCLC [360]. Some studies have focused on the clinical implications of miRNAs for radiotherapy in patients with NSCLC. miRNA-210 has been found to drive radioresistance in NSCLC via promoting HIF1α-induced glycolysis [361] and regulating IR- induced DSBs repair [362]. Furthermore, miRNA-25 has been known to lessen radiosensitivity by binding the B-cell translocation gene 2 in NSCLC cells [363], whereas miRNA-1323 has been reported to decrease radiosensitivity of NSCLC by inducing the expression of protein kinase, DNA-activated, catalytic polypeptide [364]. The reduced expression of tumor protein p53-inducible protein 3, a downstream mediator of the DDR, in IR-surviving H460R cells has been shown to be greatly involved in acquired RR [365]. MMPs has found to play an undeniable role in tumor extracellular matrix (ECM) invasion [366]. It has been demonstrated that IR-surviving NSCLC cells, after exposure to 10 Gy of, show increased motility and increased expression of MMP-2/-9 [367]. It has been suggested that the detaching soluble natural killer group 2 member D ligands in NCI-H23 cells can be a result of IR-induced MMP-2 [368]. Using a 3D NSCLC model, IR with a dose of 5 Gy has been found to increase the growth of tumor tissue analogs containing CSCs and enhance the expression of cytokines (regulated upon activation, normal T cell expressed, and secreted, epithelial-neutrophil activating peptide, and TGF-α) and factors (MMP, vimentin, and tissue inhibitors of metalloproteinase (TIMP)) [369]. It has been indicated that the level of IR-induced apoptosis decreases in those NSCLC cells exhibiting BCL-2 overexpression [370]. Our previous experimental data have reported that ABCG2 expression markedly increases in multifractionated radiotherapy-surviving NSCLC cells at a total dose of 60 Gy, conferring these cells a radioresistant phenotype [170]. Silencing MITF has been reported to promote migration, invasion, colony formation, metastasis, and tumorigenesis in CL1-0, CL1-1, and CL1-5 cell lines [341]. Overexpression of SOX2 in IR-surviving NSCLC cells has been revealed to stimulate cellular migration and anchorage-independent growth, while SOX-2 knockdown has been reported to impair their growth [324,371,372]. It has been demonstrated that inhibition of Poly (ADP-ribose) polymerase-1 (PARP-1), a well-known active candidate in DNA repair, separately diminishes proliferation, migration, EMT, phosphorylation of EGFR, Akt, p38, NF-kB, and ERK in treated NSCLC with ^{12}C [373,374]. Several signaling pathways, such as PI3K, MEK [375], Notch [376], Nrf2 [377], WNT/β-catenin [378], and Hh [379], have been described to regulate the behavior of LCSCs and contribute to radioresistance in NSCLC. It has been reported that PI3K kinase inhibition can play a role in boosting the radiosensitivity of NSCLC cells via immune evasion [380] and resistance to IR-induced apoptosis [381]. Overwhelming data have indicated that the dysregulated expression of the Notch signaling pathway is a frequent event in NSCLC [382,383]. It has been shown that high Notch pathway activity has an unequivocal role in survival, poor prognosis, and radioresistance in NSCLC patients through the inhibition of apoptosis, suggesting its potential as a therapeutic target [384,385]. Moreover, Notch-1 has been reported to increase NSCLC cells' survival under hypoxic conditions by activating the insulin-like growth factor (IGF) pathway [386]. Additionally, inhibiting IR-induced Notch-1 signaling has been found to enhance the radiotherapy efficacy in H1299 and H460 cell lines [376]. It has been reported that Nrf2 expression is significantly elevated in NSCLC cells at 4 h after IR exposure [387], as well as it has been observed to regulate the cellular antioxidant system and crosstalk with Notch1 signaling pathway in response to IR [387]. It was reviewed by Heavey et al. that inhibition of the Akt/mTOR/4EBP/eIF4E pathway in NSCLC cells might result in the development of radiotherapy and overcome radioresistance [388]. The Sonic Hh-Gli pathway has been found to promote the migrative and invasive abilities of NSCLC cells by regulating EMT [389]. The aberrant activation of the WNT/β-catenin signaling in NSCLC has been reported to correlate closely with self-renewal, proliferation, tumorigenesis, progression, and radioresistance [182,390]. Increased PI3K/AKT/mTOR activation has been shown to lead to radioresistance in NSCLC cells [301]. Previously, we have reported that residual γH2AX/53BP1 foci number decreases in multifractionated radiotherapy surviving NSCLC cells compared to parental cells post-IR at extra single doses of 2, 4, and 6 Gy. Furthermore, our previous data have detected that Rad51 protein expression might play a key role in enhancing DNA DSB repair by the HR pathway in multifractionated radiotherapy survival of p53 null NSCLC cells [391].

4. Epithelial-to-Mesenchymal Transition and Migratory Activity in Glioblastoma and Non-Small-Cell Lung Cancer

The heterogeneity of tumor cell populations allows for the movements of either individual cells or clusters of cells. EMT, a reversible molecular and cellular process, has been invoked as a mechanism by which immotile tumor cells can acquire a migratory, invasive, and motile phenotype by attenuating adherens junction and avoiding anoikis in the TME [392,393]. The reverse process is termed mesenchymal-to-epithelial transition (MET) [394]. MET and EMT have been closely linked to the acquisition of stemness characteristics in tumorigenesis [28,30,50,395–397]. Tumor cells undergoing EMT have been observed to lose their apical basal cell polarity and acquire a more spindle-shaped form [398], facilitating their dissemination into the blood circulation [28]. Moreover, EMT allows tumor cells to degrade basal extracellular matrix by MMPs activation to help these transformed cells to migrate [399,400]. A partial EMT observed among tumor cells can be explicated by the different tumorigenic capabilities of tumor cells from various niches inside tumor. Tumor cells with a partial EMT have been found to be more efficient in tumor budding, invasion, and metastasis because these processes evidently require both EMT and MET [401]. Loss of expression of tight junction proteins, including E-cadherin, and upregulation of mesenchymal markers, such as N-cadherin, Vimentin, and Fibronectin, have been considered as the key molecular events of EMT [402]. EMT-inducing TFs, such as basic helix–loop–helix (bHLH) factors (e.g., E2A, an inhibitor of DNA binding (Id2, Id3), and Twist 1/2), Snail family members (e.g., Snail and Slug), finger E-box-binding homeobox factor (ZEB) family members (e.g., ZEB1/2, SMAD interacting protein-1 (SIP1)) [403,404], Goosecoid [405], ZNF281 [406], Brachyury, sine oculis homeobox homolog 1 (SIX1), transcription factor 4, FOXC2, paired related homeobox 1 [407], and others, have been demonstrated to enhance the expression of genes associated with the mesenchymal state, such as N-cadherin, Vimentin, Fibronectin, β-integrins, and ECM-cleaving proteases [407] and directly repress mediators of epithelial adhesion proteins, such as E-Cadherin, Occludins, Claudins, Desmosomes, and cytokeratins [274,403,404,408,409]. Several EMT-related signaling pathways have been identified, including signaling pathways mediated by TGF-β [410,411], bone morphogenetic proteins, WNT–β-catenin, Notch, Hh, RTKs [402], SMADs, STATs, PI3K/Akt, MAPKs [412,413], JAK/STAT3 [414], NFkB [415], Src, and Ras [407,416]. It has been reported that radiotherapy induces tumor cells to undergo EMT, resulting in marked radioresistance [417–419]. Moreover, EMT can be induced by TME stresses (e.g., hypoxia) [420,421]. EMT has been shown to confer tumor cells' resistance to apoptotic stimuli [50]. EMT has known to be a motor of cellular plasticity [422] since it is accompanied by immunosuppressive TME [400,423,424], tumor-initiation potential [425], cell proliferation [426,427], and cellular senescence [428]. Furthermore, EMT has been shown to be associated with catabolic reprogramming for tumor cell survival during metabolic stress [429]. A high infiltrative nature and an increased migratory potential of GBM and NSCLC have been shown to be tightly associated with relapse [430,431]. EMT has been pointed out as one of the mechanisms that confer invasive and metastatic property to GBM and NSCLC after exposure to IR [432,433]. The most important adhesion and cell–cell contact factors, E-cadherin and β-catenin [434,435], have been found to be rarely expressed in GBM cells [50]. Sublethal doses of IR have been reported to induce cell migration and invasiveness of GBM [436]. Furthermore, multifractionated radiotherapy has been found to enhance the migratory capability of GBM cells in vivo [437]. STAT3/NF-κB and Slug signaling activation has been reported to enhance IR-induced tumor migration, invasion, and EMT properties in GBM via the upregulation of ICAM-1 [438]. NSCLC cells have been found to possess a spindle or rounded morphology and express high levels of EMT markers after prolonged exposure to IR [439]. It has been demonstrated that IR can increase EMT phenotype in NSCLC cells by regulating EMT markers via activating the JAK2 tyrosine kinase phosphorylates PAK1 (JAK2–PAK1)–Snail signaling pathway [440]. IR-surviving A549 and H460 cells at a dose of 5 Gy have been reported to express significantly higher levels of EMT markers (Snail1, Vimentin, and N-cadherin) compared to non-irradiated NSCLC cells [324]. Furthermore, it has been observed that the expression of Oct-4, SOX2, and β-catenin proteins markedly increases in adherent H460 cells maintained in a monolayer after IR at a dose of 5 Gy [324]. Our previous data have suggested that a fraction dose escalation regimen at a total dose of 60 Gy probably causes partial (or hybrid) EMT program activation in multifractionated radiotherapy surviving NSCLC cells through either Vimentin upregulation in p53null or an aberrant N-cadherin upregulation in p53wt cells [441]. Moreover, we have indicated previously that the hypofractionation regimen IR does not significantly influence horizontal 1D cell migration of multifractionated radiotherapy surviving NSCLC cells, though promoting their migration by 24 h after scratching [441].

5. Radiation-Induced Dormancy

Tumor niches, including metastatic, perivascular, and bone marrow cells, have been found to harbor dormant tumor cells [23]. Cellular dormancy can be reached in one of two ways: either each tumor cell arrests its cell cycling or the entire neoplasm exhibits balanced growth/apoptosis rates, but too often discussed in terms of two growth arrest mechanisms: **cellular quiescence** (G0), in which cells are in a non-proliferative/slow-cycling state with a reversible growth arrest [442,443], and **cellular senescence**, in which cell cycle arrest is largely irreversible [444–448]. Therefore, mechanisms of tumor relapse induced by the reactivation of dormant tumor cells depend on whether the cells became dormant via quiescence or senescence [449]. Many cues have been known to induce cellular dormancy, such as endoplasmic reticulum stress [450], angiogenic switching, immunological surveillance, anoikis, autophagy, senescence [23], TME (e.g., extracellular matrix, inflammatory signals, genetic, and epigenetics alterations) [445], and IR [24]. In tumor cells, including CSCs, dormancy has been shown to be critical for adaptation and protection against environmental stress and toxicity [451], leading to a tumor relapse [23]. However, several lines of evidence have reported that CSCs can contain heterogeneous subpopulations that either include rapid-cycling or quiescent subpopulations [452].

5.1. Quiescence-Associated Radioresistance

Quiescence is defined as a sleep-like state in which cells cease to divide but retain their ability to re-enter a novel cell cycle readily and rapidly [453,454]. It has been reported that tumor cells switch between phases of growth and quiescence to gain the genetic and epigenetic modifications that are imperative for survival [451]. Cellular radiosensitivity shows a heterogeneous pattern through different cell cycle phases [455,456]. Quiescent cancer cells also referred to as slow-proliferating/slow-cycling cancer cells, are considered an attractive therapeutic target for tumor treatment since they are significantly resistant to conventional radiotherapy with a higher repair capacity than cycling cells [443,457–459]. It has been confirmed that Ki-67 is degraded constantly in G0/G1 and accumulates in S/M phases [460]. Moreover, Ki-67 levels during G0/G1 have been found to indicate how long a cell has spent in these phases [460]. It has been shown that the more protracted a cell has spent in quiescence, the lower the Ki-67 level will be upon re-entering the cell cycle [460]. Furthermore, quiescent cancer cells have been known to display a low rate of BrdU incorporation [461] and a low ERK 1/2: p38 MAPK ratio [462]. The entrance into the quiescence state allows tumor cells to hamper stress and toxic stimuli. After repairing the cellular damage, the cells may re-enter the cell cycle upon stimulation by specific growth factors, such as E2F and CDK2 [463]. It has been shown that, after IR, GSCs are more quiescent than GBM cells that express elevated levels of glycolysis and oxidative phosphorylation, the so-called "Warburg effect", whereas GSCs show metabolic signs of quiescence, such as a diminished non-essential amino-acid synthesis, and unchanged levels of glycolytic and oxidative metabolites [251]. Earlier studies have demonstrated that Ras-related C3 botulinum toxin substrate 2 induces aberrant proliferation of quiescent NSCLC after IR exposure to a single dose of 2 Gy via promoting JUN-B expression through megakaryoblastic leukemia 1—serum response factor (MAL-SRF) pathway [464].

5.2. Radiation-Induced Senescence

Therapy-induced senescence (TIS), a prolonged state of cell-cycle arrest, is reported in tumor cells treated by various therapeutic agents, including IR [465]. Senescent cells have been reported to contribute to the composition of pre-malignant [466–468] and malignant lesions [469]; thus, they play an indubitable role in tumor cell fate [470,471]. Cellular senescence can be triggered by short or dysfunctional telomeres, known as replicative senescence, but also prematurely, by a variety of stress signals [472]. Interestingly, IR prematurely promotes the same phenotypes as replicative senescence prior to the Hayflick limit. This process is known as stress-induced premature senescence (SIPS) [473]. Unlike in apoptosis, cells that enter senescence are not killed; they retain some metabolic activities and secretory activity despite not undergoing cell division [474]. TIS state is accompanied by induced lysosomal biogenesis [475], macromolecular [476,477] and transcriptomic alterations [478], often leading to the synthesis and secretion of a wide spectrum of mediators, a phenomenon termed the senescence-associated secretory phenotype (SASP) [479–482]. SASP-related biomarkers include: 1- soluble factors, such as growth factors (e.g., amphiregulin, epiregulin, heregulin, EGF, basic fibroblast growth factor (bFGF), FGF7, hepatocyte growth factor, VEGF, angiogenin, stem cell factor, stromal cell-derived factor-1, placental growth factor, nerve growth factor, IGFBP-2, -3, -4, -6, -7), cytokines (e.g., IL-6, IL-7, IL-1a, -1b, IL-13, IL-15), chemokines (e.g., IL-8, CXCL1, -b, -gc, monocyte chemoattractant protein 2 (MCP-2, MCP-4, MIP-1a, MIP-3a), hepatocellular carcinoma-4, Eotaxin, Eotaxin-3, epithelial neutrophil activating peptide, I-309, interferon–inducible T cell alpha chemoattractant), other inflammatory factors (e.g., interferon -γ, CXCL13, glycosylation-inhibiting factor), proteases and regulators (e.g., MMP-1, -3, -10, -12, -13, -14, TIMP-1, TIMP-2, serpin E1) [482], receptors shedding or ligands (e.g., ICAM-1, -3, osteoprotegerin, soluble tumor necrosis factor receptor I, CD263, CD120, CD95, urokinase plasminogen activator surface receptor, soluble gp130, EGF-R), nonprotein soluble factors (e.g., prostaglandin E2, nitric oxide, ROS); 2- insoluble factors (ECM) (Fibronectin, Collagens, Laminin) [482]. Upon secretion from senescent cells, these SASP factors usually act in a paracrine manner to stimulate the proliferation and/or transformation of adjacent immortalized cancer cells or even can trigger the senescence of other cells in the TME [483]. This SASP induces an EMT and invasiveness, hallmarks of malignancy, by a paracrine mechanism that depends largely on the SASP factors IL-6 and IL-8 [484]. Senescent cells have been reported to show morphological alterations, such as an enlarged, flattened, and irregular shape with increased cytoplasmic granularity bearing more vacuoles, an increase in senescence-associated -galactosidase (SA-Gal) activity, altered mitochondria in terms of both morphology (e.g., increased mass [485]) and function [486], the expression of the pH-restricted (pH 6) [487–489], and an altered chromatin organization known as senescence-associated heterochromatin foci (SAHF) [490] contributing to the silencing of proliferation-promoting genes, including E2F target genes, such as cyclin A [491]. Senescence-associated cell enlargement is ascribed to several mechanisms, and one of them is cellular hypertrophy, in which a cell gets bigger due to an accumulation of proteins [492]. Senescent cells also lose monolayer integrity, which may result from the downregulation of intercellular junctions [493,494]. Unfortunately, TIS is reversible state for only some subsets of the senescent cell population, leading to cellular re-proliferation and, ultimately, tumor progression [444,495,496]. For example, several studies on various tumor types, including GBM and NSCLC, have shown that therapy-induced senescent cells can re-enter the cell cycle to trigger relapse [465,496–498]. It has been demonstrated that, after IR, senescent non-CSCs secrete chemokines contributing to the maintenance and migration of CSCs [499]. It has been noted that the long-term G2 arrest and subsequent senescence by G2-slippage are more preponderate at a high dose of IR than at a moderate dose [500,501]. TIS has a profound influence on the radiotherapeutic outcome, particularly in multifractionated regimens where the IR dose is increased incrementally. Because every single dose of IR will convert some tumor cells into senescent cells, thus treatment may not contribute to the anticipated antitumor effect by the time a patient receives the highest doses of IR. An emerging body of evidence has also confirmed that "irreversible" senescence can be overcome following radiotherapy. Of note, tumor suppressor proteins, such as PTEN, p53, or hypo-phosphorylated Rb, can be used to detect cellular senescence. Even the absence of markers can be used, including the absence of Ki-67 or the lack of bromodeoxyuridine (BrdU) incorporation [483]. It has been reported that the conditional expression of p53, p16^{INK4A}, or p21$^{waf1/cip1}$ alone in neoplastic cell lines results in irreversible growth arrest and senescence phenotype [502]. It is worth emphasizing that at present, the list of reliable markers reflecting the causes and features of cellular senescence in vitro and in vivo goes far beyond SA-β-Gal expression, including high expression levels of the CDK inhibitor, p16^{INK4A}, p21^{cip1} [503], SASP [484,504], Lipofuscin [505], Lamin B1 downregulation [488], γ-H2A.X, as well as SAHF [473]. The radiation-induced senescent cancer cells express SASP that is required for triggering the proliferation, invasion, and migration of surrounding cells in vitro [484,506]. Tumor cells can undergo senescence following radiotherapy in vitro and in vivo [507]. Further investigations have revealed that the increase in SASP-expressing senescent GBM cells is likely one of the main reasons for GBM recurrence post-radiotherapy [482,508]. It has been observed that ^{137}Cs γ-ray IR at single acute doses (0, 2, 5, 10, and 20 Gy) renders 17–20% of U87MG and LN229 cells dead but gives rise to 60–80% of growth-arrested GBM cells with elevation of senescence markers, such as SA-β-Gal+ cells, H3K9me3+ cells, and p53-p21^{cip1} + cells. Furthermore, it has been reported that 24 h after IR with a total dose of 20 Gy, expression of SIPS factors, such as IL6, IL8, IL1α, IL1β, chemokine (C-C motif) ligand 2 (CCL2), CXCL1, SASP mRNAs, and p21^{cip1}, increases significantly in irradiated U87MG and LN229 cells compared to non-irradiated counterpart cells. It has been suggested that IR likely triggers SASP induction in GBM cells via activation of NFκB signaling [508]. Upon treatment by IR, the primary response of GBM cells has been reported to be proliferation arrest. The arrested GBM cells then undergo premature senescence within 4–8 days following IR as alternative responses to apoptosis [509]. It has been demonstrated that PARP-1 activity in GBM during radiotherapy is required for residual GBM cells to escape from TIS [498]. IR has been shown to induce primarily premature senescence rather than apoptosis in human NSCLC in a dose-dependent manner [510]. The antitumor effect of IR doses (0–6 Gy) has been reported to correlate well with IR-induced premature senescence, as evidenced by increased SA-β-Gal staining, decreased BrdU incorporation, and elevated expression of p16^{INK4A} in irradiated NSCLC [510]. Previous studies have shown that IR-induced senescence in NSCLC cells is associated with p53 and p21 expression [471,511]. It has been demonstrated that IR induces the expression of phosphorylated p53 and p21 in a dose-dependent manner in H460 cells [510]. It has been reported that escape from TIS in both a p53 null NSCLC in vitro and in primary tumors is due to overexpression of CDK1 [512] and survivin [513] and that aberrant expression of CDK1 promotes the formation of polyploid senescent cells, which are an important intermediary through which escape preferentially occurs [495]. It has been demonstrated that the concurrent radiotherapy with the blockade of DNA-PK and PARP-1 enhances the senescence of irradiated H460 cells in vitro and in vivo further than that accomplished with IR alone [514].

6. Polyploid Giant Cancer Cells/Multinucleated Giant Cancer Cells in Glioblastoma and Non-Small-Cell Lung Cancer

Aneuploidy is a ubiquitous characteristic of tumors. Over 90% of human solid tumors are aneuploid [515]. A large amount of data has been provided irrefutable evidence that IR can activate cell cycle checkpoints that inhibit entrance into or progression through mitosis [516,517]. The frequency of polyploid giant cancer cells (PGCCs) and multinucleated giant cancer cells (MNGCs) have been reported to be positively correlated with high tumor recurrence, malignancy grade [518,519], poor prognosis, and resistance to tumor therapy [520–525]. PGCCs/MNGCs have been shown to contribute to solid tumor heterogeneity [526] and to be an integral part of the tumor cell life cycle [526]. PGCCs/MNGCs are not dormant as formerly thought [13,526,527]. It has been revealed that tumor cells can escape cell death following IR by endopolyploidization [41], as well as PGCCs/MNGCs have been observed to be more radioresistant than their diploid counterparts [528,529]. Polyploid tumor cells formed through IR-induced mitotic catastrophe have been demonstrated to be able to survive long enough to establish a growing population of cells (for weeks) post-IR [530–533]. PGCCs/MNGCs have been described as flattened tumor cells with extremely enlarged or multiple nuclei with an elevated genomic content when compared to other tumor cells in the same tumor [525,534,535], which confer on them the ability to generate the functions of different cell types via genetic and epigenetic modifications [40]. These cells have been shown to cease to proliferate or proliferate very slowly such that they are often considered as dead cells in the traditional colony formation assay, also referred to as "clonogenic survival", the gold standard for assessing radiosensitivity of human cells in vitro [40,42]. Several studies involving various tumor cell types have demonstrated that these giant cells are highly adaptable to hypoxic stress and acquire a mesenchymal phenotype with increased expression of CSCs markers, such as CD44, CD133, Oct4, stage-specific embryonic antigen-1 (SSEA-1), NANOG, and SOX2 [526] and ZEB1 [39,522,526,536–538]. The main mechanisms responsible for the formation of PGCCs/MNGCs appear to be associated with cell fusion [539], endoreplication/mitotic bypass [540,541], cytokinesis failure [540,541], and cell cannibalism by entosis [542]. Of note, polyploidy can either be reversible and irreversible [543]. Irreversible polyploidy has been known to occur through DNA re-replication in the absence of mitosis and can reach very high levels of genome duplication up to several thousand or more [544], while PGCCs/MNGCs, which typically do not exceed 32 n, can revert to mitosis and initial paradiploidy [38,533,545]. While most of these cells will undergo cell death following mitotic catastrophe [546], some of them can release continuously small rapidly proliferating viable para-diploid tumor cells termed "Raju, RJ" with extended mitotic life span via "neosis" or "de-polyploidization" [514,546–549]. Neosis, a novel manner of cell division in tumors, was first reported by Sundaram et al. in 2003 [548]. This peculiar parasexual pattern of somatic reduction division of PGCCs/MNGCs is characterized by karyokinesis through efficient mechanisms, such as nuclear budding/bursting, giving rise to small daughter nuclei; these nuclei then acquire cytoplasm, desperate from the giant mother cells, and exhibit long-term proliferation. The authors referred to this process as the "giant cell cycle" [550]. Additionally, it has been shown that this process involves nuclei remodeling, telomere clustering, and chromosome double loop formation [530,533]. The giant cell cycle is controlled by key regulators of stemness (e.g., Oct4), mitosis (e.g., cyclin B1 and aurora B kinase), and meiosis (e.g., MOS) [537,543,551]. Reduction division of polyploidy cells has been shown to express features of meiotic divisions in a disordered fashion and contribute to genetic diversity rendering tumor cells more apt to survive following antitumor treatments [530,552]. Several studies have demonstrated that RJ cells give rise to transformed cell lines with genomic instability and also display a phenotype and transcriptome different from the mother cell [548]. Compared to diploid cancer cells, RJ cells have been shown to express fewer epithelial markers and gain a mesenchymal phenotype [524]; thus, these cells can stimulate migration, invasion, and anchorage-independent growth [548]. Although their depolyploidization processes can occur at any time post-treatment, it can take several weeks or months until a stable population of daughter cells appears [42,526,553]. It has been found that the retreatment of the recovered cells causes the same process again [41]. In addition, the newly formed RJ cells have been reported to play a role in self-renewal in tumors [554,555] due to their stem-like traits [526,536,556]. Diaz-Carballo et al. [557] documented that PGCCs/MNGCs can confer the surrounding cells' stemness properties through lateral transfer of a sub-genome, in which PGCCs/MNGCs form intra-cytoplasmic daughter cells that express increased levels of CSCs markers and then transmit into neighboring cells via cytoplasmic tunnels [40]. It has been demonstrated that p53 deficiency is permissive for multipolar and asymmetric divisions of tetraploid cells, resulting in ample alterations in cell cycle progression and formation of aneuploid cells [41,552,553]. It has been shown that the response of radioresistant p53 mutated tumors to genotoxic damage is characterized by a failure to arrest in the G1 phase and induction of mitotic catastrophe [549]. Data on the enrichment of PGCCs/MNGCs following IR exposure were published first by Puck and Marcus for the human HeLa cervical carcinoma cell lines in 1956 [558]. The authors observed using CFA that a large proportion of HeLa cells lost their ability to produce macroscopic colonies ($\geq$50 cells) within 9 days post-IR at a single dose of 7 Gy [558]. Furthermore, they also showed that these cells remained metabolically active for long times post-IR (e.g., 3 weeks), indicating their ability to change medium pH, if the medium was periodically changed. Genotoxic treatment-induced PGCCs/ MNGCs have been demonstrated to exhibit increased resistance to DNA damage [41,42,548,553]. Increasing evidence has shown that curbing the genotoxic insults is clearly linked to reversible polyploidy, which itself is associated to a stemness phenotype induction [543]. It has been reported by Weihua et al. that grafting only a single MNGC was sufficient to produce metastatic lung tumors in murine fibrosarcoma model [13]. We have previously demonstrated that hypofractionation regimen causes an increase in the proportion of polyploidy in both p53-null and p53-wt radiotherapy surviving NSCLC sublines compared to parental cells [441]. They provide a powerful survival advantage to cells carrying DNA damage [543]. Polyploidization cycle has been shown to continue on days 3–5, ultimately leading to a polyploidization phase (8–32n). On days 5–6 post-IR, the switch from polyploidization to ploidy reduction divisions emerges [41]. Mirzayans et al. found that the lowest frequency of PGCCs/MNGCs in low-passage primary GBM cell lines was 1 in 20 cells (~5% of total cells) [40]. Based on such observation, the authors evaluated that each ~1 cm^3 of brain tumor contains at least 5 million of MNGCs/PGCCs [40]. It has been pointed out that PGCCs/MNGCs are not pre-existing giant cells from the parent population but generate via IR-induced homotypic cell fusion among radioresistant GBM cells [547]. Data from our very recent study have suggested the significance of TP53wt/PTENmut status in the maintenance of in vitro cycling and migration of radioresistant GBM cells to produce a high number of PGCCs/MNGCs in response to therapeutic IR doses (2–6 Gy). Our current general data have revealed that some TP53wt/PTENmutGBM cells-derived PGCCs/MNGCs can generate RJ cells and finally form large colonies 24 h post-IR (Figure 4). In addition, this work has indicated that differences in the proliferative activity, colony formation, and GBM cell lines radioresistance seem to be related to aneuploidy and neosis and not to a mutant p53 expression (Lina Alhaddad et al., 2022, unpublished data).

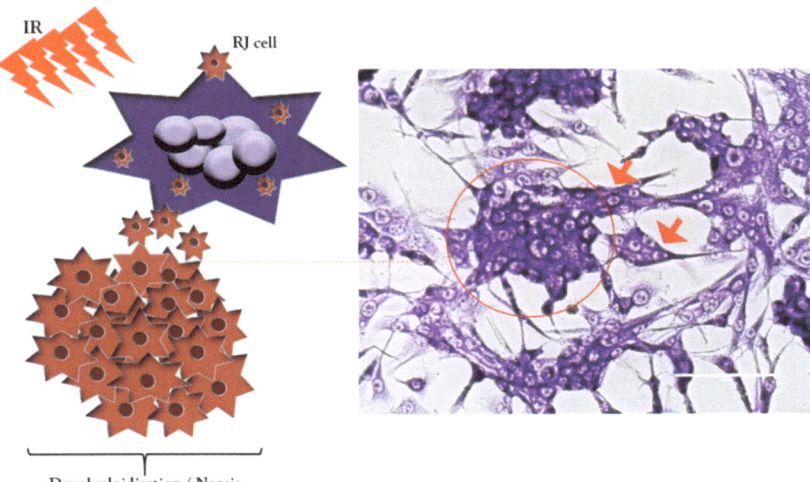

Figure 4. PGCC/MNGC-cell-derived RJ cells in X-ray irradiated GBM U-87 cells.

7. Tumor Microenvironment (TME)

Because the sites of recurrence in GBM and NSCLC following radiotherapy are located around the radiation-treated areas, it has been suggested that IR may contribute to the induction of the TME [559,560]. The TME is comprised of a variety of cell types, including proliferating tumor cells, non-neoplastic stromal cells, endothelial cells (EC), ECM, blood vessels, infiltrating immune/inflammatory cells, cancer-associated fibroblasts, myeloid suppressor cells (MSCs), regulatory T cells (T_{reg}), tumor-associated macrophages (TAMs) [137], and tumor-infiltrating lymphocytes (TILs). Furthermore, the TME also consists of various immunosuppressive factors released by all cell types within the tumor to support its growth, progression, and malignancy, such as prostaglandin E2 [561], adenosine [562], NF-κB, tumor necrosis factor-alpha (TNF-α) [563], tumor-associated gangliosides [564], immunosuppressive cytokines (for example TGF-β [565], IL-8 [566], and others [567]. All these networks of various cells and biomolecules in the TME have been shown to contribute to the radiation response [568]. The defective function of dendritic cells (DCs) has been known to represent one of the mechanisms of tumor evasion from immune system control [569]. Natural killer cells, which mediate the innate immune system and engage in reciprocal interactions with macrophages, DCs, T cells, and endothelial cells, are conspicuously absent from most tumor infiltrates [570,571]. Recent studies have pointed to the potential of the TME to initiate SC programs. TILs, containing various proportions of CD3+CD4+ and CD3+CD8+ T cells, are usually a major component of the TME [572]. TAMs have been known to be involved in inducing angiogenesis, tumor growth, migration, metastasis, invasion, immunosuppression, and resistance against radiotherapy through secreting many inhibitory chemokines and cytokines, such as IL-6, IL-8, IL-10, IL-34, colony-stimulating factor 1 (CSF-1), tumor necrosis factor, prostaglandin E2, MMPs, and CCL2, CCL5, and CCL18 [573,574]. It has been well documented that MSCs regulate the immune response under normal physiologic conditions by interacting with various immune cells [575] and the maturation, differentiation, proliferation, and functional activation of peripheral blood mononuclear cells [576], but in the tumor, presence are subverted to induce its escape [577,578]. MSCs have been shown to be increased in the peripheral blood of patients with various tumors [579]. MSCs present in the TME have been found to promote tumor growth and suppress immune cell functions, as well as display radioprotective activity through copious production of an arginase 1, an enzyme involved in the metabolism of L-arginine, which synergizes with nitric oxide synthase to increase superoxide and nitric oxide production, blunting lymphocyte responses [580,581]. MSCs also suppress T-cell responses in the TME. Tumors release TGF-β or promote TGF-β secretion from MSCs [582]. In addition, indoleamine-2,3-dioxygenase (IDO) secreted by MSCs has been reported to be involved in the breaking down of tryptophan, an essential amino acid for differentiation and T-cell proliferation [583]. Tumors produce ample factors, including IL-6, IL-10, CSF-1, granulocyte- macrophage CSF (GM-CSF), VEGF, which elicit MSC recruitment and block lymphocyte functions, as well as DCs maturation [582]. Polymorphonuclear leukocytes have been infrequently seen in tumor infiltrates [584]. Inflammatory cells present in the TME have been reported to contribute to tumor progression [577]. Tregs are a characteristic feature of the TME and represent potent mediators of dominant self-tolerance in the periphery [585,586]. Accumulations of Tregs in the TME characterized by the expression of the forkhead/winged helix transcription factor (Foxp3) have been reported to promote tumor progression and prognosis, as well as downregulate effective antitumor immune responses in tumor-bearing hosts, thereby deterring tumor immune surveillance [587–589]. In the process of tumor immune escape, Tregs have been shown to suppress antigen presentation by myeloid-derived suppressor cells [590], DCs, CD4+ T helper (Th) cells and generate tumor-specific CD8+ cytotoxic T lymphocytes through TGF-β, IL-10, and IL-35 secretion (epstein-barr virus induced 3-IL-12α heterodimer) [586,591]. Treg-expressing cytotoxic T lymphocytes associated antigen 4 have been found to combine with CD80 and CD86 on the surface of DCs, leading to reduced DCs maturation [592], as well as Tregs promote the immunosuppressive capacity of myeloid-derived suppressor cells via the programmed cell death ligand 1 (PD-L1) pathway [590]. Furthermore, it has been suggested that Tregs interfere with cell metabolism mainly in two ways: (a) IL-2 deficiency in the TME, thus inhibiting the growth of effector T cells [593]; (b) CD39 and CD73, which are constitutionally expressed in human Tregs, can hydrolyze extracellular ATP or ADP into AMP and produce adenosine [594]. Several Tregs subsets have been recognized in tumors: (a) natural Tregs (nTregs), which obstruct the proliferation of other T cells in the TME through contact-dependent mechanisms involving the CD95 or granzyme B/perforin pathways, and they have been found to be responsible for maintaining peripheral tolerance to self [595]; (b) inducible Tregs (iTregs) also referred to as type 1 regulatory T cells (Tr1), which are induced in the periphery following chronic antigenic stimulation in the presence of IL-10 derived from tolerogenic antigen-presenting cells [596]. Additionally, FOXP3+CD3+CD4+CD25+ phenotype has been found to occur in nTreg [597], while CD4+CD25lowCD132+TGF-β+IL-10+IL-4- phenotype has been considered to be a classical combined marker of Tr1 [586]. The GBM TME has been shown to be more immunosuppressive compared to other malignancies due to the release of potent immunosuppressive cytokines (e.g., IL-10 and TGF-β) [598]), negative regulators of effector cell functions (e.g., programmed death-ligand 1 and IDO), and oncometabolites (e.g., (R)-2-hydroxyglutarate6 and O6-methylguanine-DNA methyltransferase promoter methylation) [599]. It has been demonstrated that tumor-infiltrating neutrophils facilitate GSCs accumulation through S100A41 upregulation [600]. It has been shown that soluble factors secreted by endothelial cells maintain the self-renewal of GSCs and facilitate the initiation and growth of tumors [601]. It has been indicated that IR enhances the invasiveness of NSCLC via GM-CSF [602]. The expression level of IL-23 has been reported to be elevated in NSCLC patients after radiotherapy in response to the secretion of growth factors, signaling molecules, and anti-apoptosis factors compared to non-irradiated serum samples [333].

8. The Potential Treatment of Radioresistance in Glioblastoma and Non-Small-Cell Lung Cancer

Radiotherapy is a modality of oncologic treatment that can be used to treat about 50% of all cancer patients either alone or in combination with other treatment modalities such as chemotherapy, surgery, immunotherapy, and therapeutic targeting. Standard radiotherapy for GBM and NSCLC malignancies is not target-specific against them and is often not fully effective. The need to improve additional strategies for the treatment of these cancers is urgent. As mentioned previously, a major factor related to radioresistance is the existence of CSCs inside tumors, which are responsible for metastases, relapses, and radiotherapy failure. The intrinsic radioresistance of CSCs reveals the need to reassess the underlying mechanisms of the response of tumors to conventional and novel radiotherapy with a specific focus on CSCs. The identification of molecular targets that control CSCs can contribute to the development of novel chemotherapeutic drugs able to eliminate and prevent new CSCs growth in patients. This will help prevent metastasis and tumor relapse with a reduction of morbidity and toxicity, ultimately improving the outcomes in cancer patients. In order to conquer CSCs' radioresistance to conventional radiotherapy, different strategies such as immunotherapy, gene therapy, molecular inhibition, and combination therapy have been widely investigated. Moreover, although many patients are still treated with conventional radiotherapy, other modern radiotherapy techniques have been developed, such as stereotactic body radiotherapy, hadron, and ultra-high dose-rate radiation therapy, which delivers precise high doses of radiation to target local tumors.

9. Conclusions and Perspectives

Collectively, the unique proprieties of CSCs, such as the ability to sustain a pool of undifferentiated stem cells through self-renewal, a high level of plasticity due to their adaptation to the TME pressures, including oxidative stress and immunosuppression, remarkable tumorigenic and metastatic capabilities, and an efficient DNA damage repair, make them the root of tumor relapse. The identification of CSCs within GBM and NSCLC may therefore be critical to hinder tumor radioresistance. IR-induced proliferation arrest and polyploidy can favor the emergence of highly tolerable stem-like phenotype and self-renewal potential in these tumors, thereby targeting quiescent cancer cells, prematurely senescent, and PGCCs/MNGCs in conjunction with radiotherapy for patients diagnosed with GBM and NSCLC may also represent an attractive avenue to circumvent their advanced malignancy and recurrence.

Author Contributions: Conceptualization, L.A.; data acquisition, L.A.; writing—original draft preparation, L.A.; visualization, L.A.; writing—review and editing, L.A., S.L., and A.N.O.; supervision S.L. and A.N.O. All authors have read and agreed to the published version of the manuscript.

Funding: The studies were supported by the Russian Foundation for Basic Research (RFBR) project # 20-34-90035. The S.L. work was supported by the strategic academic leadership program 'Priority 2030' (Agreement 075-02-2021-1316 30 September 2021).

Institutional Review Board Statement: Not applicable.

Informed Consent Statement: Not applicable.

Data Availability Statement: Not applicable.

Conflicts of Interest: The authors declare no conflict of interest.

References

1. Berger, F.; Gay, E.; Pelletier, L.; Tropel, P.; Wion, D. Development of gliomas: Potential role of asymmetrical cell division of neural stem cells. *Lancet Oncol.* **2004**, *5*, 511–514. [CrossRef]
2. Brandes, A.A. State-of-the-art treatment of high-grade brain tumors. *Semin. Oncol.* **2003**, *30*, 4–9. [CrossRef] [PubMed]
3. Kleihues, P.; Louis, D.N.; Scheithauer, B.W.; Rorke, L.B.; Reifenberger, G.; Burger, P.C.; Cavenee, W.K. The WHO classification of tumors of the nervous system. *J. Neuropathol. Exp. Neurol.* **2002**, *61*, 215–225; discussion 219–226. [CrossRef] [PubMed]

4. Keles, G.E.; Anderson, B.; Berger, M.S. The effect of extent of resection on time to tumor progression and survival in patients with glioblastoma multiforme of the cerebral hemisphere. *Surg. Neurol.* **1999**, *52*, 371–379. [CrossRef]
5. Furnari, F.B.; Fenton, T.; Bachoo, R.M.; Mukasa, A.; Stommel, J.M.; Stegh, A.; Hahn, W.C.; Ligon, K.L.; Louis, D.N.; Brennan, C.; et al. Malignant astrocytic glioma: Genetics, biology, and paths to treatment. *Genes Dev.* **2007**, *21*, 2683–2710. [CrossRef] [PubMed]
6. Gridelli, C.; Rossi, A.; Carbone, D.P.; Guarize, J.; Karachaliou, N.; Mok, T.; Petrella, F.; Spaggiari, L.; Rosell, R. Non-small-cell lung cancer. *Nat. Rev. Dis. Prim.* **2015**, *1*, 15009. [CrossRef]
7. Ko, E.C.; Raben, D.; Formenti, S.C. The Integration of Radiotherapy with Immunotherapy for the Treatment of Non–Small Cell Lung Cancer. *Clin. Cancer Res.* **2018**, *24*, 5792–5806. [CrossRef]
8. Liu, C.; Sarkaria, J.N.; Petell, C.A.; Paraskevakou, G.; Zollman, P.J.; Schroeder, M.; Carlson, B.; Decker, P.A.; Wu, W.; James, C.D.; et al. Combination of Measles Virus Virotherapy and Radiation Therapy Has Synergistic Activity in the Treatment of Glioblastoma Multiforme. *Clin. Cancer Res.* **2007**, *13*, 7155–7165. [CrossRef]
9. Hegi, M.E.; Diserens, A.-C.; Gorlia, T.; Hamou, M.-F.; de Tribolet, N.; Weller, M.; Kros, J.M.; Hainfellner, J.A.; Mason, W.; Mariani, L.; et al. MGMTGene Silencing and Benefit from Temozolomide in Glioblastoma. *N. Engl. J. Med.* **2005**, *352*, 997–1003. [CrossRef]
10. Rich, J.N. Cancer Stem Cells in Radiation Resistance. *Cancer Res.* **2007**, *67*, 8980–8984. [CrossRef]
11. Perry, J.R.; Laperriere, N.; O'Callaghan, C.J.; Brandes, A.A.; Menten, J.; Phillips, C.; Fay, M.; Nishikawa, R.; Cairncross, J.G.; Roa, W.; et al. Short-Course Radiation plus Temozolomide in Elderly Patients with Glioblastoma. *N. Engl. J. Med.* **2017**, *376*, 1027–1037. [CrossRef] [PubMed]
12. Wisnivesky, J.P.; Bonomi, M.; Henschke, C.; Iannuzzi, M.; McGinn, T. Radiation Therapy for the Treatment of Unresected Stage I-II Non-small Cell Lung Cancer. *Chest* **2005**, *128*, 1461–1467. [CrossRef] [PubMed]
13. Weihua, Z.; Lin, Q.; Ramoth, A.J.; Fan, D.; Fidler, I.J. Formation of solid tumors by a single multinucleated cancer cell. *Cancer* **2011**, *117*, 4092–4099. [CrossRef] [PubMed]
14. Ishii, H.; Iwatsuki, M.; Ieta, K.; Ohta, D.; Haraguchi, N.; Mimori, K.; Mori, M. Cancer stem cells and chemoradiation resistance. *Cancer Sci.* **2008**, *99*, 1871–1877. [CrossRef] [PubMed]
15. Tu, S.-M.; Lin, S.-H.; Logothetis, C.J. Stem-cell origin of metastasis and heterogeneity in solid tumours. *Lancet Oncol.* **2002**, *3*, 508–513. [CrossRef]
16. Passegué, E.; Jamieson, C.H.M.; Ailles, L.E.; Weissman, I.L. Normal and leukemic hematopoiesis: Are leukemias a stem cell disorder or a reacquisition of stem cell characteristics? *Proc. Natl. Acad. Sci. USA* **2003**, *100*, 11842–11849. [CrossRef]
17. Maugeri-Saccà, M.; Vigneri, P.; De Maria, R. Cancer Stem Cells and Chemosensitivity. *Clin. Cancer Res.* **2011**, *17*, 4942–4947. [CrossRef]
18. Arnold, C.R.; Mangesius, J.; Skvortsova, I.-I.; Ganswindt, U. The Role of Cancer Stem Cells in Radiation Resistance. *Front. Oncol.* **2020**, *10*, 164. [CrossRef]
19. Jordan, C.T.; Guzman, M.L.; Noble, M. Cancer Stem Cells. *N. Engl. J. Med.* **2006**, *355*, 1253–1261. [CrossRef]
20. Creighton, C.J.; Li, X.; Landis, M.; Dixon, J.M.; Neumeister, V.M.; Sjolund, A.; Rimm, D.L.; Wong, H.; Rodriguez, A.; Herschkowitz, J.I.; et al. Residual breast cancers after conventional therapy display mesenchymal as well as tumor-initiating features. *Proc. Natl. Acad. Sci. USA* **2009**, *106*, 13820–13825. [CrossRef]
21. Han, J.; Won, M.; Kim, J.H.; Jung, E.; Min, K.; Jangili, P.; Kim, J.S. Cancer stem cell-targeted bio-imaging and chemotherapeutic perspective. *Chem. Soc. Rev.* **2020**, *49*, 7856–7878. [CrossRef] [PubMed]
22. Plaks, V.; Kong, N.; Werb, Z. The Cancer Stem Cell Niche: How Essential Is the Niche in Regulating Stemness of Tumor Cells? *Cell Stem Cell* **2015**, *16*, 225–238. [CrossRef] [PubMed]
23. Talukdar, S.; Bhoopathi, P.; Emdad, L.; Das, S.; Sarkar, D.; Fisher, P.B. Dormancy and cancer stem cells: An enigma for cancer therapeutic targeting. *Adv. Cancer Res.* **2019**, *141*, 43–84. [PubMed]
24. Liang, H.; Deng, L.; Burnette, B.; Weichselbaum, R.R.; Fu, Y.X. Radiation-induced tumor dormancy reflects an equilibrium between the proliferation and T lymphocyte-mediated death of malignant cells. *Oncoimmunology* **2013**, *2*, e25668. [CrossRef] [PubMed]
25. Vollmann-Zwerenz, A.; Leidgens, V.; Feliciello, G.; Klein, C.A.; Hau, P. Tumor Cell Invasion in Glioblastoma. *Int. J. Mol. Sci.* **2020**, *21*, 1932. [CrossRef]
26. Wang, W.; Xiong, Y.; Ding, X.; Wang, L.; Zhao, Y.; Fei, Y.; Zhu, Y.; Shen, X.; Tan, C.; Liang, Z. Cathepsin L activated by mutant p53 and Egr-1 promotes ionizing radiation-induced EMT in human NSCLC. *J. Exp. Clin. Cancer Res.* **2019**, *38*, 61. [CrossRef]
27. Iser, I.C.; Pereira, M.B.; Lenz, G.; Wink, M.R. The Epithelial-to-Mesenchymal Transition-Like Process in Glioblastoma: An Updated Systematic Review and In Silico Investigation. *Med. Res. Rev.* **2017**, *37*, 271–313. [CrossRef]
28. Nieto, M.A.; Huang, R.Y.; Jackson, R.A.; Thiery, J.P. Emt: 2016. *Cell* **2016**, *166*, 21–45. [CrossRef]
29. Loh, C.-Y.; Chai, J.; Tang, T.; Wong, W.; Sethi, G.; Shanmugam, M.; Chong, P.; Looi, C. The E-Cadherin and N-Cadherin Switch in Epithelial-to-Mesenchymal Transition: Signaling, Therapeutic Implications, and Challenges. *Cells* **2019**, *8*, 1118. [CrossRef]
30. Mani, S.A.; Guo, W.; Liao, M.J.; Eaton, E.N.; Ayyanan, A.; Zhou, A.Y.; Brooks, M.; Reinhard, F.; Zhang, C.C.; Shipitsin, M.; et al. The epithelial-mesenchymal transition generates cells with properties of stem cells. *Cell* **2008**, *133*, 704–715. [CrossRef]
31. Zhang, F.; Zhang, T.; Teng, Z.-h.; Zhang, R.; Wang, J.-B.; Mei, Q.-B. Sensitization to γ-irradiation-induced cell cycle arrest and apoptosis by the histone deacetylase inhibitor trichostatin A in non-small cell lung cancer (NSCLC) cells. *Cancer Biol. Ther.* **2014**, *8*, 823–831. [CrossRef] [PubMed]

32. Madhusudan, S.; Middleton, M.R. The emerging role of DNA repair proteins as predictive, prognostic and therapeutic targets in cancer. *Cancer Treat. Rev.* **2005**, *31*, 603–617. [CrossRef] [PubMed]
33. Karagiannis, T.C.; El-Osta, A. Double-strand breaks: Signaling pathways and repair mechanisms. *Cell Mol. Life Sci.* **2004**, *61*, 2137–2147. [CrossRef] [PubMed]
34. Sikora, E.; Czarnecka-Herok, J.; Bojko, A.; Sunderland, P. Therapy-induced polyploidization and senescence: Coincidence or interconnection? *Semin. Cancer Biol.* **2022**, *81*, 83–95. [CrossRef]
35. d'Adda di Fagagna, F.; Reaper, P.M.; Clay-Farrace, L.; Fiegler, H.; Carr, P.; Von Zglinicki, T.; Saretzki, G.; Carter, N.P.; Jackson, S.P. A DNA damage checkpoint response in telomere-initiated senescence. *Nature* **2003**, *426*, 194–198. [CrossRef]
36. Shen, Z.; Huhn, S.C.; Haffty, B.G. Escaping death to quiescence: Avoiding mitotic catastrophe after DNA damage. *Cell Cycle* **2014**, *12*, 1664. [CrossRef]
37. Kodym, E.; Kodym, R.; Reis, A.E.; Habib, A.A.; Story, M.D.; Saha, D. The small-molecule CDK inhibitor, SNS-032, enhances cellular radiosensitivity in quiescent and hypoxic non-small cell lung cancer cells. *Lung Cancer* **2009**, *66*, 37–47. [CrossRef]
38. Ivanov, A.; Cragg, M.S.; Erenpreisa, J.; Emzinsh, D.; Lukman, H.; Illidge, T.M. Endopolyploid cells produced after severe genotoxic damage have the potential to repair DNA double strand breaks. *J. Cell Sci.* **2003**, *116*, 4095–4106. [CrossRef]
39. Erenpreisa, J.; Wheatley, D. Endopolyploidy in development and cancer; "survival of the fattest?". *Cell Biology Int.* **2005**, *29*, 981–982. [CrossRef]
40. Mirzayans, R.; Andrais, B.; Murray, D. Roles of Polyploid/Multinucleated Giant Cancer Cells in Metastasis and Disease Relapse Following Anticancer Treatment. *Cancers* **2018**, *10*, 118. [CrossRef]
41. Illidge, T. Polyploid giant cells provide a survival mechanism for p53 mutant cells after dna damage. *Cell Biol. Int.* **2000**, *24*, 621–633. [CrossRef] [PubMed]
42. Puig, P.-E.; Guilly, M.-N.; Bouchot, A.; Droin, N.; Cathelin, D.; Bouyer, F.; Favier, L.; Ghiringhelli, F.; Kroemer, G.; Solary, E. Tumor cells can escape DNA-damaging cisplatin through DNA endoreduplication and reversible polyploidy. *Cell Biol. Int.* **2008**, *32*, 1031–1043. [CrossRef] [PubMed]
43. Li, R.; Wang, H.; Liang, Q.; Chen, L.; Ren, J. Radiotherapy for glioblastoma: Clinical issues and nanotechnology strategies. *Biomater. Sci.* **2022**, *10*, 892–908. [CrossRef] [PubMed]
44. Li, Q.; Zong, Y.; Li, K.; Jie, X.; Hong, J.; Zhou, X.; Wu, B.; Li, Z.; Zhang, S.; Wu, G.; et al. Involvement of endothelial CK2 in the radiation induced perivascular resistant niche (PVRN) and the induction of radioresistance for non-small cell lung cancer (NSCLC) cells. *Biol. Res.* **2019**, *52*, 22. [CrossRef] [PubMed]
45. Friedmann-Morvinski, D. Glioblastoma heterogeneity and cancer cell plasticity. *Crit. Rev. Oncog.* **2014**, *19*, 327–336. [CrossRef]
46. Chen, Z.; Fillmore, C.M.; Hammerman, P.S.; Kim, C.F.; Wong, K.K. Non-small-cell lung cancers: A heterogeneous set of diseases. *Nat. Rev. Cancer* **2014**, *14*, 535–546. [CrossRef]
47. Yaes, R.J. Tumor heterogeneity, tumor size, and radioresistance. *Int. J. Radiat. Oncol. Biol. Phys.* **1989**, *17*, 993–1005. [CrossRef]
48. Lim, Z.F.; Ma, P.C. Emerging insights of tumor heterogeneity and drug resistance mechanisms in lung cancer targeted therapy. *J. Hematol. Oncol.* **2019**, *12*, 134. [CrossRef]
49. Soubannier, V.; Stifani, S. NF-kappaB Signalling in Glioblastoma. *Biomedicines* **2017**, *5*, 29. [CrossRef]
50. Iwadate, Y. Epithelial-mesenchymal transition in glioblastoma progression. *Oncol. Lett.* **2016**, *11*, 1615–1620. [CrossRef]
51. Dagogo-Jack, I.; Shaw, A.T. Tumour heterogeneity and resistance to cancer therapies. *Nat. Rev. Clin. Oncol.* **2017**, *15*, 81–94. [CrossRef] [PubMed]
52. Chaffer, C.L.; Weinberg, R.A.; Marjanovic, N.D. Cell Plasticity and Heterogeneity in Cancer. *Clin. Chem.* **2013**, *59*, 168–179. [CrossRef]
53. Nowell, P.C. The Clonal Evolution of Tumor Cell Populations. *Science* **1976**, *194*, 23–28. [CrossRef] [PubMed]
54. Lovly, C.M.; Salama, A.K.; Salgia, R. Tumor Heterogeneity and Therapeutic Resistance. *Am. Soc. Clin. Oncol. Educ. Book* **2016**, *35*, e585–e593. [CrossRef]
55. Rich, J.N. Cancer stem cells. *Medicine* **2016**, *95*, S2–S7. [CrossRef] [PubMed]
56. Bonnet, D.; Dick, J.E. Human acute myeloid leukemia is organized as a hierarchy that originates from a primitive hematopoietic cell. *Nat. Med.* **1997**, *3*, 730–737. [CrossRef]
57. Jin, D.-Y.; Leung, E.L.-H.; Fiscus, R.R.; Tung, J.W.; Tin, V.P.-C.; Cheng, L.C.; Sihoe, A.D.-L.; Fink, L.M.; Ma, Y.; Wong, M.P. Non-Small Cell Lung Cancer Cells Expressing CD44 Are Enriched for Stem Cell-Like Properties. *PLoS ONE* **2010**, *5*, e14062. [CrossRef]
58. Visvader, J.E.; Lindeman, G.J. Cancer stem cells in solid tumours: Accumulating evidence and unresolved questions. *Nat. Rev. Cancer* **2008**, *8*, 755–768. [CrossRef]
59. Alamgeer, M.; Peacock, C.D.; Matsui, W.; Ganju, V.; Watkins, D.N. Cancer stem cells in lung cancer: Evidence and controversies. *Respirology* **2013**, *18*, 757–764. [CrossRef]
60. Ghisolfi, L.; Keates, A.C.; Hu, X.; Lee, D.K.; Li, C.J. Ionizing radiation induces stemness in cancer cells. *PLoS ONE* **2012**, *7*, e43628. [CrossRef]
61. Liu, Y.; Yang, M.; Luo, J.; Zhou, H. Radiotherapy targeting cancer stem cells "awakens" them to induce tumour relapse and metastasis in oral cancer. *Int. J. Oral Sci.* **2020**, *12*, 19. [CrossRef] [PubMed]
62. Koury, J.; Zhong, L.; Hao, J. Targeting Signaling Pathways in Cancer Stem Cells for Cancer Treatment. *Stem Cells Int.* **2017**, *2017*, 2925869. [CrossRef] [PubMed]

63. Najafi, M.; Farhood, B.; Mortezaee, K. Cancer stem cells (CSCs) in cancer progression and therapy. *J. Cell. Physiol.* **2018**, *234*, 8381–8395. [CrossRef] [PubMed]
64. Liu, G.; Yuan, X.; Zeng, Z.; Tunici, P.; Ng, H.; Abdulkadir, I.R.; Lu, L.; Irvin, D.; Black, K.L.; Yu, J.S. Analysis of gene expression and chemoresistance of CD133+ cancer stem cells in glioblastoma. *Mol. Cancer* **2006**, *5*, 67. [CrossRef]
65. Zou, Y.M.; Hu, G.Y.; Zhao, X.Q.; Lu, T.; Zhu, F.; Yu, S.Y.; Xiong, H. Hypoxia-induced autophagy contributes to radioresistance via c-Jun-mediated Beclin1 expression in lung cancer cells. *J. Huazhong Univ. Sci. Technol. Med. Sci.* **2014**, *34*, 761–767. [CrossRef]
66. Li, F.; Zhou, K.; Gao, L.; Zhang, B.; Li, W.; Yan, W.; Song, X.; Yu, H.; Wang, S.; Yu, N.; et al. Radiation induces the generation of cancer stem cells: A novel mechanism for cancer radioresistance. *Oncol. Lett.* **2016**, *12*, 3059–3065. [CrossRef]
67. Yu, Z.; Pestell, T.G.; Lisanti, M.P.; Pestell, R.G. Cancer stem cells. *Int. J. Biochem. Cell Biol.* **2012**, *44*, 2144–2151. [CrossRef]
68. Tabu, K.; Kimura, T.; Sasai, K.; Wang, L.; Bizen, N.; Nishihara, H.; Taga, T.; Tanaka, S. Analysis of an alternative human CD133 promoter reveals the implication of Ras/ERK pathway in tumor stem-like hallmarks. *Mol. Cancer* **2010**, *9*, 39. [CrossRef]
69. Isobe, T.; Hisamori, S.; Hogan, D.J.; Zabala, M.; Hendrickson, D.G.; Dalerba, P.; Cai, S.; Scheeren, F.; Kuo, A.H.; Sikandar, S.S.; et al. miR-142 regulates the tumorigenicity of human breast cancer stem cells through the canonical WNT signaling pathway. *eLife* **2014**, *3*, e01977. [CrossRef]
70. Shimono, Y.; Zabala, M.; Cho, R.W.; Lobo, N.; Dalerba, P.; Qian, D.; Diehn, M.; Liu, H.; Panula, S.P.; Chiao, E.; et al. Downregulation of miRNA-200c links breast cancer stem cells with normal stem cells. *Cell* **2009**, *138*, 592–603. [CrossRef]
71. Huntly, B.J.; Gilliland, D.G. Leukaemia stem cells and the evolution of cancer-stem-cell research. *Nat. Rev. Cancer* **2005**, *5*, 311–321. [CrossRef] [PubMed]
72. Fiala, S. The cancer cell as a stem cell unable to differentiate. A theory of carcinogenesis. *Neoplasma* **1968**, *15*, 607–622. [PubMed]
73. Clarkson, B.; Fried, J.; Strife, A.; Sakai, Y.; Ota, K.; Ohkita, T. Studies of cellular proliferation in human leukemia.III. Behavior of leukemic cells in three adults with acute leukemia given continuous infusions of3H-thymidine for 8 or 10 days. *Cancer* **1970**, *25*, 1237–1260. [CrossRef]
74. Clarkson, B.D.; Dowling, M.D.; Gee, T.S.; Cunningham, I.B.; Burchenal, J.H. Treatment of acute leukemia in adults. *Cancer* **1975**, *36*, 775–795. [CrossRef]
75. Hamburger, A.W.; Salmon, S.E. Primary Bioassay of Human Tumor Stem Cells. *Science* **1977**, *197*, 461–463. [CrossRef]
76. Lapidot, T.; Sirard, C.; Vormoor, J.; Murdoch, B.; Hoang, T.; Caceres-Cortes, J.; Minden, M.; Paterson, B.; Caligiuri, M.A.; Dick, J.E. A cell initiating human acute myeloid leukaemia after transplantation into SCID mice. *Nature* **1994**, *367*, 645–648. [CrossRef]
77. Lessard, J.; Sauvageau, G. Bmi-1 determines the proliferative capacity of normal and leukaemic stem cells. *Nature* **2003**, *423*, 255–260. [CrossRef]
78. Al-Hajj, M.; Wicha, M.S.; Benito-Hernandez, A.; Morrison, S.J.; Clarke, M.F. Prospective identification of tumorigenic breast cancer cells. *Proc. Natl. Acad. Sci. USA* **2003**, *100*, 3983–3988. [CrossRef]
79. Ailles, L.E.; Weissman, I.L. Cancer stem cells in solid tumors. *Curr. Opin. Biotechnol.* **2007**, *18*, 460–466. [CrossRef]
80. Singh, S.K.; Clarke, I.D.; Terasaki, M.; Bonn, V.E.; Hawkins, C.; Squire, J.; Dirks, P.B. Identification of a cancer stem cell in human brain tumors. *Cancer Res.* **2003**, *63*, 5821–5828.
81. Matsui, W.; Huff, C.A.; Wang, Q.; Malehorn, M.T.; Barber, J.; Tanhehco, Y.; Smith, B.D.; Civin, C.I.; Jones, R.J. Characterization of clonogenic multiple myeloma cells. *Blood* **2004**, *103*, 2332–2336. [CrossRef] [PubMed]
82. Clarke, M.F.; Dick, J.E.; Dirks, P.B.; Eaves, C.J.; Jamieson, C.H.; Jones, D.L.; Visvader, J.; Weissman, I.L.; Wahl, G.M. Cancer stem cells–perspectives on current status and future directions: AACR Workshop on cancer stem cells. *Cancer Res.* **2006**, *66*, 9339–9344. [CrossRef] [PubMed]
83. Zhang, W.C.; Shyh-Chang, N.; Yang, H.; Rai, A.; Umashankar, S.; Ma, S.; Soh, B.S.; Sun, L.L.; Tai, B.C.; Nga, M.E.; et al. Glycine decarboxylase activity drives non-small cell lung cancer tumor-initiating cells and tumorigenesis. *Cell* **2012**, *148*, 259–272. [CrossRef] [PubMed]
84. Li, C.; Heidt, D.G.; Dalerba, P.; Burant, C.F.; Zhang, L.; Adsay, V.; Wicha, M.; Clarke, M.F.; Simeone, D.M. Identification of pancreatic cancer stem cells. *Cancer Res.* **2007**, *67*, 1030–1037. [CrossRef]
85. Collins, A.T.; Berry, P.A.; Hyde, C.; Stower, M.J.; Maitland, N.J. Prospective identification of tumorigenic prostate cancer stem cells. *Cancer Res.* **2005**, *65*, 10946–10951. [CrossRef]
86. Aguglia, U.; Gambarelli, D.; Farnarier, G.; Quattrone, A. Different susceptibilities of the geniculate and extrageniculate visual pathways to human Creutzfeldt-Jakob disease (a combined neurophysiological-neuropathological study). *Electroencephalogr. Clin. Neurophysiol.* **1991**, *78*, 413–423. [CrossRef]
87. Terris, B.; Cavard, C.; Perret, C. EpCAM, a new marker for cancer stem cells in hepatocellular carcinoma. *J. Hepatol.* **2010**, *52*, 280–281. [CrossRef]
88. Zou, G.M. Cancer stem cells in leukemia, recent advances. *J. Cell Physiol.* **2007**, *213*, 440–444. [CrossRef]
89. Boiko, A.D.; Razorenova, O.V.; van de Rijn, M.; Swetter, S.M.; Johnson, D.L.; Ly, D.P.; Butler, P.D.; Yang, G.P.; Joshua, B.; Kaplan, M.J.; et al. Human melanoma-initiating cells express neural crest nerve growth factor receptor CD271. *Nature* **2010**, *466*, 133–137. [CrossRef]
90. Liang, M.H.; Robb-Nicholson, C. Health status and utility measurement viewed from the right brain: Experience from the rheumatic diseases. *J. Chronic. Dis.* **1987**, *40*, 579–583. [CrossRef]
91. Organista-Nava, J.; Gomez-Gomez, Y.; Garibay-Cerdenares, O.L.; Leyva-Vazquez, M.A.; Illades-Aguiar, B. Cervical cancer stem cell-associated genes: Prognostic implications in cervical cancer. *Oncol. Lett.* **2019**, *18*, 7–14. [CrossRef] [PubMed]

92. Curley, M.D.; Therrien, V.A.; Cummings, C.L.; Sergent, P.A.; Koulouris, C.R.; Friel, A.M.; Roberts, D.J.; Seiden, M.V.; Scadden, D.T.; Rueda, B.R.; et al. CD133 expression defines a tumor initiating cell population in primary human ovarian cancer. *Stem Cells* **2009**, *27*, 2875–2883. [CrossRef] [PubMed]
93. Takaishi, S.; Okumura, T.; Tu, S.; Wang, S.S.; Shibata, W.; Vigneshwaran, R.; Gordon, S.A.; Shimada, Y.; Wang, T.C. Identification of gastric cancer stem cells using the cell surface marker CD44. *Stem Cells* **2009**, *27*, 1006–1020. [CrossRef]
94. Eramo, A.; Lotti, F.; Sette, G.; Pilozzi, E.; Biffoni, M.; Di Virgilio, A.; Conticello, C.; Ruco, L.; Peschle, C.; De Maria, R. Identification and expansion of the tumorigenic lung cancer stem cell population. *Cell Death Differ.* **2007**, *15*, 504–514. [CrossRef] [PubMed]
95. Dubrovska, A. Report on the International Workshop 'Cancer stem cells: The mechanisms of radioresistance and biomarker discovery'. *Int. J. Radiat. Biol.* **2014**, *90*, 607–614. [CrossRef]
96. Peitzsch, C.; Nathansen, J.; Schniewind, S.I.; Schwarz, F.; Dubrovska, A. Cancer Stem Cells in Head and Neck Squamous Cell Carcinoma: Identification, Characterization and Clinical Implications. *Cancers* **2019**, *11*, 616. [CrossRef]
97. Gilbert, C.A.; Ross, A.H. Cancer stem cells: Cell culture, markers, and targets for new therapies. *J. Cell Biochem.* **2009**, *108*, 1031–1038. [CrossRef]
98. Vlashi, E.; Pajonk, F. The metabolic state of cancer stem cells—A valid target for cancer therapy? *Free Radic. Biol. Med.* **2015**, *79*, 264–268. [CrossRef]
99. Siegel, R.L.; Miller, K.D.; Jemal, A. Cancer statistics, 2019. *CA Cancer J. Clin.* **2019**, *69*, 7–34. [CrossRef]
100. Prieto-Vila, M.; Takahashi, R.U.; Usuba, W.; Kohama, I.; Ochiya, T. Drug Resistance Driven by Cancer Stem Cells and Their Niche. *Int. J. Mol. Sci.* **2017**, *18*, 2574. [CrossRef]
101. Rycaj, K.; Tang, D.G. Cancer stem cells and radioresistance. *Int. J. Radiat. Biol.* **2014**, *90*, 615–621. [CrossRef] [PubMed]
102. Eyler, C.E.; Rich, J.N. Survival of the fittest: Cancer stem cells in therapeutic resistance and angiogenesis. *J. Clin. Oncol.* **2008**, *26*, 2839–2845. [CrossRef] [PubMed]
103. Borah, A.; Raveendran, S.; Rochani, A.; Maekawa, T.; Kumar, D.S. Targeting self-renewal pathways in cancer stem cells: Clinical implications for cancer therapy. *Oncogenesis* **2015**, *4*, e177. [CrossRef] [PubMed]
104. Zhang, M.; Atkinson, R.L.; Rosen, J.M. Selective targeting of radiation-resistant tumor-initiating cells. *Proc. Natl. Acad. Sci. USA* **2010**, *107*, 3522–3527. [CrossRef] [PubMed]
105. Talukdar, S.; Pradhan, A.K.; Bhoopathi, P.; Shen, X.-N.; August, L.A.; Windle, J.J.; Sarkar, D.; Furnari, F.B.; Cavenee, W.K.; Das, S.K.; et al. MDA-9/Syntenin regulates protective autophagy in anoikis-resistant glioma stem cells. *Proc. Natl. Acad. Sci. USA* **2018**, *115*, 5768–5773. [CrossRef] [PubMed]
106. Talukdar, S.; Emdad, L.; Das, S.K.; Sarkar, D.; Fisher, P.B. Evolving Strategies for Therapeutically Targeting Cancer Stem Cells. *Adv. Cancer Res.* **2016**, *131*, 159–191.
107. Lyakhovich, A.; Lleonart, M.E. Bypassing Mechanisms of Mitochondria-Mediated Cancer Stem Cells Resistance to Chemo- and Radiotherapy. *Oxidative Med. Cell. Longev.* **2016**, *2016*, 1716341. [CrossRef]
108. Kurth, I.; Hein, L.; Mäbert, K.; Peitzsch, C.; Koi, L.; Cojoc, M.; Kunz-Schughart, L.; Baumann, M.; Dubrovska, A. Cancer stem cell related markers of radioresistance in head and neck squamous cell carcinoma. *Oncotarget* **2015**, *6*, 34494–34509. [CrossRef]
109. Chang, L.; Graham, P.; Hao, J.; Ni, J.; Deng, J.; Bucci, J.; Malouf, D.; Gillatt, D.; Li, Y. Cancer stem cells and signaling pathways in radioresistance. *Oncotarget* **2016**, *7*, 11002–11017. [CrossRef]
110. Cojoc, M.; Mäbert, K.; Muders, M.H.; Dubrovska, A. A role for cancer stem cells in therapy resistance: Cellular and molecular mechanisms. *Semin. Cancer Biol.* **2015**, *31*, 16–27. [CrossRef]
111. Shin, M.K.; Cheong, J.H. Mitochondria-centric bioenergetic characteristics in cancer stem-like cells. *Arch. Pharm. Res.* **2019**, *42*, 113–127. [CrossRef] [PubMed]
112. Dayem, A.A.; Choi, H.Y.; Kim, J.H.; Cho, S.G. Role of oxidative stress in stem, cancer, and cancer stem cells. *Cancers* **2010**, *2*, 859–884. [CrossRef] [PubMed]
113. Dando, I.; Cordani, M.; Dalla Pozza, E.; Biondani, G.; Donadelli, M.; Palmieri, M. Antioxidant Mechanisms and ROS-Related MicroRNAs in Cancer Stem Cells. *Oxid. Med. Cell Longev.* **2015**, *2015*, 425708. [CrossRef] [PubMed]
114. Diehn, M.; Cho, R.W.; Lobo, N.A.; Kalisky, T.; Dorie, M.J.; Kulp, A.N.; Qian, D.; Lam, J.S.; Ailles, L.E.; Wong, M.; et al. Association of reactive oxygen species levels and radioresistance in cancer stem cells. *Nature* **2009**, *458*, 780–783. [CrossRef]
115. Mondal, S.; Bhattacharya, K.; Mandal, C. Nutritional stress reprograms dedifferention in glioblastoma multiforme driven by PTEN/Wnt/Hedgehog axis: A stochastic model of cancer stem cells. *Cell Death Discov.* **2018**, *4*, 110. [CrossRef]
116. Szotek, P.P.; Pieretti-Vanmarcke, R.; Masiakos, P.T.; Dinulescu, D.M.; Connolly, D.; Foster, R.; Dombkowski, D.; Preffer, F.; Maclaughlin, D.T.; Donahoe, P.K. Ovarian cancer side population defines cells with stem cell-like characteristics and Mullerian Inhibiting Substance responsiveness. *Proc. Natl. Acad. Sci. USA* **2006**, *103*, 11154–11159. [CrossRef]
117. Müller, E.; Ansorge, M.; Werner, C.; Pompe, T. Mimicking the Hematopoietic Stem Cell Niche by Biomaterials. In *Bio-Inspired Materials for Biomedical Engineering*; John Wiley & Sons: Hoboken, NJ, USA, 2014; pp. 309–326.
118. Bissell, M.J.; Labarge, M.A. Context, tissue plasticity, and cancer: Are tumor stem cells also regulated by the microenvironment? *Cancer Cell* **2005**, *7*, 17–23. [CrossRef]
119. Li, Z.; Bao, S.; Wu, Q.; Wang, H.; Eyler, C.; Sathornsumetee, S.; Shi, Q.; Cao, Y.; Lathia, J.; McLendon, R.E.; et al. Hypoxia-Inducible Factors Regulate Tumorigenic Capacity of Glioma Stem Cells. *Cancer Cell* **2009**, *15*, 501–513. [CrossRef]
120. Korkaya, H.; Liu, S.; Wicha, M.S. Regulation of cancer stem cells by cytokine networks: Attacking cancer's inflammatory roots. *Clin. Cancer Res.* **2011**, *17*, 6125–6129. [CrossRef]

121. Fukumura, D.; Xu, L.; Chen, Y.; Gohongi, T.; Seed, B.; Jain, R.K. Hypoxia and acidosis independently up-regulate vascular endothelial growth factor transcription in brain tumors in vivo. *Cancer Res.* **2001**, *61*, 6020–6024.
122. Hjelmeland, A.B.; Wu, Q.; Heddleston, J.M.; Choudhary, G.S.; MacSwords, J.; Lathia, J.D.; McLendon, R.; Lindner, D.; Sloan, A.; Rich, J.N. Acidic stress promotes a glioma stem cell phenotype. *Cell Death Differ.* **2010**, *18*, 829–840. [CrossRef] [PubMed]
123. Liu, J.; Xiao, Z.; Wong, S.K.; Tin, V.P.; Ho, K.Y.; Wang, J.; Sham, M.H.; Wong, M.P. Lung cancer tumorigenicity and drug resistance are maintained through ALDH(hi)CD44(hi) tumor initiating cells. *Oncotarget* **2013**, *4*, 1698–1711. [CrossRef] [PubMed]
124. Lee, C.J.; Li, C.; Simeone, D.M. Human Pancreatic Cancer Stem Cells: Implications for How We Treat Pancreatic Cancer. *Transl. Oncol.* **2008**, *1*, 14–18. [CrossRef]
125. Vail, D.M. (Ed.) *Withrow and MacEwen's Small Animal Clinical Oncology*; Elsevier: Amsterdam, The Netherlands, 2013.
126. Ho, M.M.; Ng, A.V.; Lam, S.; Hung, J.Y. Side population in human lung cancer cell lines and tumors is enriched with stem-like cancer cells. *Cancer Res.* **2007**, *67*, 4827–4833. [CrossRef] [PubMed]
127. Kim, W.T.; Ryu, C.J. Cancer stem cell surface markers on normal stem cells. *BMB Rep.* **2017**, *50*, 285–298. [CrossRef] [PubMed]
128. Tan, D.; Roth, I.; Wickremesekera, A.; Davis, P.; Kaye, A.; Mantamadiotis, T.; Stylli, S.; Tan, S. Therapeutic Targeting of Cancer Stem Cells in Human Glioblastoma by Manipulating the Renin-Angiotensin System. *Cells* **2019**, *8*, 1364. [CrossRef] [PubMed]
129. Zhang, X.; Zhao, W.; Li, Y. Stemness-related markers in cancer. *Cancer Transl. Med.* **2017**, *3*, 87–95. [CrossRef]
130. Klonisch, T.; Wiechec, E.; Hombach-Klonisch, S.; Ande, S.R.; Wesselborg, S.; Schulze-Osthoff, K.; Los, M. Cancer stem cell markers in common cancers—Therapeutic implications. *Trends Mol. Med.* **2008**, *14*, 450–460. [CrossRef]
131. Reya, T.; Morrison, S.J.; Clarke, M.F.; Weissman, I.L. Stem cells, cancer, and cancer stem cells. *Nature* **2001**, *414*, 105–111. [CrossRef]
132. Shackleton, M.; Vaillant, F.; Simpson, K.J.; Stingl, J.; Smyth, G.K.; Asselin-Labat, M.-L.; Wu, L.; Lindeman, G.J.; Visvader, J.E. Generation of a functional mammary gland from a single stem cell. *Nature* **2006**, *439*, 84–88. [CrossRef]
133. Redmer, T.; Walz, I.; Klinger, B.; Khouja, S.; Welte, Y.; Schäfer, R.; Regenbrecht, C. The role of the cancer stem cell marker CD271 in DNA damage response and drug resistance of melanoma cells. *Oncogenesis* **2017**, *6*, e291. [CrossRef] [PubMed]
134. Lupia, M.; Angiolini, F.; Bertalot, G.; Freddi, S.; Sachsenmeier, K.F.; Chisci, E.; Kutryb-Zajac, B.; Confalonieri, S.; Smolenski, R.T.; Giovannoni, R.; et al. CD73 Regulates Stemness and Epithelial-Mesenchymal Transition in Ovarian Cancer-Initiating Cells. *Stem Cell Rep.* **2018**, *10*, 1412–1425. [CrossRef] [PubMed]
135. Taddei, A.; Giampietro, C.; Conti, A.; Orsenigo, F.; Breviario, F.; Pirazzoli, V.; Potente, M.; Daly, C.; Dimmeler, S.; Dejana, E. Endothelial adherens junctions control tight junctions by VE-cadherin-mediated upregulation of claudin-5. *Nat. Cell Biol.* **2008**, *10*, 923–934. [CrossRef] [PubMed]
136. Medema, J.P. Cancer stem cells: The challenges ahead. *Nat. Cell Biol.* **2013**, *15*, 338–344. [CrossRef] [PubMed]
137. Begicevic, R.-R.; Falasca, M. ABC Transporters in Cancer Stem Cells: Beyond Chemoresistance. *Int. J. Mol. Sci.* **2017**, *18*, 2362. [CrossRef]
138. Padmanabhan, R.; Chen, K.G.; Gottesman, M.M. Lost in Translation: Regulation of ABCG2 Expression in Human Embryonic Stem Cells. *J. Stem Cell Res.* **2014**, *4*, 3. [CrossRef] [PubMed]
139. Markovsky, E.; Vax, E.; Ben-Shushan, D.; Eldar-Boock, A.; Shukrun, R.; Yeini, E.; Barshack, I.; Caspi, R.; Harari-Steinberg, O.; Pode-Shakked, N.; et al. Wilms Tumor NCAM-Expressing Cancer Stem Cells as Potential Therapeutic Target for Polymeric Nanomedicine. *Mol. Cancer Ther.* **2017**, *16*, 2462–2472. [CrossRef]
140. Pustovalova, M.; Blokhina, T.; Alhaddad, L.; Chigasova, A.; Chuprov-Netochin, R.; Veviorskiy, A.; Filkov, G.; Osipov, A.N.; Leonov, S. CD44+ and CD133+ Non-Small Cell Lung Cancer Cells Exhibit DNA Damage Response Pathways and Dormant Polyploid Giant Cancer Cell Enrichment Relating to Their p53 Status. *Int. J. Mol. Sci.* **2022**, *23*, 4922. [CrossRef]
141. Roy, S.K.; Shrivastava, A.; Srivastav, S.; Shankar, S.; Srivastava, R.K. SATB2 is a novel biomarker and therapeutic target for cancer. *J. Cell. Mol. Med.* **2020**, *24*, 11064–11069. [CrossRef]
142. Bao, B.; Wang, Z.; Ali, S.; Kong, D.; Banerjee, S.; Ahmad, A.; Li, Y.; Azmi, A.S.; Miele, L.; Sarkar, F.H. Over-expression of FoxM1 leads to epithelial-mesenchymal transition and cancer stem cell phenotype in pancreatic cancer cells. *J. Cell. Biochem.* **2011**, *112*, 2296–2306. [CrossRef]
143. Qi, Y.; Wei, J.; Zhang, X. Requirement of transcription factor NME2 for the maintenance of the stemness of gastric cancer stem-like cells. *Cell Death Dis.* **2021**, *12*, 924. [CrossRef] [PubMed]
144. Zhang, Q.; Han, Z.; Zhu, Y.; Chen, J.; Li, W. Role of hypoxia inducible factor-1 in cancer stem cells (Review). *Mol. Med. Rep.* **2021**, *23*, 17. [CrossRef] [PubMed]
145. Liu, A.; Yu, X.; Liu, S. Pluripotency transcription factors and cancer stem cells: Small genes make a big difference. *Chin. J. Cancer* **2013**. [CrossRef] [PubMed]
146. Pandit, H.; Li, Y.; Li, X.; Zhang, W.; Li, S.; Martin, R.C.G. Enrichment of cancer stem cells via beta-catenin contributing to the tumorigenesis of hepatocellular carcinoma. *BMC Cancer* **2018**, *18*, 783. [CrossRef] [PubMed]
147. Wurdak, H.; Zhu, S.; Romero, A.; Lorger, M.; Watson, J.; Chiang, C.Y.; Zhang, J.; Natu, V.S.; Lairson, L.L.; Walker, J.R.; et al. An RNAi screen identifies TRRAP as a regulator of brain tumor-initiating cell differentiation. *Cell Stem Cell* **2010**, *6*, 37–47. [CrossRef]
148. Hao, J.; Zhang, Y.; Jing, D.; Li, Y.; Li, J.; Zhao, Z. Role of Hippo Signaling in Cancer Stem Cells. *J. Cell. Physiol.* **2014**, *229*, 266–270. [CrossRef]
149. Safa, A.R. Resistance to Cell Death and Its Modulation in Cancer Stem Cells. *Crit. Rev. Oncog.* **2016**, *21*, 203–219. [CrossRef]
150. Hong, M.; Tan, H.; Li, S.; Cheung, F.; Wang, N.; Nagamatsu, T.; Feng, Y. Cancer Stem Cells: The Potential Targets of Chinese Medicines and Their Active Compounds. *Int. J. Mol. Sci.* **2016**, *17*, 893. [CrossRef]

151. Zakaria, N.; Mohd Yusoff, N.; Zakaria, Z.; Widera, D.; Yahaya, B.H. Inhibition of NF-kappaB Signaling Reduces the Stemness Characteristics of Lung Cancer Stem Cells. *Front. Oncol.* **2018**, *8*, 166. [CrossRef]
152. Kelly, P.N.; Strasser, A. The role of Bcl-2 and its pro-survival relatives in tumourigenesis and cancer therapy. *Cell Death Differ.* **2011**, *18*, 1414–1424. [CrossRef]
153. Visvader, J.E.; Lindeman, G.J. Cancer stem cells: Current status and evolving complexities. *Cell Stem Cell* **2012**, *10*, 717–728. [CrossRef] [PubMed]
154. Badve, S.; Nakshatri, H. Breast-cancer stem cells-beyond semantics. *Lancet Oncol.* **2012**, *13*, e43–e48. [CrossRef]
155. Liu, S.; Cong, Y.; Wang, D.; Sun, Y.; Deng, L.; Liu, Y.; Martin-Trevino, R.; Shang, L.; McDermott, S.P.; Landis, M.D.; et al. Breast Cancer Stem Cells Transition between Epithelial and Mesenchymal States Reflective of their Normal Counterparts. *Stem Cell Rep.* **2014**, *2*, 78–91. [CrossRef] [PubMed]
156. Aghajani, M.; Mansoori, B.; Mohammadi, A.; Asadzadeh, Z.; Baradaran, B. New emerging roles of CD133 in cancer stem cell: Signaling pathway and miRNA regulation. *J. Cell. Physiol.* **2019**, *234*, 21642–21661. [CrossRef]
157. Desai, A.; Webb, B.; Gerson, S.L. CD133+ cells contribute to radioresistance via altered regulation of DNA repair genes in human lung cancer cells. *Radiother. Oncol.* **2014**, *110*, 538–545. [CrossRef]
158. Levina, V.; Marrangoni, A.; Wang, T.; Parikh, S.; Su, Y.; Herberman, R.; Lokshin, A.; Gorelik, E. Elimination of Human Lung Cancer Stem Cells through Targeting of the Stem Cell Factor–c-kit Autocrine Signaling Loop. *Cancer Res.* **2010**, *70*, 338–346. [CrossRef]
159. Saya, H. MS 26.01 Therapeutic Strategies Targeting Cancer Stem Cells. *J. Thorac. Oncol.* **2017**, *12*, S1725–S1726. [CrossRef]
160. Tsubouchi, K.; Minami, K.; Hayashi, N.; Yokoyama, Y.; Mori, S.; Yamamoto, H.; Koizumi, M. The CD44 standard isoform contributes to radioresistance of pancreatic cancer cells. *J. Radiat. Res.* **2017**, *58*, 816–826. [CrossRef]
161. Kaidi, A.; Williams, A.C.; Paraskeva, C. Interaction between β-catenin and HIF-1 promotes cellular adaptation to hypoxia. *Nat. Cell Biol.* **2007**, *9*, 210–217. [CrossRef]
162. Moeller, B.J.; Dreher, M.R.; Rabbani, Z.N.; Schroeder, T.; Cao, Y.; Li, C.Y.; Dewhirst, M.W. Pleiotropic effects of HIF-1 blockade on tumor radiosensitivity. *Cancer Cell* **2005**, *8*, 99–110. [CrossRef]
163. Dimri, G.P.; Martinez, J.L.; Jacobs, J.J.; Keblusek, P.; Itahana, K.; Van Lohuizen, M.; Campisi, J.; Wazer, D.E.; Band, V. The Bmi-1 oncogene induces telomerase activity and immortalizes human mammary epithelial cells. *Cancer Res.* **2002**, *62*, 4736–4745. [PubMed]
164. Tao, W.; Zhang, A.; Zhai, K.; Huang, Z.; Huang, H.; Zhou, W.; Huang, Q.; Fang, X.; Prager, B.C.; Wang, X.; et al. SATB2 drives glioblastoma growth by recruiting CBP to promote FOXM1 expression in glioma stem cells. *EMBO Mol. Med.* **2020**, *12*, e12291. [CrossRef] [PubMed]
165. Gottesman, M.M.; Fojo, T.; Bates, S.E. Multidrug resistance in cancer: Role of ATP-dependent transporters. *Nat. Rev. Cancer* **2002**, *2*, 48–58. [CrossRef] [PubMed]
166. Copsel, S.; Garcia, C.; Diez, F.; Vermeulem, M.; Baldi, A.; Bianciotti, L.G.; Russel, F.G.; Shayo, C.; Davio, C. Multidrug resistance protein 4 (MRP4/ABCC4) regulates cAMP cellular levels and controls human leukemia cell proliferation and differentiation. *J. Biol. Chem.* **2011**, *286*, 6979–6988. [CrossRef]
167. Glavinas, H.; Krajcsi, P.; Cserepes, J.; Sarkadi, B. The role of ABC transporters in drug resistance, metabolism and toxicity. *Curr. Drug Deliv.* **2004**, *1*, 27–42. [CrossRef]
168. Bleau, A.-M.; Hambardzumyan, D.; Ozawa, T.; Fomchenko, E.I.; Huse, J.T.; Brennan, C.W.; Holland, E.C. PTEN/PI3K/Akt Pathway Regulates the Side Population Phenotype and ABCG2 Activity in Glioma Tumor Stem-like Cells. *Cell Stem Cell* **2009**, *4*, 226–235. [CrossRef]
169. Moitra, K. Overcoming Multidrug Resistance in Cancer Stem Cells. *BioMed Res. Int.* **2015**, *2015*, 635745. [CrossRef]
170. Pustovalova, M.; Alhaddad, L.; Smetanina, N.; Chigasova, A.; Blokhina, T.; Chuprov-Netochin, R.; Osipov, A.N.; Leonov, S. The p53-53BP1-Related Survival of A549 and H1299 Human Lung Cancer Cells after Multifractionated Radiotherapy Demonstrated Different Response to Additional Acute X-ray Exposure. *Int. J. Mol. Sci.* **2020**, *21*, 3342. [CrossRef]
171. Castellan, M.; Guarnieri, A.; Fujimura, K.; Zanconato, F.; Battilana, G.; Panciera, T.; Sladitschek, H.L.; Contessotto, P.; Citron, A.; Grilli, A.; et al. Single-cell analyses reveal YAP/TAZ as regulators of stemness and cell plasticity in glioblastoma. *Nat. Cancer* **2020**, *2*, 174–188. [CrossRef]
172. Benham-Pyle, B.W.; Pruitt, B.L.; Nelson, W.J. Cell adhesion. Mechanical strain induces E-cadherin-dependent Yap1 and beta-catenin activation to drive cell cycle entry. *Science* **2015**, *348*, 1024–1027. [CrossRef]
173. Shreberk-Shaked, M.; Dassa, B.; Sinha, S.; Di Agostino, S.; Azuri, I.; Mukherjee, S.; Aylon, Y.; Blandino, G.; Ruppin, E.; Oren, M. A Division of Labor between YAP and TAZ in Non-Small Cell Lung Cancer. *Cancer Res.* **2020**, *80*, 4145–4157. [CrossRef] [PubMed]
174. Overholtzer, M.; Zhang, J.; Smolen, G.A.; Muir, B.; Li, W.; Sgroi, D.C.; Deng, C.X.; Brugge, J.S.; Haber, D.A. Transforming properties of YAP, a candidate oncogene on the chromosome 11q22 amplicon. *Proc. Natl. Acad. Sci. USA* **2006**, *103*, 12405–12410. [CrossRef] [PubMed]
175. Neradil, J.; Veselska, R. Nestin as a marker of cancer stem cells. *Cancer Sci.* **2015**, *106*, 803–811. [CrossRef] [PubMed]
176. O'Brien, C.A.; Kreso, A.; Jamieson, C.H. Cancer stem cells and self-renewal. *Clin. Cancer Res.* **2010**, *16*, 3113–3120. [CrossRef] [PubMed]

177. Stahl, S.; Fung, E.; Adams, C.; Lengqvist, J.; Mork, B.; Stenerlow, B.; Lewensohn, R.; Lehtio, J.; Zubarev, R.; Viktorsson, K. Proteomics and pathway analysis identifies JNK signaling as critical for high linear energy transfer radiation-induced apoptosis in non-small lung cancer cells. *Mol. Cell Proteom.* **2009**, *8*, 1117–1129. [CrossRef] [PubMed]
178. Yang, L.; Shi, P.; Zhao, G.; Xu, J.; Peng, W.; Zhang, J.; Zhang, G.; Wang, X.; Dong, Z.; Chen, F.; et al. Targeting cancer stem cell pathways for cancer therapy. *Signal Transduct. Target. Ther.* **2020**, *5*, 8. [CrossRef]
179. Khan, A.Q.; Ahmed, E.I.; Elareer, N.R.; Junejo, K.; Steinhoff, M.; Uddin, S. Role of miRNA-Regulated Cancer Stem Cells in the Pathogenesis of Human Malignancies. *Cells* **2019**, *8*, 840. [CrossRef]
180. Correnti, M.; Booijink, R.; Di Maira, G.; Raggi, C.; Marra, F. Stemness features in liver cancer. *Hepatoma Res.* **2018**, *4*, 69. [CrossRef]
181. Kim, K.W.; Kim, J.Y.; Qiao, J.; Clark, R.A.; Powers, C.M.; Correa, H.; Chung, D.H. Dual-Targeting AKT2 and ERK in cancer stem-like cells in neuroblastoma. *Oncotarget* **2019**, *10*, 5645–5659. [CrossRef]
182. Wang, J.; Wakeman, T.P.; Lathia, J.D.; Hjelmeland, A.B.; Wang, X.F.; White, R.R.; Rich, J.N.; Sullenger, B.A. Notch promotes radioresistance of glioma stem cells. *Stem Cells* **2010**, *28*, 17–28. [CrossRef]
183. Stewart, D.J. Wnt signaling pathway in non-small cell lung cancer. *J. Natl. Cancer Inst.* **2014**, *106*, djt356. [CrossRef] [PubMed]
184. Matsui, W.H. Cancer stem cell signaling pathways. *Medicine* **2016**, *95*, S8–S19. [CrossRef] [PubMed]
185. Schreck, K.C.; Taylor, P.; Marchionni, L.; Gopalakrishnan, V.; Bar, E.E.; Gaiano, N.; Eberhart, C.G. The Notch target Hes1 directly modulates Gli1 expression and Hedgehog signaling: A potential mechanism of therapeutic resistance. *Clin. Cancer Res.* **2010**, *16*, 6060–6070. [CrossRef] [PubMed]
186. Vlashi, E.; Pajonk, F. Cancer stem cells, cancer cell plasticity and radiation therapy. *Semin. Cancer Biol.* **2015**, *31*, 28–35. [CrossRef] [PubMed]
187. Yang, Y.; Zhou, H.; Zhang, G.; Xue, X. Targeting the canonical Wnt/beta-catenin pathway in cancer radioresistance: Updates on the molecular mechanisms. *J. Cancer Res. Ther.* **2019**, *15*, 272–277. [CrossRef]
188. Liu, C.; Wang, R. The Roles of Hedgehog Signaling Pathway in Radioresistance of Cervical Cancer. *Dose-Response* **2019**, *17*, 1559325819885293. [CrossRef]
189. Kim, R.K.; Kaushik, N.; Suh, Y.; Yoo, K.C.; Cui, Y.H.; Kim, M.J.; Lee, H.J.; Kim, I.G.; Lee, S.J. Radiation driven epithelial-mesenchymal transition is mediated by Notch signaling in breast cancer. *Oncotarget* **2016**, *7*, 53430–53442. [CrossRef]
190. Kong, D.; Banerjee, S.; Ahmad, A.; Li, Y.; Wang, Z.; Sethi, S.; Sarkar, F.H. Epithelial to mesenchymal transition is mechanistically linked with stem cell signatures in prostate cancer cells. *PLoS ONE* **2010**, *5*, e12445. [CrossRef]
191. Hassan, K.A.; Wang, L.; Korkaya, H.; Chen, G.; Maillard, I.; Beer, D.G.; Kalemkerian, G.P.; Wicha, M.S. Notch pathway activity identifies cells with cancer stem cell-like properties and correlates with worse survival in lung adenocarcinoma. *Clin. Cancer Res.* **2013**, *19*, 1972–1980. [CrossRef]
192. Park, J.H.; Shin, J.E.; Park, H.W. The Role of Hippo Pathway in Cancer Stem Cell Biology. *Mol. Cells* **2018**, *41*, 83–92. [CrossRef]
193. Zhang, Y.; Wang, Y.; Zhou, D.; Wang, K.; Wang, X.; Wang, X.; Jiang, Y.; Zhao, M.; Yu, R.; Zhou, X. Radiation-induced YAP activation confers glioma radioresistance via promoting FGF2 transcription and DNA damage repair. *Oncogene* **2021**, *40*, 4580–4591. [CrossRef] [PubMed]
194. Yang, K.; Zhao, Y.; Du, Y.; Tang, R. Evaluation of Hippo Pathway and CD133 in Radiation Resistance in Small-Cell Lung Cancer. *J. Oncol.* **2021**, *2021*, 8842554. [CrossRef] [PubMed]
195. Krause, M.; Dubrovska, A.; Linge, A.; Baumann, M. Cancer stem cells: Radioresistance, prediction of radiotherapy outcome and specific targets for combined treatments. *Adv. Drug Deliv. Rev.* **2017**, *109*, 63–73. [CrossRef] [PubMed]
196. Maugeri-Saccà, M.; Bartucci, M.; De Maria, R. DNA Damage Repair Pathways in Cancer Stem Cells. *Mol. Cancer Ther.* **2012**, *11*, 1627–1636. [CrossRef] [PubMed]
197. Eriksson, D.; Stigbrand, T. Radiation-induced cell death mechanisms. *Tumor Biol.* **2010**, *31*, 363–372. [CrossRef] [PubMed]
198. Babayan, N.; Vorobyeva, N.; Grigoryan, B.; Grekhova, A.; Pustovalova, M.; Rodneva, S.; Fedotov, Y.; Tsakanova, G.; Aroutiounian, R.; Osipov, A. Low Repair Capacity of DNA Double-Strand Breaks Induced by Laser-Driven Ultrashort Electron Beams in Cancer Cells. *Int. J. Mol. Sci.* **2020**, *21*, 9488. [CrossRef] [PubMed]
199. Mladenov, E.; Magin, S.; Soni, A.; Iliakis, G. DNA Double-Strand Break Repair as Determinant of Cellular Radiosensitivity to Killing and Target in Radiation Therapy. *Front. Oncol.* **2013**, *3*, 113. [CrossRef]
200. Bushmanov, A.; Vorobyeva, N.; Molodtsova, D.; Osipov, A.N. Utilization of DNA double-strand breaks for biodosimetry of ionizing radiation exposure. *Environ. Adv.* **2022**, *8*, 100207. [CrossRef]
201. Biau, J.; Chautard, E.; Berthault, N.; de Koning, L.; Court, F.; Pereira, B.; Verrelle, P.; Dutreix, M. Combining the DNA Repair Inhibitor Dbait With Radiotherapy for the Treatment of High Grade Glioma: Efficacy and Protein Biomarkers of Resistance in Preclinical Models. *Front. Oncol.* **2019**, *9*, 549. [CrossRef]
202. Wyman, C.; Kanaar, R. DNA double-strand break repair: All's well that ends well. *Annu. Rev. Genet.* **2006**, *40*, 363–383. [CrossRef]
203. Morgan, M.A.; Lawrence, T.S. Molecular Pathways: Overcoming Radiation Resistance by Targeting DNA Damage Response Pathways. *Clin. Cancer Res.* **2015**, *21*, 2898–2904. [CrossRef] [PubMed]
204. Biau, J.; Chautard, E.; Verrelle, P.; Dutreix, M. Altering DNA Repair to Improve Radiation Therapy: Specific and Multiple Pathway Targeting. *Front. Oncol.* **2019**, *9*, 1009. [CrossRef] [PubMed]
205. Ulyanenko, S.; Pustovalova, M.; Koryakin, S.; Beketov, E.; Lychagin, A.; Ulyanenko, L.; Kaprin, A.; Grekhova, A.; Ozerova, A.M.; Ozerov, I.V.; et al. Formation of gammaH2AX and pATM Foci in Human Mesenchymal Stem Cells Exposed to Low Dose-Rate Gamma-Radiation. *Int. J. Mol. Sci.* **2019**, *20*, 2645. [CrossRef] [PubMed]

206. Britton, S.; Coates, J.; Jackson, S.P. A new method for high-resolution imaging of Ku foci to decipher mechanisms of DNA double-strand break repair. *J. Cell Biol.* **2013**, *202*, 579–595. [CrossRef]
207. Park, E.J.; Chan, D.W.; Park, J.H.; Oettinger, M.A.; Kwon, J. DNA-PK is activated by nucleosomes and phosphorylates H2AX within the nucleosomes in an acetylation-dependent manner. *Nucleic Acids Res.* **2003**, *31*, 6819–6827. [CrossRef]
208. Ma, Y.; Pannicke, U.; Schwarz, K.; Lieber, M.R. Hairpin Opening and Overhang Processing by an Artemis/DNA-Dependent Protein Kinase Complex in Nonhomologous End Joining and V(D)J Recombination. *Cell* **2002**, *108*, 781–794. [CrossRef]
209. Nick McElhinny, S.A.; Snowden, C.M.; McCarville, J.; Ramsden, D.A. Ku Recruits the XRCC4-Ligase IV Complex to DNA Ends. *Mol. Cell. Biol.* **2000**, *20*, 2996–3003. [CrossRef]
210. Ahnesorg, P.; Smith, P.; Jackson, S.P. XLF Interacts with the XRCC4-DNA Ligase IV Complex to Promote DNA Nonhomologous End-Joining. *Cell* **2006**, *124*, 301–313. [CrossRef]
211. Belyaev, I.Y. Radiation-induced DNA repair foci: Spatio-temporal aspects of formation, application for assessment of radiosensitivity and biological dosimetry. *Mutat. Res./Rev. Mutat. Res.* **2010**, *704*, 132–141. [CrossRef]
212. Tsvetkova, A.; Ozerov, I.V.; Pustovalova, M.; Grekhova, A.; Eremin, P.; Vorobyeva, N.; Eremin, I.; Pulin, A.; Zorin, V.; Kopnin, P.; et al. γH2AX, 53BP1 and Rad51 protein foci changes in mesenchymal stem cells during prolonged X-ray irradiation. *Oncotarget* **2017**, *8*, 64317–64329. [CrossRef]
213. Mao, Z.; Bozzella, M.; Seluanov, A.; Gorbunova, V. DNA repair by nonhomologous end joining and homologous recombination during cell cycle in human cells. *Cell Cycle* **2014**, *7*, 2902–2906. [CrossRef] [PubMed]
214. Kakarougkas, A.; Jeggo, P.A. DNA DSB repair pathway choice: An orchestrated handover mechanism. *Br. J. Radiol.* **2014**, *87*, 20130685. [CrossRef] [PubMed]
215. Safa, A.R.; Saadatzadeh, M.R.; Cohen-Gadol, A.A.; Pollok, K.E.; Bijangi-Vishehsaraei, K. Glioblastoma stem cells (GSCs) epigenetic plasticity and interconversion between differentiated non-GSCs and GSCs. *Genes Dis.* **2015**, *2*, 152–163. [CrossRef] [PubMed]
216. Vlashi, E.; Lagadec, C.; Vergnes, L.; Matsutani, T.; Masui, K.; Poulou, M.; Popescu, R.; Della Donna, L.; Evers, P.; Dekmezian, C.; et al. Metabolic state of glioma stem cells and nontumorigenic cells. *Proc. Natl. Acad. Sci. USA* **2011**, *108*, 16062–16067. [CrossRef]
217. Ogden, A.T.; Waziri, A.E.; Lochhead, R.A.; Fusco, D.; Lopez, K.; Ellis, J.A.; Kang, J.; Assanah, M.; McKhann, G.M.; Sisti, M.B.; et al. Identification of A2b5+Cd133− Tumor-Initiating Cells in Adult Human Gliomas. *Neurosurgery* **2008**, *62*, 505–515. [CrossRef]
218. Aum, D.J.; Kim, D.H.; Beaumont, T.L.; Leuthardt, E.C.; Dunn, G.P.; Kim, A.H. Molecular and cellular heterogeneity: The hallmark of glioblastoma. *Neurosurg. Focus* **2014**, *37*, E11. [CrossRef]
219. Nakano, I. Stem cell signature in glioblastoma: Therapeutic development for a moving target. *J. Neurosurg.* **2015**, *122*, 324–330. [CrossRef]
220. Jackson, E.L.; Alvarez-Buylla, A. Characterization of adult neural stem cells and their relation to brain tumors. *Cells Tissues Organs* **2008**, *188*, 212–224. [CrossRef]
221. Zhu, Y.; Guignard, F.; Zhao, D.; Liu, L.; Burns, D.K.; Mason, R.P.; Messing, A.; Parada, L.F. Early inactivation of p53 tumor suppressor gene cooperating with NF1 loss induces malignant astrocytoma. *Cancer Cell* **2005**, *8*, 119–130. [CrossRef]
222. Kondo, T.; Setoguchi, T.; Taga, T. Persistence of a small subpopulation of cancer stem-like cells in the C6 glioma cell line. *Proc. Natl. Acad. Sci. USA* **2004**, *101*, 781–786. [CrossRef]
223. Goodell, M.A.; Brose, K.; Paradis, G.; Conner, A.S.; Mulligan, R.C. Isolation and functional properties of murine hematopoietic stem cells that are replicating in vivo. *J. Exp. Med.* **1996**, *183*, 1797–1806. [CrossRef] [PubMed]
224. Lathia, J.D.; Mack, S.C.; Mulkearns-Hubert, E.E.; Valentim, C.L.; Rich, J.N. Cancer stem cells in glioblastoma. *Genes Dev.* **2015**, *29*, 1203–1217. [CrossRef] [PubMed]
225. Bao, S.; Wu, Q.; McLendon, R.E.; Hao, Y.; Shi, Q.; Hjelmeland, A.B.; Dewhirst, M.W.; Bigner, D.D.; Rich, J.N. Glioma stem cells promote radioresistance by preferential activation of the DNA damage response. *Nature* **2006**, *444*, 756–760. [CrossRef] [PubMed]
226. Lim, Y.C.; Roberts, T.L.; Day, B.W.; Harding, A.; Kozlov, S.; Kijas, A.W.; Ensbey, K.S.; Walker, D.G.; Lavin, M.F. A role for homologous recombination and abnormal cell-cycle progression in radioresistance of glioma-initiating cells. *Mol. Cancer Ther.* **2012**, *11*, 1863–1872. [CrossRef] [PubMed]
227. Son, M.J.; Woolard, K.; Nam, D.H.; Lee, J.; Fine, H.A. SSEA-1 is an enrichment marker for tumor-initiating cells in human glioblastoma. *Cell Stem Cell* **2009**, *4*, 440–452. [CrossRef]
228. Patru, C.; Romao, L.; Varlet, P.; Coulombel, L.; Raponi, E.; Cadusseau, J.; Renault-Mihara, F.; Thirant, C.; Leonard, N.; Berhneim, A.; et al. CD133, CD15/SSEA-1, CD34 or side populations do not resume tumor-initiating properties of long-term cultured cancer stem cells from human malignant glio-neuronal tumors. *BMC Cancer* **2010**, *10*, 66. [CrossRef]
229. Singh, S.K.; Hawkins, C.; Clarke, I.D.; Squire, J.A.; Bayani, J.; Hide, T.; Henkelman, R.M.; Cusimano, M.D.; Dirks, P.B. Identification of human brain tumour initiating cells. *Nature* **2004**, *432*, 396–401. [CrossRef]
230. Huang, Z.; Cheng, L.; Guryanova, O.A.; Wu, Q.; Bao, S. Cancer stem cells in glioblastoma—molecular signaling and therapeutic targeting. *Protein Cell* **2010**, *1*, 638–655. [CrossRef]
231. Mao, X.G.; Zhang, X.; Xue, X.Y.; Guo, G.; Wang, P.; Zhang, W.; Fei, Z.; Zhen, H.N.; You, S.W.; Yang, H. Brain Tumor Stem-Like Cells Identified by Neural Stem Cell Marker CD15. *Transl. Oncol.* **2009**, *2*, 247–257. [CrossRef]
232. Jijiwa, M.; Demir, H.; Gupta, S.; Leung, C.; Joshi, K.; Orozco, N.; Huang, T.; Yildiz, V.O.; Shibahara, I.; de Jesus, J.A.; et al. CD44v6 regulates growth of brain tumor stem cells partially through the AKT-mediated pathway. *PLoS ONE* **2011**, *6*, e24217. [CrossRef]
233. Bao, S.; Wu, Q.; Li, Z.; Sathornsumetee, S.; Wang, H.; McLendon, R.E.; Hjelmeland, A.B.; Rich, J.N. Targeting cancer stem cells through L1CAM suppresses glioma growth. *Cancer Res.* **2008**, *68*, 6043–6048. [CrossRef]

234. Lathia, J.D.; Gallagher, J.; Heddleston, J.M.; Wang, J.; Eyler, C.E.; Macswords, J.; Wu, Q.; Vasanji, A.; McLendon, R.E.; Hjelmeland, A.B.; et al. Integrin alpha 6 regulates glioblastoma stem cells. *Cell Stem Cell* **2010**, *6*, 421–432. [CrossRef]
235. Yoo, K.C.; Kang, J.H.; Choi, M.Y.; Suh, Y.; Zhao, Y.; Kim, M.J.; Chang, J.H.; Shim, J.K.; Yoon, S.J.; Kang, S.G.; et al. Soluble ICAM-1 a Pivotal Communicator between Tumors and Macrophages, Promotes Mesenchymal Shift of Glioblastoma. *Adv. Sci.* **2022**, *9*, e2102768. [CrossRef]
236. Reifenberger, G.; Szymas, J.; Wechsler, W. Differential expression of glial- and neuronal-associated antigens in human tumors of the central and peripheral nervous system. *Acta Neuropathol.* **1987**, *74*, 105–123. [CrossRef] [PubMed]
237. Hagiwara, H.; Aotsuka, Y.; Yamamoto, Y.; Miyahara, J.; Mitoh, Y. Determination of the antigen/epitope that is recognized by human monoclonal antibody CLN-IgG. *Hum. Antibodies* **2001**, *10*, 77–82. [CrossRef] [PubMed]
238. Babic, B.; Matthias Corvinus, F.; Hadjijusufovic, E.; Tagkalos, E.; Lang, H.; Grimminger, P. Ps01.162: Is There a Difference in Survival between Younger and Older Gastric Cancer (Including Aeg Ii and Aeg Iii) Patients after Gastrectomy? *Dis. Esophagus* **2018**, *31*, 95. [CrossRef]
239. Hugwil, A.V. The meaning of the anti-cancer antibody CLN-IgG (Pritumumab) generated by human×human hybridoma technology against the cyto-skeletal protein, vimentin, in the course of the treatment of malignancy. *Med. Hypotheses* **2013**, *81*, 489–495. [CrossRef] [PubMed]
240. Clement, V.; Sanchez, P.; de Tribolet, N.; Radovanovic, I.; Ruiz i Altaba, A. HEDGEHOG-GLI1 Signaling Regulates Human Glioma Growth, Cancer Stem Cell Self-Renewal, and Tumorigenicity. *Curr. Biol.* **2007**, *17*, 165–172. [CrossRef] [PubMed]
241. Zhu, J.; Wang, H.; Sun, Q.; Ji, X.; Zhu, L.; Cong, Z.; Zhou, Y.; Liu, H.; Zhou, M. Nrf2 is required to maintain the self-renewal of glioma stem cells. *BMC Cancer* **2013**, *13*, 380. [CrossRef]
242. Zhu, J.; Wang, H.; Fan, Y.; Lin, Y.; Zhang, L.; Ji, X.; Zhou, M. Targeting the NF-E2-related factor 2 pathway: A novel strategy for glioblastoma (review). *Oncol. Rep.* **2014**, *32*, 443–450. [CrossRef]
243. Leelatian, N.; Ihrie, R.A. Head of the Class: OLIG2 and Glioblastoma Phenotype. *Cancer Cell* **2016**, *29*, 613–615. [CrossRef] [PubMed]
244. Liu, M.; Dai, B.; Kang, S.H.; Ban, K.; Huang, F.J.; Lang, F.F.; Aldape, K.D.; Xie, T.X.; Pelloski, C.E.; Xie, K.; et al. FoxM1B is overexpressed in human glioblastomas and critically regulates the tumorigenicity of glioma cells. *Cancer Res.* **2006**, *66*, 3593–3602. [CrossRef] [PubMed]
245. Li, X.T.; Li, J.C.; Feng, M.; Zhou, Y.X.; Du, Z.W. Novel lncRNA-ZNF281 regulates cell growth, stemness and invasion of glioma stem-like U251s cells. *Neoplasma* **2019**, *66*, 118–127. [CrossRef] [PubMed]
246. Suva, M.L.; Rheinbay, E.; Gillespie, S.M.; Patel, A.P.; Wakimoto, H.; Rabkin, S.D.; Riggi, N.; Chi, A.S.; Cahill, D.P.; Nahed, B.V.; et al. Reconstructing and reprogramming the tumor-propagating potential of glioblastoma stem-like cells. *Cell* **2014**, *157*, 580–594. [CrossRef] [PubMed]
247. Qiang, L.; Wu, T.; Zhang, H.W.; Lu, N.; Hu, R.; Wang, Y.J.; Zhao, L.; Chen, F.H.; Wang, X.T.; You, Q.D.; et al. HIF-1alpha is critical for hypoxia-mediated maintenance of glioblastoma stem cells by activating Notch signaling pathway. *Cell Death Differ.* **2012**, *19*, 284–294. [CrossRef]
248. Dahlrot, R.H.; Hermansen, S.K.; Hansen, S.; Kristensen, B.W. What is the clinical value of cancer stem cell markers in gliomas? *Int. J. Clin. Exp. Pathol.* **2013**, *6*, 334–348.
249. Banelli, B.; Forlani, A.; Allemanni, G.; Morabito, A.; Pistillo, M.P.; Romani, M. MicroRNA in Glioblastoma: An Overview. *Int. J. Genom.* **2017**, *2017*, 7639084. [CrossRef]
250. Charles, N.A.; Holland, E.C. TRRAP and the maintenance of stemness in gliomas. *Cell Stem Cell* **2010**, *6*, 6–7. [CrossRef]
251. Spehalski, E.I.; Peters, C.; Camphausen, K.A.; Tofilon, P. Distinctions Between the Metabolic Changes in Glioblastoma Cells and Glioma Stem-like Cells Following Irradiation. *Int. J. Radiat. Oncol. Biol. Phys.* **2017**, *99*, e617. [CrossRef]
252. Godoy, P.R.D.V.; Mello, S.S.; Magalhães, D.A.R.; Donaires, F.S.; Nicolucci, P.; Donadi, E.A.; Passos, G.A.; Sakamoto-Hojo, E.T. Ionizing radiation-induced gene expression changes in TP53 proficient and deficient glioblastoma cell lines. *Mutat. Res./Genet. Toxicol. Environ. Mutagen.* **2013**, *756*, 46–55. [CrossRef]
253. Camphausen, K.; Purow, B.; Sproull, M.; Scott, T.; Ozawa, T.; Deen, D.F.; Tofilon, P.J. Orthotopic Growth of Human Glioma Cells Quantitatively and Qualitatively Influences Radiation-Induced Changes in Gene Expression. *Cancer Res.* **2005**, *65*, 10389–10393. [CrossRef] [PubMed]
254. Tsai, M.-H.; Cook, J.A.; Chandramouli, G.V.R.; DeGraff, W.; Yan, H.; Zhao, S.; Coleman, C.N.; Mitchell, J.B.; Chuang, E.Y. Gene Expression Profiling of Breast, Prostate, and Glioma Cells following Single versus Fractionated Doses of Radiation. *Cancer Res.* **2007**, *67*, 3845–3852. [CrossRef] [PubMed]
255. Zhang, L.; Cheng, F.; Wei, Y.; Zhang, L.; Guo, D.; Wang, B.; Li, W. Inhibition of TAZ contributes radiation-induced senescence and growth arrest in glioma cells. *Oncogene* **2018**, *38*, 2788–2799. [CrossRef] [PubMed]
256. Behrooz, A.B.; Syahir, A. Could We Address the Interplay Between CD133, Wnt/beta-Catenin, and TERT Signaling Pathways as a Potential Target for Glioblastoma Therapy? *Front. Oncol.* **2021**, *11*, 642719. [CrossRef] [PubMed]
257. Olive, P.L. DNA damage and repair in individual cells: Applications of the comet assay in radiobiology. *Int. J. Radiat. Biol.* **1999**, *75*, 395–405. [CrossRef]
258. Legler, J.M.; Ries, L.A.; Smith, M.A.; Warren, J.L.; Heineman, E.F.; Kaplan, R.S.; Linet, M.S. Cancer surveillance series [corrected]: Brain and other central nervous system cancers: Recent trends in incidence and mortality. *J. Natl. Cancer Inst.* **1999**, *91*, 1382–1390. [CrossRef]

259. Beier, D.; Hau, P.; Proescholdt, M.; Lohmeier, A.; Wischhusen, J.; Oefner, P.J.; Aigner, L.; Brawanski, A.; Bogdahn, U.; Beier, C.P. CD133(+) and CD133(-) glioblastoma-derived cancer stem cells show differential growth characteristics and molecular profiles. *Cancer Res.* **2007**, *67*, 4010–4015. [CrossRef]
260. Campos, B.; Zeng, L.; Daotrong, P.H.; Eckstein, V.; Unterberg, A.; Mairbaurl, H.; Herold-Mende, C. Expression and regulation of AC133 and CD133 in glioblastoma. *Glia* **2011**, *59*, 1974–1986. [CrossRef]
261. Gambelli, F.; Sasdelli, F.; Manini, I.; Gambarana, C.; Oliveri, G.; Miracco, C.; Sorrentino, V. Identification of cancer stem cells from human glioblastomas: Growth and differentiation capabilities and CD133/prominin-1 expression. *Cell Biol. Int.* **2012**, *36*, 29–38. [CrossRef]
262. Brown, D.V.; Filiz, G.; Daniel, P.M.; Hollande, F.; Dworkin, S.; Amiridis, S.; Kountouri, N.; Ng, W.; Morokoff, A.F.; Mantamadiotis, T. Expression of CD133 and CD44 in glioblastoma stem cells correlates with cell proliferation, phenotype stability and intra-tumor heterogeneity. *PLoS ONE* **2017**, *12*, e0172791. [CrossRef]
263. Kowalski-Chauvel, A.; Modesto, A.; Gouaze-Andersson, V.; Baricault, L.; Gilhodes, J.; Delmas, C.; Lemarie, A.; Toulas, C.; Cohen-Jonathan-Moyal, E.; Seva, C. Alpha-6 integrin promotes radioresistance of glioblastoma by modulating DNA damage response and the transcription factor Zeb1. *Cell Death Dis.* **2018**, *9*, 872. [CrossRef] [PubMed]
264. Halliday, J.; Helmy, K.; Pattwell, S.S.; Pitter, K.L.; LaPlant, Q.; Ozawa, T.; Holland, E.C. In vivo radiation response of proneural glioma characterized by protective p53 transcriptional program and proneural-mesenchymal shift. *Proc. Natl. Acad. Sci. USA* **2014**, *111*, 5248–5253. [CrossRef] [PubMed]
265. Trog, D.; Moenkemann, H.; Haertel, N.; Schuller, H.; Golubnitschaja, O. Expression of ABC-1 transporter is elevated in human glioma cells under irradiation and temozolomide treatment. *Amino Acids* **2005**, *28*, 213–219. [CrossRef] [PubMed]
266. Ray, S.K. The Transcription Regulator Kruppel-Like Factor 4 and Its Dual Roles of Oncogene in Glioblastoma and Tumor Suppressor in Neuroblastoma. *Immunopathol. Dis Ther.* **2016**, *7*, 127–139. [CrossRef]
267. Hayes, J.D.; Dinkova-Kostova, A.T. The Nrf2 regulatory network provides an interface between redox and intermediary metabolism. *Trends Biochem. Sci.* **2014**, *39*, 199–218. [CrossRef]
268. Dreger, H.; Westphal, K.; Weller, A.; Baumann, G.; Stangl, V.; Meiners, S.; Stangl, K. Nrf2-dependent upregulation of antioxidative enzymes: A novel pathway for proteasome inhibitor-mediated cardioprotection. *Cardiovasc. Res.* **2009**, *83*, 354–361. [CrossRef]
269. Singh, A.; Bodas, M.; Wakabayashi, N.; Bunz, F.; Biswal, S. Gain of Nrf2 function in non-small-cell lung cancer cells confers radioresistance. *Antioxid. Redox. Signal.* **2010**, *13*, 1627–1637. [CrossRef]
270. Suzuki, T.; Yamamoto, M. Molecular basis of the Keap1-Nrf2 system. *Free Radic. Biol. Med.* **2015**, *88*, 93–100. [CrossRef]
271. Shibata, T.; Ohta, T.; Tong, K.I.; Kokubu, A.; Odogawa, R.; Tsuta, K.; Asamura, H.; Yamamoto, M.; Hirohashi, S. Cancer related mutations in NRF2 impair its recognition by Keap1-Cul3 E3 ligase and promote malignancy. *Proc. Natl. Acad. Sci. USA* **2008**, *105*, 13568–13573. [CrossRef]
272. Facchino, S.; Abdouh, M.; Chatoo, W.; Bernier, G. BMI1 confers radioresistance to normal and cancerous neural stem cells through recruitment of the DNA damage response machinery. *J. Neurosci.* **2010**, *30*, 10096–10111. [CrossRef]
273. Mukherjee, B.; McEllin, B.; Camacho, C.V.; Tomimatsu, N.; Sirasanagandala, S.; Nannepaga, S.; Hatanpaa, K.J.; Mickey, B.; Madden, C.; Maher, E.; et al. EGFRvIII and DNA double-strand break repair: A molecular mechanism for radioresistance in glioblastoma. *Cancer Res.* **2009**, *69*, 4252–4259. [CrossRef] [PubMed]
274. Majc, B.; Sever, T.; Zaric, M.; Breznik, B.; Turk, B.; Lah, T.T. Epithelial-to-mesenchymal transition as the driver of changing carcinoma and glioblastoma microenvironment. *Biochim. Biophys. Acta Mol. Cell Res.* **2020**, *1867*, 118782. [CrossRef] [PubMed]
275. Hovinga, K.E.; Stalpers, L.J.; van Bree, C.; Donker, M.; Verhoeff, J.J.; Rodermond, H.M.; Bosch, D.A.; van Furth, W.R. Radiation-enhanced vascular endothelial growth factor (VEGF) secretion in glioblastoma multiforme cell lines-a clue to radioresistance? *J. Neurooncol.* **2005**, *74*, 99–103. [CrossRef] [PubMed]
276. Lee, C.G.; Heijn, M.; di Tomaso, E.; Griffon-Etienne, G.; Ancukiewicz, M.; Koike, C.; Park, K.R.; Ferrara, N.; Jain, R.K.; Suit, H.D.; et al. Anti-Vascular endothelial growth factor treatment augments tumor radiation response under normoxic or hypoxic conditions. *Cancer Res.* **2000**, *60*, 5565–5570. [PubMed]
277. Maachani, U.B.; Shankavaram, U.; Kramp, T.; Tofilon, P.J.; Camphausen, K.; Tandle, A.T. FOXM1 and STAT3 interaction confers radioresistance in glioblastoma cells. *Oncotarget* **2016**, *7*, 77365–77377. [CrossRef]
278. Povlsen, L.K.; Beli, P.; Wagner, S.A.; Poulsen, S.L.; Sylvestersen, K.B.; Poulsen, J.W.; Nielsen, M.L.; Bekker-Jensen, S.; Mailand, N.; Choudhary, C. Systems-wide analysis of ubiquitylation dynamics reveals a key role for PAF15 ubiquitylation in DNA-damage bypass. *Nat. Cell Biol.* **2012**, *14*, 1089–1098. [CrossRef]
279. Lee, H.C.; Kim, D.W.; Jung, K.Y.; Park, I.C.; Park, M.J.; Kim, M.S.; Woo, S.H.; Rhee, C.H.; Yoo, H.; Lee, S.H.; et al. Increased expression of antioxidant enzymes in radioresistant variant from U251 human glioblastoma cell line. *Int. J. Mol. Med.* **2004**, *13*, 883–887. [CrossRef]
280. Flor, S.; Oliva, C.R.; Ali, M.Y.; Coleman, K.L.; Greenlee, J.D.; Jones, K.A.; Monga, V.; Griguer, C.E. Catalase Overexpression Drives an Aggressive Phenotype in Glioblastoma. *Antioxidants* **2021**, *10*, 1988. [CrossRef]
281. Pang, L.Y.; Hurst, E.A.; Argyle, D.J. Cyclooxygenase-2: A Role in Cancer Stem Cell Survival and Repopulation of Cancer Cells during Therapy. *Stem Cells Int.* **2016**, *2016*, 2048731. [CrossRef]
282. Ma, H.I.; Chiou, S.H.; Hueng, D.Y.; Tai, L.K.; Huang, P.I.; Kao, C.L.; Chen, Y.W.; Sytwu, H.K. Celecoxib and radioresistant glioblastoma-derived CD133+ cells: Improvement in radiotherapeutic effects. Laboratory investigation. *J. Neurosurg.* **2011**, *114*, 651–662. [CrossRef]

283. Wang, W.; Long, L.; Wang, L.; Tan, C.; Fei, X.; Chen, L.; Huang, Q.; Liang, Z. Knockdown of Cathepsin L promotes radiosensitivity of glioma stem cells both in vivo and in vitro. *Cancer Lett.* **2016**, *371*, 274–284. [CrossRef] [PubMed]
284. Wang, J.; Yang, T.; Xu, G.; Liu, H.; Ren, C.; Xie, W.; Wang, M. Cyclin-Dependent Kinase 2 Promotes Tumor Proliferation and Induces Radio Resistance in Glioblastoma. *Transl. Oncol.* **2016**, *9*, 548–556. [CrossRef] [PubMed]
285. Marampon, F.; Megiorni, F.; Camero, S.; Crescioli, C.; McDowell, H.P.; Sferra, R.; Vetuschi, A.; Pompili, S.; Ventura, L.; De Felice, F.; et al. HDAC4 and HDAC6 sustain DNA double strand break repair and stem-like phenotype by promoting radioresistance in glioblastoma cells. *Cancer Lett.* **2017**, *397*, 1–11. [CrossRef]
286. Deng, X.; Ma, L.; Wu, M.; Zhang, G.; Jin, C.; Guo, Y.; Liu, R. miR-124 radiosensitizes human glioma cells by targeting CDK4. *J. Neurooncol.* **2013**, *114*, 263–274. [CrossRef] [PubMed]
287. Moskwa, P.; Zinn, P.O.; Choi, Y.E.; Shukla, S.A.; Fendler, W.; Chen, C.C.; Lu, J.; Golub, T.R.; Hjelmeland, A.; Chowdhury, D. A functional screen identifies miRs that induce radioresistance in glioblastomas. *Mol. Cancer Res.* **2014**, *12*, 1767–1778. [CrossRef] [PubMed]
288. Alkhaibary, A.; Alassiri, A.H.; AlSufiani, F.; Alharbi, M.A. Ki-67 labeling index in glioblastoma; does it really matter? *Hematol./Oncol. Stem Cell Ther.* **2019**, *12*, 82–88. [CrossRef]
289. Mastronardi, L.; Guiducci, A.; Puzzilli, F.; Ruggeri, A. Relationship between Ki-67 labeling index and survival in high-grade glioma patients treated after surgery with tamoxifen. *J. Neurosurg. Sci.* **1999**, *43*, 263–270.
290. Tamura, K.; Aoyagi, M.; Ando, N.; Ogishima, T.; Wakimoto, H.; Yamamoto, M.; Ohno, K. Expansion of CD133-positive glioma cells in recurrent de novo glioblastomas after radiotherapy and chemotherapy. *J. Neurosurg.* **2013**, *119*, 1145–1155. [CrossRef]
291. Zottel, A.; Jovcevska, I.; Samec, N.; Komel, R. Cytoskeletal proteins as glioblastoma biomarkers and targets for therapy: A systematic review. *Crit. Rev. Oncol. Hematol.* **2021**, *160*, 103283. [CrossRef]
292. Nguemgo Kouam, P.; Rezniczek, G.A.; Kochanneck, A.; Priesch-Grzeszkowiak, B.; Hero, T.; Adamietz, I.A.; Buhler, H. Robo1 and vimentin regulate radiation-induced motility of human glioblastoma cells. *PLoS ONE* **2018**, *13*, e0198508. [CrossRef]
293. Chakravarti, A.; Zhai, G.G.; Zhang, M.; Malhotra, R.; Latham, D.E.; Delaney, M.A.; Robe, P.; Nestler, U.; Song, Q.; Loeffler, J. Survivin enhances radiation resistance in primary human glioblastoma cells via caspase-independent mechanisms. *Oncogene* **2004**, *23*, 7494–7506. [CrossRef] [PubMed]
294. Yu, H.; Zhang, S.; Ibrahim, A.N.; Wang, J.; Deng, Z.; Wang, M. RCC2 promotes proliferation and radio-resistance in glioblastoma via activating transcription of DNMT1. *Biochem. Biophys. Res. Commun.* **2019**, *516*, 999–1006. [CrossRef] [PubMed]
295. Han, X.; Xue, X.; Zhou, H.; Zhang, G. A molecular view of the radioresistance of gliomas. *Oncotarget* **2017**, *8*, 100931–100941. [CrossRef] [PubMed]
296. Marampon, F.; Gravina, G.L.; Zani, B.M.; Popov, V.M.; Fratticci, A.; Cerasani, M.; Di Genova, D.; Mancini, M.; Ciccarelli, C.; Ficorella, C.; et al. Hypoxia sustains glioblastoma radioresistance through ERKs/DNA-PKcs/HIF-1alpha functional interplay. *Int. J. Oncol.* **2014**, *44*, 2121–2131. [CrossRef] [PubMed]
297. Marwick, C. Pharmaceutical industry commission, government agencies seek to expedite new addiction therapy. *JAMA* **1991**, *265*, 841. [CrossRef] [PubMed]
298. Kim, S.H.; Ezhilarasan, R.; Phillips, E.; Gallego-Perez, D.; Sparks, A.; Taylor, D.; Ladner, K.; Furuta, T.; Sabit, H.; Chhipa, R.; et al. Serine/Threonine Kinase MLK4 Determines Mesenchymal Identity in Glioma Stem Cells in an NF-kappaB-dependent Manner. *Cancer Cell* **2016**, *29*, 201–213. [CrossRef]
299. Bar, E.E.; Chaudhry, A.; Lin, A.; Fan, X.; Schreck, K.; Matsui, W.; Piccirillo, S.; Vescovi, A.L.; DiMeco, F.; Olivi, A.; et al. Cyclopamine-mediated hedgehog pathway inhibition depletes stem-like cancer cells in glioblastoma. *Stem Cells* **2007**, *25*, 2524–2533. [CrossRef]
300. Zhang, N.; Wei, P.; Gong, A.; Chiu, W.T.; Lee, H.T.; Colman, H.; Huang, H.; Xue, J.; Liu, M.; Wang, Y.; et al. FoxM1 promotes beta-catenin nuclear localization and controls Wnt target-gene expression and glioma tumorigenesis. *Cancer Cell* **2011**, *20*, 427–442. [CrossRef]
301. Burris, H.A., III. Overcoming acquired resistance to anticancer therapy: Focus on the PI3K/AKT/mTOR pathway. *Cancer Chemother. Pharm.* **2013**, *71*, 829–842. [CrossRef]
302. Ashton, C.H.; Rawlins, M.D.; Tyrer, S.P. Buspirone in benzodiazepine withdrawal. *Br. J. Psychiatry* **1991**, *158*, 283–284. [CrossRef]
303. Cao, Y.; Lathia, J.D.; Eyler, C.E.; Wu, Q.; Li, Z.; Wang, H.; McLendon, R.E.; Hjelmeland, A.B.; Rich, J.N. Erythropoietin Receptor Signaling Through STAT3 Is Required for Glioma Stem Cell Maintenance. *Genes Cancer* **2010**, *1*, 50–61. [CrossRef] [PubMed]
304. Ali, M.Y.; Oliva, C.R.; Noman, A.S.M.; Allen, B.G.; Goswami, P.C.; Zakharia, Y.; Monga, V.; Spitz, D.R.; Buatti, J.M.; Griguer, C.E. Radioresistance in Glioblastoma and the Development of Radiosensitizers. *Cancers* **2020**, *12*, 2511. [CrossRef]
305. Farooqi, A.A.; Siddik, Z.H. Platelet-derived growth factor (PDGF) signalling in cancer: Rapidly emerging signalling landscape. *Cell Biochem. Funct.* **2015**, *33*, 257–265. [CrossRef] [PubMed]
306. Godlewski, J.; Nowicki, M.O.; Bronisz, A.; Williams, S.; Otsuki, A.; Nuovo, G.; Raychaudhury, A.; Newton, H.B.; Chiocca, E.A.; Lawler, S. Targeting of the Bmi-1 oncogene/stem cell renewal factor by microRNA-128 inhibits glioma proliferation and self-renewal. *Cancer Res.* **2008**, *68*, 9125–9130. [CrossRef] [PubMed]
307. Koul, D. PTEN signaling pathways in glioblastoma. *Cancer Biol. Ther.* **2008**, *7*, 1321–1325. [CrossRef] [PubMed]
308. Morgenroth, A.; Vogg, A.T.; Ermert, K.; Zlatopolskiy, B.; Mottaghy, F.M. Hedgehog signaling sensitizes glioma stem cells to endogenous nano-irradiation. *Oncotarget* **2014**, *5*, 5483–5493. [CrossRef] [PubMed]

309. Han, N.; Hu, G.; Shi, L.; Long, G.; Yang, L.; Xi, Q.; Guo, Q.; Wang, J.; Dong, Z.; Zhang, M. Notch1 ablation radiosensitizes glioblastoma cells. *Oncotarget* **2017**, *8*, 88059–88068. [CrossRef]
310. Bhat, K.P.L.; Balasubramaniyan, V.; Vaillant, B.; Ezhilarasan, R.; Hummelink, K.; Hollingsworth, F.; Wani, K.; Heathcock, L.; James, J.D.; Goodman, L.D.; et al. Mesenchymal differentiation mediated by NF-kappaB promotes radiation resistance in glioblastoma. *Cancer Cell* **2013**, *24*, 331–346. [CrossRef]
311. Xu, R.X.; Liu, R.Y.; Wu, C.M.; Zhao, Y.S.; Li, Y.; Yao, Y.Q.; Xu, Y.H. DNA damage-induced NF-kappaB activation in human glioblastoma cells promotes miR-181b expression and cell proliferation. *Cell Physiol. Biochem.* **2015**, *35*, 913–925. [CrossRef]
312. Huang, T.T.; Wuerzberger-Davis, S.M.; Seufzer, B.J.; Shumway, S.D.; Kurama, T.; Boothman, D.A.; Miyamoto, S. NF-kappaB activation by camptothecin. A linkage between nuclear DNA damage and cytoplasmic signaling events. *J. Biol. Chem.* **2000**, *275*, 9501–9509. [CrossRef]
313. McCool, K.W.; Miyamoto, S. DNA damage-dependent NF-kappaB activation: NEMO turns nuclear signaling inside out. *Immunol. Rev.* **2012**, *246*, 311–326. [CrossRef] [PubMed]
314. Volcic, M.; Karl, S.; Baumann, B.; Salles, D.; Daniel, P.; Fulda, S.; Wiesmuller, L. NF-kappaB regulates DNA double-strand break repair in conjunction with BRCA1-CtIP complexes. *Nucleic Acids Res.* **2012**, *40*, 181–195. [CrossRef] [PubMed]
315. Wu, K.; Jiang, S.W.; Thangaraju, M.; Wu, G.; Couch, F.J. Induction of the BRCA2 promoter by nuclear factor-kappa B. *J. Biol. Chem.* **2000**, *275*, 35548–35556. [CrossRef] [PubMed]
316. Miyamoto, S. Nuclear initiated NF-kappaB signaling: NEMO and ATM take center stage. *Cell Res.* **2011**, *21*, 116–130. [CrossRef]
317. Wu, J.K.; Ye, Z.; Darras, B.T. Frequency of p53 tumor suppressor gene mutations in human primary brain tumors. *Neurosurgery* **1993**, *33*, 824–830; discussion 821–830. [CrossRef]
318. Chen, P.; Iavarone, A.; Fick, J.; Edwards, M.; Prados, M.; Israel, M.A. Constitutional p53 mutations associated with brain tumors in young adults. *Cancer Genet. Cytogenet.* **1995**, *82*, 106–115. [CrossRef]
319. Shu, H.K.; Kim, M.M.; Chen, P.; Furman, F.; Julin, C.M.; Israel, M.A. The intrinsic radioresistance of glioblastoma-derived cell lines is associated with a failure of p53 to induce p21(BAX) expression. *Proc. Natl. Acad. Sci. USA* **1998**, *95*, 14453–14458. [CrossRef]
320. Jiang, Z.; Pore, N.; Cerniglia, G.J.; Mick, R.; Georgescu, M.M.; Bernhard, E.J.; Hahn, S.M.; Gupta, A.K.; Maity, A. Phosphatase and tensin homologue deficiency in glioblastoma confers resistance to radiation and temozolomide that is reversed by the protease inhibitor nelfinavir. *Cancer Res.* **2007**, *67*, 4467–4473. [CrossRef]
321. Li, L.; Liu, F.; Salmonsen, R.A.; Turner, T.K.; Litofsky, N.S.; Di Cristofano, A.; Pandolfi, P.P.; Jones, S.N.; Recht, L.D.; Ross, A.H. PTEN in neural precursor cells: Regulation of migration, apoptosis, and proliferation. *Mol. Cell Neurosci.* **2002**, *20*, 21–29. [CrossRef]
322. Lomonaco, S.L.; Finniss, S.; Xiang, C.; Decarvalho, A.; Umansky, F.; Kalkanis, S.N.; Mikkelsen, T.; Brodie, C. The induction of autophagy by gamma-radiation contributes to the radioresistance of glioma stem cells. *Int. J. Cancer* **2009**, *125*, 717–722. [CrossRef]
323. Zhuang, W.; Qin, Z.; Liang, Z. The role of autophagy in sensitizing malignant glioma cells to radiation therapy. *Acta Biochim. Biophys. Sin.* **2009**, *41*, 341–351. [CrossRef] [PubMed]
324. Gomez-Casal, R.; Bhattacharya, C.; Ganesh, N.; Bailey, L.; Basse, P.; Gibson, M.; Epperly, M.; Levina, V. Non-small cell lung cancer cells survived ionizing radiation treatment display cancer stem cell and epithelial-mesenchymal transition phenotypes. *Mol. Cancer* **2013**, *12*, 94. [CrossRef] [PubMed]
325. Shien, K.; Toyooka, S.; Ichimura, K.; Soh, J.; Furukawa, M.; Maki, Y.; Muraoka, T.; Tanaka, N.; Ueno, T.; Asano, H.; et al. Prognostic impact of cancer stem cellTransporters in Cancer non-small cell lung cancer patients treated with induction chemoradiotherapy. *Lung Cancer* **2012**, *77*, 162–167. [CrossRef] [PubMed]
326. Zakaria, N.; Yusoff, N.M.; Zakaria, Z.; Lim, M.N.; Baharuddin, P.J.; Fakiruddin, K.S.; Yahaya, B. Human non-small cell lung cancer expresses putative cancer stem cell markers and exhibits the transcriptomic profile of multipotent cells. *BMC Cancer* **2015**, *15*, 84. [CrossRef]
327. Lee, H.J.; Choe, G.; Jheon, S.; Sung, S.W.; Lee, C.T.; Chung, J.H. CD24, a novel cancer biomarker, predicting disease-free survival of non-small cell lung carcinomas: A retrospective study of prognostic factor analysis from the viewpoint of forthcoming (seventh) new TNM classification. *J. Thorac. Oncol.* **2010**, *5*, 649–657. [CrossRef] [PubMed]
328. Karimi-Busheri, F.; Rasouli-Nia, A.; Zadorozhny, V.; Fakhrai, H. CD24+/CD38- as new prognostic marker for non-small cell lung cancer. *Multidiscip. Respir. Med.* **2013**, *8*, 65. [CrossRef]
329. Summer, R.; Kotton, D.N.; Sun, X.; Ma, B.; Fitzsimmons, K.; Fine, A. Side population cells and Bcrp1 expression in lung. *Am. J. Physiol. Lung Cell Mol. Physiol.* **2003**, *285*, L97–L104. [CrossRef]
330. Editors, P.O. Retraction: Identification and Characterization of Cells with Cancer Stem Cell Properties in Human Primary Lung Cancer Cell Lines. *PLoS ONE* **2020**, *15*, e0232726. [CrossRef]
331. Jiang, F.; Qiu, Q.; Khanna, A.; Todd, N.W.; Deepak, J.; Xing, L.; Wang, H.; Liu, Z.; Su, Y.; Stass, S.A.; et al. Aldehyde dehydrogenase 1 is a tumor stem cell-associated marker in lung cancer. *Mol. Cancer Res.* **2009**, *7*, 330–338. [CrossRef]
332. Liang, D.; Shi, Y. Aldehyde dehydrogenase-1 is a specific marker for stem cells in human lung adenocarcinoma. *Med. Oncol.* **2012**, *29*, 633–639. [CrossRef]
333. Kiziltunc Ozmen, H.; Simsek, M. Serum IL-23, E-selectin and sICAM levels in non-small cell lung cancer patients before and after radiotherapy. *J. Int. Med. Res.* **2020**, *48*, 300060520923493. [CrossRef] [PubMed]
334. Li, F.; Zeng, H.; Ying, K. The combination of stem cell markers CD133 and ABCG2 predicts relapse in stage I non-small cell lung carcinomas. *Med. Oncol.* **2011**, *28*, 1458–1462. [CrossRef] [PubMed]

335. Kwa, H.B.; Michalides, R.J.A.M.; Dijkman, J.H.; Mooi, W.J. The prognostic value of NCAM, p53 and cyclin D1 in resected non-small cell lung cancer. *Lung Cancer* **1996**, *14*, 207–217. [CrossRef]
336. Zhang, X.-Y.; Dong, Q.-G.; Huang, J.-S.; Huang, A.-M.; Shi, C.-L.; Jin, B.; Sha, H.-F.; Feng, J.-X.; Geng, Q.; Zhou, J.; et al. The expression of stem cell-related indicators as a prognostic factor in human lung adenocarcinoma. *J. Surg. Oncol.* **2010**, *102*, 856–862. [CrossRef]
337. Shao, W.; Chen, H.; He, J. The role of SOX-2 on the survival of patients with non-small cell lung cancer. *J. Thorac. Dis.* **2015**, *7*, 1113–1118. [CrossRef]
338. Fadous-Khalife, M.C.; Aloulou, N.; Jalbout, M.; Hadchity, J.; Aftimos, G.; Paris, F.; Hadchity, E. Kruppel-like factor 4: A new potential biomarker of lung cancer. *Mol. Clin. Oncol.* **2016**, *5*, 35–40. [CrossRef]
339. Chanvorachote, P.; Sriratanasak, N.; Nonpanya, N. C-myc Contributes to Malignancy of Lung Cancer: A Potential Anticancer Drug Target. *Anticancer Res.* **2020**, *40*, 609–618. [CrossRef]
340. Ma, Y.N.; Zhang, H.Y.; Fei, L.R.; Zhang, M.Y.; Wang, C.C.; Luo, Y.; Han, Y.C. SATB2 suppresses non-small cell lung cancer invasiveness by G9a. *Clin. Exp. Med.* **2018**, *18*, 37–44. [CrossRef]
341. Hsiao, Y.J.; Chang, W.H.; Chen, H.Y.; Hsu, Y.C.; Chiu, S.C.; Chiang, C.C.; Chang, G.C.; Chen, Y.J.; Wang, C.Y.; Chen, Y.M.; et al. MITF functions as a tumor suppressor in non-small cell lung cancer beyond the canonically oncogenic role. *Aging* **2020**, *13*, 646–674. [CrossRef]
342. Harada, D.; Takigawa, N.; Kiura, K. The Role of STAT3 in Non-Small Cell Lung Cancer. *Cancers* **2014**, *6*, 708–722. [CrossRef]
343. Wang, G.; Xiao, L.; Wang, F.; Yang, J.; Yang, L.; Zhao, Y.; Jin, W. Hypoxia inducible factor-1alpha/B-cell lymphoma 2 signaling impacts radiosensitivity of H1299 non-small cell lung cancer cells in a normoxic environment. *Radiat. Environ. Biophys.* **2019**, *58*, 439–448. [CrossRef]
344. Lu, J.; Zhan, Y.; Feng, J.; Luo, J.; Fan, S. MicroRNAs associated with therapy of non-small cell lung cancer. *Int. J. Biol. Sci.* **2018**, *14*, 390–397. [CrossRef] [PubMed]
345. Sone, K.; Maeno, K.; Masaki, A.; Kunii, E.; Takakuwa, O.; Kagawa, Y.; Takeuchi, A.; Fukuda, S.; Uemura, T.; Fukumitsu, K.; et al. Nestin Expression Affects Resistance to Chemotherapy and Clinical Outcome in Small Cell Lung Cancer. *Front. Oncol.* **2020**, *10*, 1367. [CrossRef] [PubMed]
346. Zhang, X.; Tian, T.; Sun, W.; Liu, C.; Fang, X. Bmi-1 overexpression as an efficient prognostic marker in patients with nonsmall cell lung cancer. *Medicine* **2017**, *96*, e7346. [CrossRef] [PubMed]
347. Lang, Y.; Kong, X.; He, C.; Wang, F.; Liu, B.; Zhang, S.; Ning, J.; Zhu, K.; Xu, S. Musashi1 Promotes Non-Small Cell Lung Carcinoma Malignancy and Chemoresistance via Activating the Akt Signaling Pathway. *Cell Physiol. Biochem.* **2017**, *44*, 455–466. [CrossRef] [PubMed]
348. Kumar, M.; Jaiswal, R.K.; Prasad, R.; Yadav, S.S.; Kumar, A.; Yadava, P.K.; Singh, R.P. PARP-1 induces EMT in non-small cell lung carcinoma cells via modulating the transcription factors Smad4, p65 and ZEB1. *Life Sci.* **2021**, *269*, 118994. [CrossRef]
349. Jafarian, A.H.; Kooshki Forooshani, M.; Reisi, H.; Mohamadian Roshan, N. Matrix metalloproteinase-9 (MMP-9) Expression in Non-Small Cell Lung Carcinoma and Its Association with Clinicopathologic Factors. *Iran. J. Pathol.* **2020**, *15*, 326–333. [CrossRef]
350. Merchant, N.; Nagaraju, G.P.; Rajitha, B.; Lammata, S.; Jella, K.K.; Buchwald, Z.S.; Lakka, S.S.; Ali, A.N. Matrix metalloproteinases: Their functional role in lung cancer. *Carcinogenesis* **2017**, *38*, 766–780. [CrossRef]
351. Byers, L.A.; Heymach, J.V. Dual targeting of the vascular endothelial growth factor and epidermal growth factor receptor pathways: Rationale and clinical applications for non-small-cell lung cancer. *Clin. Lung Cancer* **2007**, *8* (Suppl. 2), S79–S85. [CrossRef]
352. Otsuka, S.; Bebb, G. The CXCR4/SDF-1 chemokine receptor axis: A new target therapeutic for non-small cell lung cancer. *J. Thorac. Oncol.* **2008**, *3*, 1379–1383. [CrossRef]
353. Kristiansen, G.; Schluns, K.; Yongwei, Y.; Denkert, C.; Dietel, M.; Petersen, I. CD24 is an independent prognostic marker of survival in nonsmall cell lung cancer patients. *Br. J. Cancer* **2003**, *88*, 231–236. [CrossRef] [PubMed]
354. Hu, B.; Ma, Y.; Yang, Y.; Zhang, L.; Han, H.; Chen, J. CD44 promotes cell proliferation in non-small cell lung cancer. *Oncol. Lett.* **2018**, *15*, 5627–5633. [CrossRef] [PubMed]
355. Tirino, V.; Camerlingo, R.; Franco, R.; Malanga, D.; La Rocca, A.; Viglietto, G.; Rocco, G.; Pirozzi, G. The role of CD133 in the identification and characterisation of tumour-initiating cells in non-small-cell lung cancer. *Eur. J. Cardiothorac. Surg.* **2009**, *36*, 446–453. [CrossRef] [PubMed]
356. Ko, T.Y.; Kim, J.I.; Lee, S.H. Relationship between Cancer Stem Cell Marker CD133 and Cancer Germline Antigen Genes in NCI-H292 Lung Cancer Cells. *Korean J. Thorac. Cardiovasc. Surg.* **2020**, *53*, 22–27. [CrossRef]
357. Kim, W.Y.; Oh, S.H.; Woo, J.K.; Hong, W.K.; Lee, H.Y. Targeting heat shock protein 90 overrides the resistance of lung cancer cells by blocking radiation-induced stabilization of hypoxia-inducible factor-1alpha. *Cancer Res.* **2009**, *69*, 1624–1632. [CrossRef]
358. Akakura, N.; Kobayashi, M.; Horiuchi, I.; Suzuki, A.; Wang, J.; Chen, J.; Niizeki, H.; Kawamura, K.; Hosokawa, M.; Asaka, M. Constitutive expression of hypoxia-inducible factor-1alpha renders pancreatic cancer cells resistant to apoptosis induced by hypoxia and nutrient deprivation. *Cancer Res.* **2001**, *61*, 6548–6554.
359. Kim, J.Y.; Kim, H.J.; Jung, C.W.; Lee, T.S.; Kim, E.H.; Park, M.J. CXCR4 uses STAT3-mediated slug expression to maintain radioresistance of non-small cell lung cancer cells: Emerges as a potential prognostic biomarker for lung cancer. *Cell Death Dis.* **2021**, *12*, 48. [CrossRef]

360. Loriot, Y.; Mordant, P.; Dorvault, N.; De la motte Rouge, T.; Bourhis, J.; Soria, J.C.; Deutsch, E. BMS-690514, a VEGFR and EGFR tyrosine kinase inhibitor, shows anti-tumoural activity on non-small-cell lung cancer xenografts and induces sequence-dependent synergistic effect with radiation. *Br. J. Cancer* **2010**, *103*, 347–353. [CrossRef]
361. Jiang, S.; Wang, R.; Yan, H.; Jin, L.; Dou, X.; Chen, D. MicroRNA-21 modulates radiation resistance through upregulation of hypoxia-inducible factor-1alpha-promoted glycolysis in non-small cell lung cancer cells. *Mol. Med. Rep.* **2016**, *13*, 4101–4107. [CrossRef]
362. Grosso, S.; Doyen, J.; Parks, S.K.; Bertero, T.; Paye, A.; Cardinaud, B.; Gounon, P.; Lacas-Gervais, S.; Noel, A.; Pouyssegur, J.; et al. MiR-210 promotes a hypoxic phenotype and increases radioresistance in human lung cancer cell lines. *Cell Death Dis.* **2013**, *4*, e544. [CrossRef]
363. He, Z.; Liu, Y.; Xiao, B.; Qian, X. miR-25 modulates NSCLC cell radio-sensitivity through directly inhibiting BTG2 expression. *Biochem. Biophys. Res. Commun.* **2015**, *457*, 235–241. [CrossRef] [PubMed]
364. Li, Y.; Han, W.; Ni, T.T.; Lu, L.; Huang, M.; Zhang, Y.; Cao, H.; Zhang, H.Q.; Luo, W.; Li, H. Knockdown of microRNA-1323 restores sensitivity to radiation by suppression of PRKDC activity in radiation-resistant lung cancer cells. *Oncol. Rep.* **2015**, *33*, 2821–2828. [CrossRef] [PubMed]
365. Lee, Y.S.; Oh, J.H.; Yoon, S.; Kwon, M.S.; Song, C.W.; Kim, K.H.; Cho, M.J.; Mollah, M.L.; Je, Y.J.; Kim, Y.D.; et al. Differential gene expression profiles of radioresistant non-small-cell lung cancer cell lines established by fractionated irradiation: Tumor protein p53-inducible protein 3 confers sensitivity to ionizing radiation. *Int. J. Radiat. Oncol. Biol. Phys.* **2010**, *77*, 858–866. [CrossRef] [PubMed]
366. Davidson, B.; Goldberg, I.; Kopolovic, J.; Lerner-Geva, L.; Gotlieb, W.H.; Ben-Baruch, G.; Reich, R. MMP-2 and TIMP-2 expression correlates with poor prognosis in cervical carcinoma–a clinicopathologic study using immunohistochemistry and mRNA in situ hybridization. *Gynecol. Oncol.* **1999**, *73*, 372–382. [CrossRef] [PubMed]
367. Tsutsumi, K.; Tsuda, M.; Yazawa, N.; Nakamura, H.; Ishihara, S.; Haga, H.; Yasuda, M.; Yamazaki, R.; Shirato, H.; Kawaguchi, H.; et al. Increased motility and invasiveness in tumor cells that survive 10 Gy irradiation. *Cell Struct. Funct.* **2009**, *34*, 89–96. [CrossRef] [PubMed]
368. Heo, W.; Lee, Y.S.; Son, C.H.; Yang, K.; Park, Y.S.; Bae, J. Radiation-induced matrix metalloproteinases limit natural killer cell-mediated anticancer immunity in NCI-H23 lung cancer cells. *Mol. Med. Rep.* **2015**, *11*, 1800–1806. [CrossRef]
369. Zhuang, X.; Qiao, T.; Xu, G.; Yuan, S.; Zhang, Q.; Chen, X. Combination of nadroparin with radiotherapy results in powerful synergistic antitumor effects in lung adenocarcinoma A549 cells. *Oncol. Rep.* **2016**, *36*, 2200–2206. [CrossRef]
370. Swinson, D.E.; Jones, J.L.; Cox, G.; Richardson, D.; Harris, A.L.; O'Byrne, K.J. Hypoxia-inducible factor-1 alpha in non small cell lung cancer: Relation to growth factor, protease and apoptosis pathways. *Int. J. Cancer* **2004**, *111*, 43–50. [CrossRef]
371. Hussenet, T.; Dali, S.; Exinger, J.; Monga, B.; Jost, B.; Dembele, D.; Martinet, N.; Thibault, C.; Huelsken, J.; Brambilla, E.; et al. SOX2 is an oncogene activated by recurrent 3q26.3 amplifications in human lung squamous cell carcinomas. *PLoS ONE* **2010**, *5*, e8960. [CrossRef]
372. Bass, A.J.; Watanabe, H.; Mermel, C.H.; Yu, S.; Perner, S.; Verhaak, R.G.; Kim, S.Y.; Wardwell, L.; Tamayo, P.; Gat-Viks, I.; et al. SOX2 is an amplified lineage-survival oncogene in lung and esophageal squamous cell carcinomas. *Nat. Genet.* **2009**, *41*, 1238–1242. [CrossRef]
373. Chowdhury, P.; Dey, P.; Ghosh, S.; Sarma, A.; Ghosh, U. Reduction of metastatic potential by inhibiting EGFR/Akt/p38/ERK signaling pathway and epithelial-mesenchymal transition after carbon ion exposure is potentiated by PARP-1 inhibition in non-small-cell lung cancer. *BMC Cancer* **2019**, *19*, 829. [CrossRef] [PubMed]
374. Guster, J.D.; Weissleder, S.V.; Busch, C.J.; Kriegs, M.; Petersen, C.; Knecht, R.; Dikomey, E.; Rieckmann, T. The inhibition of PARP but not EGFR results in the radiosensitization of HPV/p16-positive HNSCC cell lines. *Radiother. Oncol.* **2014**, *113*, 345–351. [CrossRef] [PubMed]
375. Toulany, M.; Iida, M.; Keinath, S.; Iyi, F.F.; Mueck, K.; Fehrenbacher, B.; Mansour, W.Y.; Schaller, M.; Wheeler, D.L.; Rodemann, H.P. Dual targeting of PI3K and MEK enhances the radiation response of K-RAS mutated non-small cell lung cancer. *Oncotarget* **2016**, *7*, 43746–43761. [CrossRef] [PubMed]
376. Kang, J.; Kim, E.; Kim, W.; Seong, K.M.; Youn, H.; Kim, J.W.; Kim, J.; Youn, B. Rhamnetin and cirsiliol induce radiosensitization and inhibition of epithelial-mesenchymal transition (EMT) by miR-34a-mediated suppression of Notch-1 expression in non-small cell lung cancer cell lines. *J. Biol. Chem.* **2013**, *288*, 27343–27357. [CrossRef] [PubMed]
377. Tian, Y.; Liu, Q.; He, X.; Yuan, X.; Chen, Y.; Chu, Q.; Wu, K. Emerging roles of Nrf2 signal in non-small cell lung cancer. *J. Hematol. Oncol.* **2016**, *9*, 14. [CrossRef] [PubMed]
378. Wu, D.; Li, L.; Yan, W. Knockdown of TC-1 enhances radiosensitivity of non-small cell lung cancer via the Wnt/beta-catenin pathway. *Biol. Open* **2016**, *5*, 492–498. [CrossRef]
379. Zeng, J.; Aziz, K.; Chettiar, S.T.; Aftab, B.T.; Armour, M.; Gajula, R.; Gandhi, N.; Salih, T.; Herman, J.M.; Wong, J.; et al. Hedgehog pathway inhibition radiosensitizes non-small cell lung cancers. *Int. J. Radiat. Oncol. Biol. Phys.* **2013**, *86*, 143–149. [CrossRef]
380. Heavey, S.; O'Byrne, K.J.; Gately, K. Strategies for co-targeting the PI3K/AKT/mTOR pathway in NSCLC. *Cancer Treat. Rev.* **2014**, *40*, 445–456. [CrossRef]
381. Zhang, T.; Cui, G.B.; Zhang, J.; Zhang, F.; Zhou, Y.A.; Jiang, T.; Li, X.F. Inhibition of PI3 kinases enhances the sensitivity of non-small cell lung cancer cells to ionizing radiation. *Oncol. Rep.* **2010**, *24*, 1683–1689. [CrossRef]

382. Zagouras, P.; Stifani, S.; Blaumueller, C.M.; Carcangiu, M.L.; Artavanis-Tsakonas, S. Alterations in Notch signaling in neoplastic lesions of the human cervix. *Proc. Natl. Acad. Sci. USA* **1995**, *92*, 6414–6418. [CrossRef]
383. Grabher, C.; von Boehmer, H.; Look, A.T. Notch 1 activation in the molecular pathogenesis of T-cell acute lymphoblastic leukaemia. *Nat. Rev. Cancer* **2006**, *6*, 347–359. [CrossRef] [PubMed]
384. Theys, J.; Yahyanejad, S.; Habets, R.; Span, P.; Dubois, L.; Paesmans, K.; Kattenbeld, B.; Cleutjens, J.; Groot, A.J.; Schuurbiers, O.C.J.; et al. High NOTCH activity induces radiation resistance in non small cell lung cancer. *Radiother. Oncol.* **2013**, *108*, 440–445. [CrossRef] [PubMed]
385. Zou, B.; Zhou, X.L.; Lai, S.Q.; Liu, J.C. Notch signaling and non-small cell lung cancer. *Oncol. Lett.* **2018**, *15*, 3415–3421. [CrossRef] [PubMed]
386. Eliasz, S.; Liang, S.; Chen, Y.; De Marco, M.A.; Machek, O.; Skucha, S.; Miele, L.; Bocchetta, M. Notch-1 stimulates survival of lung adenocarcinoma cells during hypoxia by activating the IGF-1R pathway. *Oncogene* **2010**, *29*, 2488–2498. [CrossRef]
387. Zhao, Q.; Mao, A.; Yan, J.; Sun, C.; Di, C.; Zhou, X.; Li, H.; Guo, R.; Zhang, H. Downregulation of Nrf2 promotes radiation-induced apoptosis through Nrf2 mediated Notch signaling in non-small cell lung cancer cells. *Int. J. Oncol.* **2016**, *48*, 765–773. [CrossRef]
388. Chen, Y.H.; Pan, S.L.; Wang, J.C.; Kuo, S.H.; Cheng, J.C.; Teng, C.M. Radiation-induced VEGF-C expression and endothelial cell proliferation in lung cancer. *Strahlenther. Onkol.* **2014**, *190*, 1154–1162. [CrossRef]
389. Jiang, L.; Huang, J.; Hu, Y.; Lu, P.; Luo, Q.; Wang, L. Gli promotes tumor progression through regulating epithelial-mesenchymal transition in non-small-cell lung cancer. *J. Cardiothorac. Surg.* **2020**, *15*, 18. [CrossRef]
390. Garcia Campelo, M.R.; Alonso Curbera, G.; Aparicio Gallego, G.; Grande Pulido, E.; Anton Aparicio, L.M. Stem cell and lung cancer development: Blaming the Wnt, Hh and Notch signalling pathway. *Clin. Transl. Oncol.* **2011**, *13*, 77–83. [CrossRef]
391. Pustovalova, M.; Alhaddad, L.; Blokhina, T.; Smetanina, N.; Chigasova, A.; Chuprov-Netochin, R.; Eremin, P.; Gilmutdinova, I.; Osipov, A.N.; Leonov, S. The CD44high Subpopulation of Multifraction Irradiation-Surviving NSCLC Cells Exhibits Partial EMT-Program Activation and DNA Damage Response Depending on Their p53 Status. *Int. J. Mol. Sci.* **2021**, *22*, 2369. [CrossRef]
392. Cao, Z.; Livas, T.; Kyprianou, N. Anoikis and EMT: Lethal "Liaisons" during Cancer Progression. *Crit. Rev. Oncog.* **2016**, *21*, 155–168. [CrossRef]
393. Thiery, J.P.; Acloque, H.; Huang, R.Y.; Nieto, M.A. Epithelial-mesenchymal transitions in development and disease. *Cell* **2009**, *139*, 871–890. [CrossRef] [PubMed]
394. Lah, T.T.; Novak, M.; Breznik, B. Brain malignancies: Glioblastoma and brain metastases. *Semin. Cancer Biol.* **2020**, *60*, 262–273. [CrossRef] [PubMed]
395. Mittal, V. Epithelial Mesenchymal Transition in Tumor Metastasis. *Annu. Rev. Pathol.* **2018**, *13*, 395–412. [CrossRef] [PubMed]
396. Das, R.; Gregory, P.A.; Hollier, B.G.; Tilley, W.D.; Selth, L.A. Epithelial plasticity in prostate cancer: Principles and clinical perspectives. *Trends Mol. Med.* **2014**, *20*, 643–651. [CrossRef]
397. Ansieau, S.; Bastid, J.; Doreau, A.; Morel, A.P.; Bouchet, B.P.; Thomas, C.; Fauvet, F.; Puisieux, I.; Doglioni, C.; Piccinin, S.; et al. Induction of EMT by twist proteins as a collateral effect of tumor-promoting inactivation of premature senescence. *Cancer Cell* **2008**, *14*, 79–89. [CrossRef]
398. Odero-Marah, V.; Hawsawi, O.; Henderson, V.; Sweeney, J. Epithelial-Mesenchymal Transition (EMT) and Prostate Cancer. *Adv. Exp. Med. Biol.* **2018**, *1095*, 101–110. [CrossRef]
399. Radisky, E.S.; Radisky, D.C. Matrix metalloproteinase-induced epithelial-mesenchymal transition in breast cancer. *J. Mammary Gland Biol. Neoplasia* **2010**, *15*, 201–212. [CrossRef]
400. Lu, W.; Kang, Y. Epithelial-Mesenchymal Plasticity in Cancer Progression and Metastasis. *Dev. Cell* **2019**, *49*, 361–374. [CrossRef]
401. Jolly, M.K.; Mani, S.A.; Levine, H. Hybrid epithelial/mesenchymal phenotype(s): The 'fittest' for metastasis? *Biochim. Biophys. Acta Rev. Cancer* **2018**, *1870*, 151–157. [CrossRef]
402. Gonzalez, D.M.; Medici, D. Signaling mechanisms of the epithelial-mesenchymal transition. *Sci. Signal.* **2014**, *7*, re8. [CrossRef]
403. Huber, M.A.; Kraut, N.; Beug, H. Molecular requirements for epithelial-mesenchymal transition during tumor progression. *Curr. Opin. Cell Biol.* **2005**, *17*, 548–558. [CrossRef] [PubMed]
404. Peinado, H.; Olmeda, D.; Cano, A. Snail, Zeb and bHLH factors in tumour progression: An alliance against the epithelial phenotype? *Nat. Rev. Cancer* **2007**, *7*, 415–428. [CrossRef] [PubMed]
405. Kuner, R.; Muley, T.; Meister, M.; Ruschhaupt, M.; Buness, A.; Xu, E.C.; Schnabel, P.; Warth, A.; Poustka, A.; Sultmann, H.; et al. Global gene expression analysis reveals specific patterns of cell junctions in non-small cell lung cancer subtypes. *Lung Cancer* **2009**, *63*, 32–38. [CrossRef] [PubMed]
406. Pierdomenico, M.; Palone, F.; Cesi, V.; Vitali, R.; Mancuso, A.B.; Cucchiara, S.; Oliva, S.; Aloi, M.; Stronati, L. Transcription Factor ZNF281: A Novel Player in Intestinal Inflammation and Fibrosis. *Front. Immunol.* **2018**, *9*, 2907. [CrossRef]
407. De Craene, B.; Berx, G. Regulatory networks defining EMT during cancer initiation and progression. *Nat. Rev. Cancer* **2013**, *13*, 97–110. [CrossRef]
408. Boelens, M.C.; van den Berg, A.; Vogelzang, I.; Wesseling, J.; Postma, D.S.; Timens, W.; Groen, H.J. Differential expression and distribution of epithelial adhesion molecules in non-small cell lung cancer and normal bronchus. *J. Clin. Pathol.* **2007**, *60*, 608–614. [CrossRef]
409. Scheel, C.; Weinberg, R.A. Cancer stem cells and epithelial-mesenchymal transition: Concepts and molecular links. *Semin. Cancer Biol.* **2012**, *22*, 396–403. [CrossRef]

410. Kawamoto, A.; Yokoe, T.; Tanaka, K.; Saigusa, S.; Toiyama, Y.; Yasuda, H.; Inoue, Y.; Miki, C.; Kusunoki, M. Radiation induces epithelial-mesenchymal transition in colorectal cancer cells. *Oncol. Rep.* **2012**, *27*, 51–57. [CrossRef]
411. Andarawewa, K.L.; Erickson, A.C.; Chou, W.S.; Costes, S.V.; Gascard, P.; Mott, J.D.; Bissell, M.J.; Barcellos-Hoff, M.H. Ionizing radiation predisposes nonmalignant human mammary epithelial cells to undergo transforming growth factor beta induced epithelial to mesenchymal transition. *Cancer Res.* **2007**, *67*, 8662–8670. [CrossRef]
412. Zhang, Y.E. Non-Smad pathways in TGF-beta signaling. *Cell Res.* **2009**, *19*, 128–139. [CrossRef]
413. Xu, J.; Lamouille, S.; Derynck, R. TGF-beta-induced epithelial to mesenchymal transition. *Cell Res.* **2009**, *19*, 156–172. [CrossRef] [PubMed]
414. Jin, W. Role of JAK/STAT3 Signaling in the Regulation of Metastasis, the Transition of Cancer Stem Cells, and Chemoresistance of Cancer by Epithelial-Mesenchymal Transition. *Cells* **2020**, *9*, 217. [CrossRef] [PubMed]
415. Smit, M.A.; Peeper, D.S. Epithelial-mesenchymal transition and senescence: Two cancer-related processes are crossing paths. *Aging* **2010**, *2*, 735–741. [CrossRef] [PubMed]
416. Scheel, C.; Eaton, E.N.; Li, S.H.; Chaffer, C.L.; Reinhardt, F.; Kah, K.J.; Bell, G.; Guo, W.; Rubin, J.; Richardson, A.L.; et al. Paracrine and autocrine signals induce and maintain mesenchymal and stem cell states in the breast. *Cell* **2011**, *145*, 926–940. [CrossRef]
417. Chang, L.; Graham, P.H.; Hao, J.; Bucci, J.; Cozzi, P.J.; Kearsley, J.H.; Li, Y. Emerging roles of radioresistance in prostate cancer metastasis and radiation therapy. *Cancer Metastasis Rev.* **2014**, *33*, 469–496. [CrossRef]
418. Marie-Egyptienne, D.T.; Lohse, I.; Hill, R.P. Cancer stem cells, the epithelial to mesenchymal transition (EMT) and radioresistance: Potential role of hypoxia. *Cancer Lett.* **2013**, *341*, 63–72. [CrossRef]
419. Yao, Y.H.; Cui, Y.; Qiu, X.N.; Zhang, L.Z.; Zhang, W.; Li, H.; Yu, J.M. Attenuated LKB1-SIK1 signaling promotes epithelial-mesenchymal transition and radioresistance of non-small cell lung cancer cells. *Chin. J. Cancer* **2016**, *35*, 50. [CrossRef]
420. Heddleston, J.M.; Li, Z.; McLendon, R.E.; Hjelmeland, A.B.; Rich, J.N. The hypoxic microenvironment maintains glioblastoma stem cells and promotes reprogramming towards a cancer stem cell phenotype. *Cell Cycle* **2009**, *8*, 3274–3284. [CrossRef]
421. Salnikov, A.V.; Liu, L.; Platen, M.; Gladkich, J.; Salnikova, O.; Ryschich, E.; Mattern, J.; Moldenhauer, G.; Werner, J.; Schemmer, P.; et al. Hypoxia induces EMT in low and highly aggressive pancreatic tumor cells but only cells with cancer stem cell characteristics acquire pronounced migratory potential. *PLoS ONE* **2012**, *7*, e46391. [CrossRef]
422. Brabletz, S.; Brabletz, T. The ZEB/miR-200 feedback loop—a motor of cellular plasticity in development and cancer? *EMBO Rep.* **2010**, *11*, 670–677. [CrossRef]
423. Tripathi, S.C.; Peters, H.L.; Taguchi, A.; Katayama, H.; Wang, H.; Momin, A.; Jolly, M.K.; Celiktas, M.; Rodriguez-Canales, J.; Liu, H.; et al. Immunoproteasome deficiency is a feature of non-small cell lung cancer with a mesenchymal phenotype and is associated with a poor outcome. *Proc. Natl. Acad. Sci. USA* **2016**, *113*, E1555–E1564. [CrossRef] [PubMed]
424. Chen, L.; Gibbons, D.L.; Goswami, S.; Cortez, M.A.; Ahn, Y.H.; Byers, L.A.; Zhang, X.; Yi, X.; Dwyer, D.; Lin, W.; et al. Metastasis is regulated via microRNA-200/ZEB1 axis control of tumour cell PD-L1 expression and intratumoral immunosuppression. *Nat. Commun.* **2014**, *5*, 5241. [CrossRef] [PubMed]
425. Creighton, C.J.; Chang, J.C.; Rosen, J.M. Epithelial-mesenchymal transition (EMT) in tumor-initiating cells and its clinical implications in breast cancer. *J. Mammary Gland Biol. Neoplasia* **2010**, *15*, 253–260. [CrossRef] [PubMed]
426. Vega, S.; Morales, A.V.; Ocana, O.H.; Valdes, F.; Fabregat, I.; Nieto, M.A. Snail blocks the cell cycle and confers resistance to cell death. *Genes Dev.* **2004**, *18*, 1131–1143. [CrossRef] [PubMed]
427. Comaills, V.; Kabeche, L.; Morris, R.; Buisson, R.; Yu, M.; Madden, M.W.; LiCausi, J.A.; Boukhali, M.; Tajima, K.; Pan, S.; et al. Genomic Instability Is Induced by Persistent Proliferation of Cells Undergoing Epithelial-to-Mesenchymal Transition. *Cell Rep.* **2016**, *17*, 2632–2647. [CrossRef]
428. Liu, M.; Quek, L.E.; Sultani, G.; Turner, N. Epithelial-mesenchymal transition induction is associated with augmented glucose uptake and lactate production in pancreatic ductal adenocarcinoma. *Cancer Metab.* **2016**, *4*, 19. [CrossRef]
429. Cha, Y.H.; Yook, J.I.; Kim, H.S.; Kim, N.H. Catabolic metabolism during cancer EMT. *Arch. Pharm. Res.* **2015**, *38*, 313–320. [CrossRef]
430. Chamberlain, M.C. Radiographic patterns of relapse in glioblastoma. *J. Neurooncol.* **2011**, *101*, 319–323. [CrossRef]
431. Bremnes, R.M.; Al-Shibli, K.; Donnem, T.; Sirera, R.; Al-Saad, S.; Andersen, S.; Stenvold, H.; Camps, C.; Busund, L.T. The role of tumor-infiltrating immune cells and chronic inflammation at the tumor site on cancer development, progression, and prognosis: Emphasis on non-small cell lung cancer. *J. Thorac. Oncol.* **2011**, *6*, 824–833. [CrossRef]
432. Lee, S.Y.; Jeong, E.K.; Ju, M.K.; Jeon, H.M.; Kim, M.Y.; Kim, C.H.; Park, H.G.; Han, S.I.; Kang, H.S. Induction of metastasis, cancer stem cell phenotype, and oncogenic metabolism in cancer cells by ionizing radiation. *Mol. Cancer* **2017**, *16*, 10. [CrossRef]
433. Cho, J.H.; Hong, W.G.; Jung, Y.J.; Lee, J.; Lee, E.; Hwang, S.G.; Um, H.D.; Park, J.K. Gamma-Ionizing radiation-induced activation of the EGFR-p38/ERK-STAT3/CREB-1-EMT pathway promotes the migration/invasion of non-small cell lung cancer cells and is inhibited by podophyllotoxin acetate. *Tumour Biol.* **2016**, *37*, 7315–7325. [CrossRef] [PubMed]
434. Thiery, J.P. Epithelial-mesenchymal transitions in tumour progression. *Nat. Rev. Cancer* **2002**, *2*, 442–454. [CrossRef] [PubMed]
435. Guarino, M.; Rubino, B.; Ballabio, G. The role of epithelial-mesenchymal transition in cancer pathology. *Pathology* **2007**, *39*, 305–318. [CrossRef] [PubMed]
436. Wild-Bode, C.; Weller, M.; Rimner, A.; Dichgans, J.; Wick, W. Sublethal irradiation promotes migration and invasiveness of glioma cells: Implications for radiotherapy of human glioblastoma. *Cancer Res.* **2001**, *61*, 2744–2750. [PubMed]

437. Bensimon, J.; Altmeyer-Morel, S.; Benjelloun, H.; Chevillard, S.; Lebeau, J. CD24(-/low) stem-like breast cancer marker defines the radiation-resistant cells involved in memorization and transmission of radiation-induced genomic instability. *Oncogene* **2013**, *32*, 251–258. [CrossRef] [PubMed]
438. Lin, J.C.; Tsai, J.T.; Chao, T.Y.; Ma, H.I.; Liu, W.H. The STAT3/Slug Axis Enhances Radiation-Induced Tumor Invasion and Cancer Stem-like Properties in Radioresistant Glioblastoma. *Cancers* **2018**, *10*, 512. [CrossRef] [PubMed]
439. Shintani, Y.; Okimura, A.; Sato, K.; Nakagiri, T.; Kadota, Y.; Inoue, M.; Sawabata, N.; Minami, M.; Ikeda, N.; Kawahara, K.; et al. Epithelial to mesenchymal transition is a determinant of sensitivity to chemoradiotherapy in non-small cell lung cancer. *Ann. Thorac. Surg.* **2011**, *92*, 1794–1804; discussion 1804. [CrossRef]
440. Kim, E.; Youn, H.; Kwon, T.; Son, B.; Kang, J.; Yang, H.J.; Seong, K.M.; Kim, W.; Youn, B. PAK1 tyrosine phosphorylation is required to induce epithelial-mesenchymal transition and radioresistance in lung cancer cells. *Cancer Res.* **2014**, *74*, 5520–5531. [CrossRef]
441. Alhaddad, L.; Pustovalova, M.; Blokhina, T.; Chuprov-Netochin, R.; Osipov, A.N.; Leonov, S. IR-Surviving NSCLC Cells Exhibit Different Patterns of Molecular and Cellular Reactions Relating to the Multifraction Irradiation Regimen and p53-Family Proteins Expression. *Cancers* **2021**, *13*, 2669. [CrossRef]
442. Saleh, T.; Carpenter, V.J.; Bloukh, S.; Gewirtz, D.A. Targeting tumor cell senescence and polyploidy as potential therapeutic strategies. *Semin. Cancer Biol.* **2022**, *81*, 37–47. [CrossRef]
443. Zhang, J.; Si, J.; Gan, L.; Di, C.; Xie, Y.; Sun, C.; Li, H.; Guo, M.; Zhang, H. Research progress on therapeutic targeting of quiescent cancer cells. *Artif. Cells Nanomed. Biotechnol.* **2019**, *47*, 2810–2820. [CrossRef] [PubMed]
444. Ewald, J.A.; Desotelle, J.A.; Wilding, G.; Jarrard, D.F. Therapy-induced senescence in cancer. *J. Natl. Cancer Inst.* **2010**, *102*, 1536–1546. [CrossRef] [PubMed]
445. Aguirre-Ghiso, J.A. Models, mechanisms and clinical evidence for cancer dormancy. *Nat. Rev. Cancer* **2007**, *7*, 834–846. [CrossRef] [PubMed]
446. Triana-Martinez, F.; Loza, M.I.; Dominguez, E. Beyond Tumor Suppression: Senescence in Cancer Stemness and Tumor Dormancy. *Cells* **2020**, *9*, 346. [CrossRef] [PubMed]
447. Rao, S.G.; Jackson, J.G. SASP: Tumor Suppressor or Promoter? Yes! *Trends Cancer* **2016**, *2*, 676–687. [CrossRef]
448. Sharpless, N.E.; Sherr, C.J. Forging a signature of in vivo senescence. *Nat. Rev. Cancer* **2015**, *15*, 397–408. [CrossRef]
449. Santos-de-Frutos, K.; Djouder, N. When dormancy fuels tumour relapse. *Commun. Biol.* **2021**, *4*, 747. [CrossRef]
450. Edelstein, J.E. Prosthetic feet. State of the Art. *Phys. Ther.* **1988**, *68*, 1874–1881. [CrossRef]
451. Crea, F.; Nur Saidy, N.R.; Collins, C.C.; Wang, Y. The epigenetic/noncoding origin of tumor dormancy. *Trends Mol. Med.* **2015**, *21*, 206–211. [CrossRef]
452. Meacham, C.E.; Morrison, S.J. Tumour heterogeneity and cancer cell plasticity. *Nature* **2013**, *501*, 328–337. [CrossRef]
453. Mohammad, K.; Dakik, P.; Medkour, Y.; Mitrofanova, D.; Titorenko, V.I. Quiescence Entry, Maintenance, and Exit in Adult Stem Cells. *Int. J. Mol. Sci.* **2019**, *20*, 2158. [CrossRef] [PubMed]
454. Coller, H.A.; Sang, L.; Roberts, J.M. A new description of cellular quiescence. *PLoS Biol.* **2006**, *4*, e83. [CrossRef] [PubMed]
455. Krenning, L.; van den Berg, J.; Medema, R.H. Life or Death after a Break: What Determines the Choice? *Mol. Cell* **2019**, *76*, 346–358. [CrossRef] [PubMed]
456. Shaltiel, I.A.; Krenning, L.; Bruinsma, W.; Medema, R.H. The same, only different—DNA damage checkpoints and their reversal throughout the cell cycle. *J. Cell Sci.* **2015**, *128*, 607–620. [CrossRef] [PubMed]
457. Puig, I.; Tenbaum, S.P.; Chicote, I.; Arques, O.; Martinez-Quintanilla, J.; Cuesta-Borras, E.; Ramirez, L.; Gonzalo, P.; Soto, A.; Aguilar, S.; et al. TET2 controls chemoresistant slow-cycling cancer cell survival and tumor recurrence. *J. Clin. Investig.* **2018**, *128*, 3887–3905. [CrossRef]
458. Wolter, K.; Zender, L. Therapy-induced senescence—An induced synthetic lethality in liver cancer? *Nat. Rev. Gastroenterol. Hepatol.* **2020**, *17*, 135–136. [CrossRef]
459. Masunaga, S.; Sakurai, Y.; Tanaka, H.; Hirayama, R.; Matsumoto, Y.; Uzawa, A.; Suzuki, M.; Kondo, N.; Narabayashi, M.; Maruhashi, A.; et al. Radiosensitivity of pimonidazole-unlabelled intratumour quiescent cell population to gamma-rays, accelerated carbon ion beams and boron neutron capture reaction. *Br. J. Radiol.* **2013**, *86*, 20120302. [CrossRef]
460. Miller, I.; Min, M.; Yang, C.; Tian, C.; Gookin, S.; Carter, D.; Spencer, S.L. Ki67 is a Graded Rather than a Binary Marker of Proliferation versus Quiescence. *Cell Rep.* **2018**, *24*, 1105–1112. [CrossRef]
461. Zeniou, M.; Feve, M.; Mameri, S.; Dong, J.; Salome, C.; Chen, W.; El-Habr, E.A.; Bousson, F.; Sy, M.; Obszynski, J.; et al. Chemical Library Screening and Structure-Function Relationship Studies Identify Bisacodyl as a Potent and Selective Cytotoxic Agent Towards Quiescent Human Glioblastoma Tumor Stem-Like Cells. *PLoS ONE* **2015**, *10*, e0134793. [CrossRef]
462. Yao, M.; Xie, C.; Kiang, M.Y.; Teng, Y.; Harman, D.; Tiffen, J.; Wang, Q.; Sved, P.; Bao, S.; Witting, P.; et al. Targeting of cytosolic phospholipase A2alpha impedes cell cycle re-entry of quiescent prostate cancer cells. *Oncotarget* **2015**, *6*, 34458–34474. [CrossRef]
463. Kwon, J.S.; Everetts, N.J.; Wang, X.; Wang, W.; Della Croce, K.; Xing, J.; Yao, G. Controlling Depth of Cellular Quiescence by an Rb-E2F Network Switch. *Cell Rep.* **2017**, *20*, 3223–3235. [CrossRef] [PubMed]
464. Pei, H.; Guo, Z.; Wang, Z.; Dai, Y.; Zheng, L.; Zhu, L.; Zhang, J.; Hu, W.; Nie, J.; Mao, W.; et al. RAC2 promotes abnormal proliferation of quiescent cells by enhanced JUNB expression via the MAL-SRF pathway. *Cell Cycle* **2018**, *17*, 1115–1123. [CrossRef] [PubMed]

465. Chitikova, Z.V.; Gordeev, S.A.; Bykova, T.V.; Zubova, S.G.; Pospelov, V.A.; Pospelova, T.V. Sustained activation of DNA damage response in irradiated apoptosis-resistant cells induces reversible senescence associated with mTOR downregulation and expression of stem cell markers. *Cell Cycle* **2014**, *13*, 1424–1439. [CrossRef] [PubMed]
466. Collado, M.; Gil, J.; Efeyan, A.; Guerra, C.; Schuhmacher, A.J.; Barradas, M.; Benguría, A.; Zaballos, A.; Flores, J.M.; Barbacid, M.; et al. Senescence in premalignant tumours. *Nature* **2005**, *436*, 642. [CrossRef] [PubMed]
467. He, G.; Dhar, D.; Nakagawa, H.; Font-Burgada, J.; Ogata, H.; Jiang, Y.; Shalapour, S.; Seki, E.; Yost, S.E.; Jepsen, K.; et al. Identification of Liver Cancer Progenitors Whose Malignant Progression Depends on Autocrine IL-6 Signaling. *Cell* **2013**, *155*, 384–396. [CrossRef]
468. Joselow, A.; Lynn, D.; Terzian, T.; Box, N.F. Senescence-Like Phenotypes in Human Nevi. *Methods Mol. Biol.* **2017**, *1534*, 175–184.
469. Haugstetter, A.M.; Loddenkemper, C.; Lenze, D.; Gröne, J.; Standfuß, C.; Petersen, I.; Dörken, B.; Schmitt, C.A. Cellular senescence predicts treatment outcome in metastasised colorectal cancer. *Br. J. Cancer* **2010**, *103*, 505–509. [CrossRef]
470. Kahlem, P.; Dörken, B.; Schmitt, C.A. Cellular senescence in cancer treatment: Friend or foe? *J. Clin. Investig.* **2004**, *113*, 169–174. [CrossRef]
471. Schmitt, C.A.; Fridman, J.S.; Yang, M.; Lee, S.; Baranov, E.; Hoffman, R.M.; Lowe, S.W. A Senescence Program Controlled by p53 and p16INK4a Contributes to the Outcome of Cancer Therapy. *Cell* **2002**, *109*, 335–346. [CrossRef]
472. Serrano, M.; Lin, A.W.; McCurrach, M.E.; Beach, D.; Lowe, S.W. Oncogenic ras provokes premature cell senescence associated with accumulation of p53 and p16INK4a. *Cell* **1997**, *88*, 593–602. [CrossRef]
473. Mikula-Pietrasik, J.; Niklas, A.; Uruski, P.; Tykarski, A.; Ksiazek, K. Mechanisms and significance of therapy-induced and spontaneous senescence of cancer cells. *Cell Mol. Life Sci.* **2020**, *77*, 213–229. [CrossRef] [PubMed]
474. Razmik Mirzayans, D.M. Role of Therapy-Induced Cellular Senescence in Tumor Cells and its Modification in Radiotherapy: The Good, The Bad and The Ugly. *J. Nucl. Med. Radiat. Ther.* **2013**, *s6*. [CrossRef]
475. Lee, B.Y.; Han, J.A.; Im, J.S.; Morrone, A.; Johung, K.; Goodwin, E.C.; Kleijer, W.J.; DiMaio, D.; Hwang, E.S. Senescence-associated β-galactosidase is lysosomal β-galactosidase. *Aging Cell* **2006**, *5*, 187–195. [CrossRef] [PubMed]
476. Ogrodnik, M.; Miwa, S.; Tchkonia, T.; Tiniakos, D.; Wilson, C.L.; Lahat, A.; Day, C.P.; Burt, A.; Palmer, A.; Anstee, Q.M.; et al. Cellular senescence drives age-dependent hepatic steatosis. *Nat. Commun.* **2017**, *8*, 15691. [CrossRef] [PubMed]
477. Kaushik, S.; Cuervo, A.M. Proteostasis and aging. *Nat. Med.* **2015**, *21*, 1406–1415. [CrossRef] [PubMed]
478. Hernandez-Segura, A.; de Jong, T.V.; Melov, S.; Guryev, V.; Campisi, J.; Demaria, M. Unmasking Transcriptional Heterogeneity in Senescent Cells. *Curr. Biol.* **2017**, *27*, 2652–2660.e2654. [CrossRef]
479. Suzuki, K.; Boothman, D.A. Stress-induced Premature Senescence (SIPS). *J. Radiat. Res.* **2008**, *49*, 105–112. [CrossRef]
480. Saleh, T.; Tyutyunyk-Massey, L.; Cudjoe, E.K.; Idowu, M.O.; Landry, J.W.; Gewirtz, D.A. Non-Cell Autonomous Effects of the Senescence-Associated Secretory Phenotype in Cancer Therapy. *Front. Oncol.* **2018**, *8*, 164. [CrossRef]
481. Antonangeli, F.; Soriani, A.; Ricci, B.; Ponzetta, A.; Benigni, G.; Morrone, S.; Bernardini, G.; Santoni, A. Natural killer cell recognition of in vivo drug-induced senescent multiple myeloma cells. *OncoImmunology* **2016**, *5*, e1218105. [CrossRef]
482. Coppé, J.-P.; Desprez, P.-Y.; Krtolica, A.; Campisi, J. The Senescence-Associated Secretory Phenotype: The Dark Side of Tumor Suppression. *Annu. Rev. Pathol. Mech. Dis.* **2010**, *5*, 99–118. [CrossRef]
483. Hansel, C.; Jendrossek, V.; Klein, D. Cellular Senescence in the Lung: The Central Role of Senescent Epithelial Cells. *Int. J. Mol. Sci.* **2020**, *21*, 3279. [CrossRef]
484. Coppe, J.P.; Patil, C.K.; Rodier, F.; Sun, Y.; Munoz, D.P.; Goldstein, J.; Nelson, P.S.; Desprez, P.Y.; Campisi, J. Senescence-associated secretory phenotypes reveal cell-nonautonomous functions of oncogenic RAS and the p53 tumor suppressor. *PLoS Biol.* **2008**, *6*, 2853–2868. [CrossRef] [PubMed]
485. Passos, J.F.; Nelson, G.; Wang, C.; Richter, T.; Simillion, C.; Proctor, C.J.; Miwa, S.; Olijslagers, S.; Hallinan, J.; Wipat, A.; et al. Feedback between p21 and reactive oxygen production is necessary for cell senescence. *Mol. Syst. Biol.* **2010**, *6*, 347. [CrossRef] [PubMed]
486. Wiley, C.D.; Velarde, M.C.; Lecot, P.; Liu, S.; Sarnoski, E.A.; Freund, A.; Shirakawa, K.; Lim, H.W.; Davis, S.S.; Ramanathan, A.; et al. Mitochondrial Dysfunction Induces Senescence with a Distinct Secretory Phenotype. *Cell Metab.* **2016**, *23*, 303–314. [CrossRef]
487. Chang, B.D.; Broude, E.V.; Dokmanovic, M.; Zhu, H.; Ruth, A.; Xuan, Y.; Kandel, E.S.; Lausch, E.; Christov, K.; Roninson, I.B. A senescence-like phenotype distinguishes tumor cells that undergo terminal proliferation arrest after exposure to anticancer agents. *Cancer Res.* **1999**, *59*, 3761–3767.
488. Dimri, G.P.; Lee, X.; Basile, G.; Acosta, M.; Scott, G.; Roskelley, C.; Medrano, E.E.; Linskens, M.; Rubelj, I.; Pereira-Smith, O.; et al. A biomarker that identifies senescent human cells in culture and in aging skin in vivo. *Proc. Natl. Acad. Sci. USA* **1995**, *92*, 9363–9367. [CrossRef]
489. Campisi, J. Cellular senescence as a tumor-suppressor mechanism. *Trends Cell Biol.* **2001**, *11*, S27–S31. [CrossRef]
490. Chien, Y.; Scuoppo, C.; Wang, X.; Fang, X.; Balgley, B.; Bolden, J.E.; Premsrirut, P.; Luo, W.; Chicas, A.; Lee, C.S.; et al. Control of the senescence-associated secretory phenotype by NF-kappaB promotes senescence and enhances chemosensitivity. *Genes Dev.* **2011**, *25*, 2125–2136. [CrossRef]
491. Aird, K.M.; Zhang, R. Detection of senescence-associated heterochromatin foci (SAHF). *Methods Mol. Biol.* **2013**, *965*, 185–196. [CrossRef]

492. Ksiazek, K.; Korybalska, K.; Jorres, A.; Witowski, J. Accelerated senescence of human peritoneal mesothelial cells exposed to high glucose: The role of TGF-beta1. *Lab. Investig.* **2007**, *87*, 345–356. [CrossRef]
493. Krouwer, V.J.; Hekking, L.H.; Langelaar-Makkinje, M.; Regan-Klapisz, E.; Post, J.A. Endothelial cell senescence is associated with disrupted cell-cell junctions and increased monolayer permeability. *Vasc. Cell* **2012**, *4*, 12. [CrossRef] [PubMed]
494. Statuto, M.; Bianchi, C.; Perego, R.; Del Monte, U. Drop of connexin 43 in replicative senescence of human fibroblasts HEL-299 as a possible biomarker of senescence. *Exp. Gerontol.* **2002**, *37*, 1113–1120. [CrossRef]
495. Wang, Q.; Wu, P.C.; Dong, D.Z.; Ivanova, I.; Chu, E.; Zeliadt, S.; Vesselle, H.; Wu, D.Y. Polyploidy road to therapy-induced cellular senescence and escape. *Int. J. Cancer* **2013**, *132*, 1505–1515. [CrossRef]
496. Saleh, T.; Tyutyunyk-Massey, L.; Murray, G.F.; Alotaibi, M.R.; Kawale, A.S.; Elsayed, Z.; Henderson, S.C.; Yakovlev, V.; Elmore, L.W.; Toor, A.; et al. Tumor cell escape from therapy-induced senescence. *Biochem. Pharm.* **2019**, *162*, 202–212. [CrossRef] [PubMed]
497. Yang, L.; Fang, J.; Chen, J. Tumor cell senescence response produces aggressive variants. *Cell Death Discov.* **2017**, *3*, 17049. [CrossRef] [PubMed]
498. Ghorai, A.; Mahaddalkar, T.; Thorat, R.; Dutt, S. Sustained inhibition of PARP-1 activity delays glioblastoma recurrence by enhancing radiation-induced senescence. *Cancer Lett.* **2020**, *490*, 44–53. [CrossRef]
499. Cahu, J.; Bustany, S.; Sola, B. Senescence-associated secretory phenotype favors the emergence of cancer stem-like cells. *Cell Death Dis.* **2012**, *3*, e446. [CrossRef]
500. Ye, C.; Zhang, X.; Wan, J.; Chang, L.; Hu, W.; Bing, Z.; Zhang, S.; Li, J.; He, J.; Wang, J.; et al. Radiation-induced cellular senescence results from a slippage of long-term G2 arrested cells into G1 phase. *Cell Cycle* **2013**, *12*, 1424–1432. [CrossRef]
501. He, J.; Li, J.; Ye, C.; Zhou, L.; Zhu, J.; Wang, J.; Mizota, A.; Furusawa, Y.; Zhou, G. Cell cycle suspension: A novel process lurking in G(2) arrest. *Cell Cycle* **2011**, *10*, 1468–1476. [CrossRef]
502. Sugrue, M.M.; Shin, D.Y.; Lee, S.W.; Aaronson, S.A. Wild-type p53 triggers a rapid senescence program in human tumor cells lacking functional p53. *Proc. Natl. Acad. Sci. USA* **1997**, *94*, 9648–9653. [CrossRef]
503. Calio, A.; Zamo, A.; Ponzoni, M.; Zanolin, M.E.; Ferreri, A.J.; Pedron, S.; Montagna, L.; Parolini, C.; Fraifeld, V.E.; Wolfson, M.; et al. Cellular Senescence Markers p16INK4a and p21CIP1/WAF Are Predictors of Hodgkin Lymphoma Outcome. *Clin. Cancer Res.* **2015**, *21*, 5164–5172. [CrossRef] [PubMed]
504. Gorgoulis, V.; Adams, P.D.; Alimonti, A.; Bennett, D.C.; Bischof, O.; Bishop, C.; Campisi, J.; Collado, M.; Evangelou, K.; Ferbeyre, G.; et al. Cellular Senescence: Defining a Path Forward. *Cell* **2019**, *179*, 813–827. [CrossRef] [PubMed]
505. Evangelou, K.; Lougiakis, N.; Rizou, S.V.; Kotsinas, A.; Kletsas, D.; Munoz-Espin, D.; Kastrinakis, N.G.; Pouli, N.; Marakos, P.; Townsend, P.; et al. Robust, universal biomarker assay to detect senescent cells in biological specimens. *Aging Cell* **2017**, *16*, 192–197. [CrossRef] [PubMed]
506. Liao, E.C.; Hsu, Y.T.; Chuah, Q.Y.; Lee, Y.J.; Hu, J.Y.; Huang, T.C.; Yang, P.M.; Chiu, S.J. Radiation induces senescence and a bystander effect through metabolic alterations. *Cell Death Dis.* **2014**, *5*, e1255. [CrossRef]
507. Roninson, I.B. Tumor cell senescence in cancer treatment. *Cancer Res.* **2003**, *63*, 2705–2715.
508. Jeon, H.Y.; Kim, J.K.; Ham, S.W.; Oh, S.Y.; Kim, J.; Park, J.B.; Lee, J.Y.; Kim, S.C.; Kim, H. Irradiation induces glioblastoma cell senescence and senescence-associated secretory phenotype. *Tumour Biol.* **2016**, *37*, 5857–5867. [CrossRef]
509. Quick, Q.A.; Gewirtz, D.A. An accelerated senescence response to radiation in wild-type p53 glioblastoma multiforme cells. *J. Neurosurg.* **2006**, *105*, 111–118. [CrossRef]
510. Luo, H.; Yount, C.; Lang, H.; Yang, A.; Riemer, E.C.; Lyons, K.; Vanek, K.N.; Silvestri, G.A.; Schulte, B.A.; Wang, G.Y. Activation of p53 with Nutlin-3a radiosensitizes lung cancer cells via enhancing radiation-induced premature senescence. *Lung Cancer* **2013**, *81*, 167–173. [CrossRef]
511. Jones, K.R.; Elmore, L.W.; Jackson-Cook, C.; Demasters, G.; Povirk, L.F.; Holt, S.E.; Gewirtz, D.A. p53-Dependent accelerated senescence induced by ionizing radiation in breast tumour cells. *Int. J. Radiat. Biol.* **2005**, *81*, 445–458. [CrossRef]
512. Roberson, R.S.; Kussick, S.J.; Vallieres, E.; Chen, S.Y.; Wu, D.Y. Escape from therapy-induced accelerated cellular senescence in p53-null lung cancer cells and in human lung cancers. *Cancer Res.* **2005**, *65*, 2795–2803. [CrossRef]
513. Wang, Q.; Wu, P.C.; Roberson, R.S.; Luk, B.V.; Ivanova, I.; Chu, E.; Wu, D.Y. Survivin and escaping in therapy-induced cellular senescence. *Int. J. Cancer* **2011**, *128*, 1546–1558. [CrossRef] [PubMed]
514. Azad, A.; Bukczynska, P.; Jackson, S.; Haupt, Y.; Cullinane, C.; McArthur, G.A.; Solomon, B. Co-targeting deoxyribonucleic acid-dependent protein kinase and poly(adenosine diphosphate-ribose) polymerase-1 promotes accelerated senescence of irradiated cancer cells. *Int. J. Radiat. Oncol. Biol. Phys.* **2014**, *88*, 385–394. [CrossRef] [PubMed]
515. Williams, B.R.; Amon, A. Aneuploidy: Cancer's fatal flaw? *Cancer Res.* **2009**, *69*, 5289–5291. [CrossRef] [PubMed]
516. Sudo, T.; Nitta, M.; Saya, H.; Ueno, N.T. Dependence of paclitaxel sensitivity on a functional spindle assembly checkpoint. *Cancer Res.* **2004**, *64*, 2502–2508. [CrossRef]
517. Jordan, M.A.; Wilson, L. Microtubules as a target for anticancer drugs. *Nat. Rev. Cancer* **2004**, *4*, 253–265. [CrossRef]
518. Zhang, Z.; Feng, X.; Deng, Z.; Cheng, J.; Wang, Y.; Zhao, M.; Zhao, Y.; He, S.; Huang, Q. Irradiation-induced polyploid giant cancer cells are involved in tumor cell repopulation via neosis. *Mol. Oncol.* **2021**, *15*, 2219–2234. [CrossRef]
519. Rand, C.W.; Courville, C.B. Multinucleation of cortical nerve cells at the margins of traumatic lesions of the human brain. *J. Neuropathol. Exp. Neurol.* **1947**, *6*, 1–14. [CrossRef]
520. Liu, J. The dualistic origin of human tumors. *Semin. Cancer Biol.* **2018**, *53*, 1–16. [CrossRef]

521. Barok, M.; Tanner, M.; Koninki, K.; Isola, J. Trastuzumab-DM1 causes tumour growth inhibition by mitotic catastrophe in trastuzumab-resistant breast cancer cells in vivo. *Breast Cancer Res.* **2011**, *13*, R46. [CrossRef]
522. Lin, K.C.; Torga, G.; Sun, Y.; Axelrod, R.; Pienta, K.J.; Sturm, J.C.; Austin, R.H. The role of heterogeneous environment and docetaxel gradient in the emergence of polyploid, mesenchymal and resistant prostate cancer cells. *Clin. Exp. Metastasis* **2019**, *36*, 97–108. [CrossRef]
523. Ogden, A.; Rida, P.C.; Knudsen, B.S.; Kucuk, O.; Aneja, R. Docetaxel-induced polyploidization may underlie chemoresistance and disease relapse. *Cancer Lett.* **2015**, *367*, 89–92. [CrossRef] [PubMed]
524. Zhang, S.; Zhang, D.; Yang, Z.; Zhang, X. Tumor Budding, Micropapillary Pattern, and Polyploidy Giant Cancer Cells in Colorectal Cancer: Current Status and Future Prospects. *Stem Cells Int.* **2016**, *2016*, 4810734. [CrossRef] [PubMed]
525. Fei, F.; Zhang, M.; Li, B.; Zhao, L.; Wang, H.; Liu, L.; Li, Y.; Ding, P.; Gu, Y.; Zhang, X.; et al. Formation of Polyploid Giant Cancer Cells Involves in the Prognostic Value of Neoadjuvant Chemoradiation in Locally Advanced Rectal Cancer. *J. Oncol.* **2019**, *2019*, 2316436. [CrossRef] [PubMed]
526. Zhang, S.; Mercado-Uribe, I.; Xing, Z.; Sun, B.; Kuang, J.; Liu, J. Generation of cancer stem-like cells through the formation of polyploid giant cancer cells. *Oncogene* **2014**, *33*, 116–128. [CrossRef]
527. Fujiwara, T.; Bandi, M.; Nitta, M.; Ivanova, E.V.; Bronson, R.T.; Pellman, D. Cytokinesis failure generating tetraploids promotes tumorigenesis in p53-null cells. *Nature* **2005**, *437*, 1043–1047. [CrossRef]
528. Revesz, L.; Norman, U. Chromosome ploidy and radiosensitivity of tumours. *Nature* **1960**, *187*, 861–862. [CrossRef]
529. Castedo, M.; Coquelle, A.; Vitale, I.; Vivet, S.; Mouhamad, S.; Viaud, S.; Zitvogel, L.; Kroemer, G. Selective resistance of tetraploid cancer cells against DNA damage-induced apoptosis. *Ann. N. Y. Acad. Sci.* **2006**, *1090*, 35–49. [CrossRef]
530. Ianzini, F.; Kosmacek, E.A.; Nelson, E.S.; Napoli, E.; Erenpreisa, J.; Kalejs, M.; Mackey, M.A. Activation of meiosis-specific genes is associated with depolyploidization of human tumor cells following radiation-induced mitotic catastrophe. *Cancer Res.* **2009**, *69*, 2296–2304. [CrossRef]
531. Prieur-Carrillo, G.; Chu, K.; Lindqvist, J.; Dewey, W.C. Computerized video time-lapse (CVTL) analysis of the fate of giant cells produced by X-irradiating EJ30 human bladder carcinoma cells. *Radiat Res.* **2003**, *159*, 705–712. [CrossRef]
532. Ianzini, F.; Mackey, M.A. Development of the large scale digital cell analysis system. *Radiat. Prot. Dosim.* **2002**, *99*, 289–293. [CrossRef]
533. Erenpreisa, J.A.; Cragg, M.S.; Fringes, B.; Sharakhov, I.; Illidge, T.M. Release of mitotic descendants by giant cells from irradiated Burkitt's lymphoma cell line. *Cell Biol. Int.* **2000**, *24*, 635–648. [CrossRef] [PubMed]
534. Horbay, R.; Stoika, R. Giant cell formation: The way to cell death or cell survival? *Open Life Sci.* **2011**, *6*, 675–684. [CrossRef]
535. Sliwinska, M.A.; Mosieniak, G.; Wolanin, K.; Babik, A.; Piwocka, K.; Magalska, A.; Szczepanowska, J.; Fronk, J.; Sikora, E. Induction of senescence with doxorubicin leads to increased genomic instability of HCT116 cells. *Mech. Ageing Dev.* **2009**, *130*, 24–32. [CrossRef]
536. Niu, N.; Mercado-Uribe, I.; Liu, J. Dedifferentiation into blastomere-like cancer stem cells via formation of polyploid giant cancer cells. *Oncogene* **2017**, *36*, 4887–4900. [CrossRef] [PubMed]
537. Erenpreisa, J.; Salmina, K.; Huna, A.; Jackson, T.R.; Vazquez-Martin, A.; Cragg, M.S. The "virgin birth", polyploidy, and the origin of cancer. *Oncoscience* **2015**, *2*, 3–14. [CrossRef]
538. Zhang, D.; Yang, X.; Yang, Z.; Fei, F.; Li, S.; Qu, J.; Zhang, M.; Li, Y.; Zhang, X.; Zhang, S. Daughter Cells and Erythroid Cells Budding from PGCCs and Their Clinicopathological Significances in Colorectal Cancer. *J. Cancer* **2017**, *8*, 469–478. [CrossRef]
539. Hosaka, M.; Hatori, M.; Smith, R.; Kokubun, S. Giant cell formation through fusion of cells derived from a human giant cell tumor of tendon sheath. *J. Orthop. Sci.* **2004**, *9*, 581–584. [CrossRef]
540. Brodbeck, W.G.; Anderson, J.M. Giant cell formation and function. *Curr. Opin. Hematol.* **2009**, *16*, 53–57. [CrossRef]
541. Holland, A.J.; Cleveland, D.W. Boveri revisited: Chromosomal instability, aneuploidy and tumorigenesis. *Nat. Rev. Mol. Cell Biol.* **2009**, *10*, 478–487. [CrossRef]
542. Krajcovic, M.; Overholtzer, M. Mechanisms of ploidy increase in human cancers: A new role for cell cannibalism. *Cancer Res.* **2012**, *72*, 1596–1601. [CrossRef]
543. Erenpreisa, J.; Cragg, M.S. Three steps to the immortality of cancer cells: Senescence, polyploidy and self-renewal. *Cancer Cell Int.* **2013**, *13*, 92. [CrossRef] [PubMed]
544. Beermann, W. Control of Differentiation at the Chromosomal Level. *J. Exp. Zool.* **1964**, *157*, 49–62. [CrossRef] [PubMed]
545. Erenpreisa, J.; Cragg, M.S.; Anisimov, A.P.; Illidge, T.M. Tumor cell embryonality and the ploidy number 32n: Is it a developmental checkpoint? *Cell Cycle* **2011**, *10*, 1873–1874. [CrossRef] [PubMed]
546. Vakifahmetoglu, H.; Olsson, M.; Zhivotovsky, B. Death through a tragedy: Mitotic catastrophe. *Cell Death Differ.* **2008**, *15*, 1153–1162. [CrossRef]
547. Kaur, E.; Rajendra, J.; Jadhav, S.; Shridhar, E.; Goda, J.S.; Moiyadi, A.; Dutt, S. Radiation-induced homotypic cell fusions of innately resistant glioblastoma cells mediate their sustained survival and recurrence. *Carcinogenesis* **2015**, *36*, 685–695. [CrossRef]
548. Sundaram, M.; Guernsey, D.L.; Rajaraman, M.M.; Rajaraman, R. Neosis: A novel type of cell division in cancer. *Cancer Biol. Ther.* **2004**, *3*, 207–218. [CrossRef]
549. Erenpreisa, J.; Cragg, M.S. Mitotic death: A mechanism of survival? A review. *Cancer Cell Int.* **2001**, *1*, 1. [CrossRef]
550. Niu, N.; Zhang, J.; Zhang, N.; Mercado-Uribe, I.; Tao, F.; Han, Z.; Pathak, S.; Multani, A.S.; Kuang, J.; Yao, J.; et al. Linking genomic reorganization to tumor initiation via the giant cell cycle. *Oncogenesis* **2016**, *5*, e281. [CrossRef]

551. Erenpreisa, J.; Ivanov, A.; Wheatley, S.P.; Kosmacek, E.A.; Ianzini, F.; Anisimov, A.P.; Mackey, M.; Davis, P.J.; Plakhins, G.; Illidge, T.M. Endopolyploidy in irradiated p53-deficient tumour cell lines: Persistence of cell division activity in giant cells expressing Aurora-B kinase. *Cell Biol. Int.* **2008**, *32*, 1044–1056. [CrossRef]
552. Erenpreisa, J.; Cragg, M.S.; Salmina, K.; Hausmann, M.; Scherthan, H. The role of meiotic cohesin REC8 in chromosome segregation in gamma irradiation-induced endopolyploid tumour cells. *Exp. Cell Res.* **2009**, *315*, 2593–2603. [CrossRef]
553. Vitale, I.; Senovilla, L.; Jemaa, M.; Michaud, M.; Galluzzi, L.; Kepp, O.; Nanty, L.; Criollo, A.; Rello-Varona, S.; Manic, G.; et al. Multipolar mitosis of tetraploid cells: Inhibition by p53 and dependency on Mos. *EMBO J.* **2010**, *29*, 1272–1284. [CrossRef] [PubMed]
554. Rajaraman, R.; Guernsey, D.L.; Rajaraman, M.M.; Rajaraman, S.R. Stem cells, senescence, neosis and self-renewal in cancer. *Cancer Cell Int.* **2006**, *6*, 25. [CrossRef] [PubMed]
555. Rajaraman, R.; Rajaraman, M.M.; Rajaraman, S.R.; Guernsey, D.L. Neosis–a paradigm of self-renewal in cancer. *Cell Biol. Int.* **2005**, *29*, 1084–1097. [CrossRef] [PubMed]
556. White-Gilbertson, S.; Voelkel-Johnson, C. Giants and monsters: Unexpected characters in the story of cancer recurrence. *Adv. Cancer Res.* **2020**, *148*, 201–232. [CrossRef]
557. Diaz-Carballo, D.; Saka, S.; Klein, J.; Rennkamp, T.; Acikelli, A.H.; Malak, S.; Jastrow, H.; Wennemuth, G.; Tempfer, C.; Schmitz, I.; et al. A Distinct Oncogenerative Multinucleated Cancer Cell Serves as a Source of Stemness and Tumor Heterogeneity. *Cancer Res.* **2018**, *78*, 2318–2331. [CrossRef] [PubMed]
558. Puck, T.T.; Marcus, P.I. Action of x-rays on mammalian cells. *J. Exp. Med.* **1956**, *103*, 653–666. [CrossRef] [PubMed]
559. Liang, B.C.; Thornton, A.F., Jr.; Sandler, H.M.; Greenberg, H.S. Malignant astrocytomas: Focal tumor recurrence after focal external beam radiation therapy. *J. Neurosurg.* **1991**, *75*, 559–563. [CrossRef]
560. Sneed, P.K.; Gutin, P.H.; Larson, D.A.; Malec, M.K.; Phillips, T.L.; Prados, M.D.; Scharfen, C.O.; Weaver, K.A.; Wara, W.M. Patterns of recurrence of glioblastoma multiforme after external irradiation followed by implant boost. *Int. J. Radiat. Oncol. Biol. Phys.* **1994**, *29*, 719–727. [CrossRef]
561. Sitarz, R.; Leguit, R.J.; de Leng, W.W.; Morsink, F.H.; Polkowski, W.P.; Maciejewski, R.; Offerhaus, G.J.; Milne, A.N. Cyclooxygenase-2 mediated regulation of E-cadherin occurs in conventional but not early-onset gastric cancer cell lines. *Cell Oncol.* **2009**, *31*, 475–485. [CrossRef]
562. Hoskin, D.W.; Mader, J.S.; Furlong, S.J.; Conrad, D.M.; Blay, J. Inhibition of T cell and natural killer cell function by adenosine and its contribution to immune evasion by tumor cells (Review). *Int. J. Oncol.* **2008**, *32*, 527–535. [CrossRef]
563. Malik, S.T.; Griffin, D.B.; Fiers, W.; Balkwill, F.R. Paradoxical effects of tumour necrosis factor in experimental ovarian cancer. *Int. J. Cancer* **1989**, *44*, 918–925. [CrossRef]
564. Sa, G.; Das, T.; Moon, C.; Hilston, C.M.; Rayman, P.A.; Rini, B.I.; Tannenbaum, C.S.; Finke, J.H. GD3, an overexpressed tumor-derived ganglioside, mediates the apoptosis of activated but not resting T cells. *Cancer Res.* **2009**, *69*, 3095–3104. [CrossRef] [PubMed]
565. Toutirais, O.; Chartier, P.; Dubois, D.; Bouet, F.; Leveque, J.; Catros-Quemener, V.; Genetet, N. Constitutive expression of TGF-beta1, interleukin-6 and interleukin-8 by tumor cells as a major component of immune escape in human ovarian carcinoma. *Eur. Cytokine Netw.* **2003**, *14*, 246–255. [PubMed]
566. Inoue, K.; Slaton, J.W.; Kim, S.J.; Perrotte, P.; Eve, B.Y.; Bar-Eli, M.; Radinsky, R.; Dinney, C.P. Interleukin 8 expression regulates tumorigenicity and metastasis in human bladder cancer. *Cancer Res.* **2000**, *60*, 2290–2299. [CrossRef] [PubMed]
567. Doubrovina, E.S.; Doubrovin, M.M.; Vider, E.; Sisson, R.B.; O'Reilly, R.J.; Dupont, B.; Vyas, Y.M. Evasion from NK cell immunity by MHC class I chain-related molecules expressing colon adenocarcinoma. *J. Immunol.* **2003**, *171*, 6891–6899. [CrossRef] [PubMed]
568. Mannino, M.; Chalmers, A.J. Radioresistance of glioma stem cells: Intrinsic characteristic or property of the 'microenvironment-stem cell unit'? *Mol. Oncol.* **2011**, *5*, 374–386. [CrossRef]
569. Gabrilovich, D.; Ishida, T.; Oyama, T.; Ran, S.; Kravtsov, V.; Nadaf, S.; Carbone, D.P. Vascular endothelial growth factor inhibits the development of dendritic cells and dramatically affects the differentiation of multiple hematopoietic lineages in vivo. *Blood* **1998**, *92*, 4150–4166. [CrossRef]
570. Whiteside, T.L.; Vujanovic, N.L.; Herberman, R.B. Natural killer cells and tumor therapy. *Curr. Top. Microbiol. Immunol.* **1998**, *230*, 221–244. [CrossRef]
571. Vivier, E.; Tomasello, E.; Baratin, M.; Walzer, T.; Ugolini, S. Functions of natural killer cells. *Nat. Immunol.* **2008**, *9*, 503–510. [CrossRef]
572. Kaufman, H.L.; Wolchok, J.D. *General Principles of Tumor Immunotherapy*; Springer: Berlin/Heidelberg, Germany, 2007.
573. Baay, M.; Brouwer, A.; Pauwels, P.; Peeters, M.; Lardon, F. Tumor cells and tumor-associated macrophages: Secreted proteins as potential targets for therapy. *Clin. Dev. Immunol.* **2011**, *2011*, 565187. [CrossRef]
574. Tong, H.; Ke, J.Q.; Jiang, F.Z.; Wang, X.J.; Wang, F.Y.; Li, Y.R.; Lu, W.; Wan, X.P. Tumor-associated macrophage-derived CXCL8 could induce ERalpha suppression via HOXB13 in endometrial cancer. *Cancer Lett.* **2016**, *376*, 127–136. [CrossRef] [PubMed]
575. Augello, A.; Tasso, R.; Negrini, S.M.; Amateis, A.; Indiveri, F.; Cancedda, R.; Pennesi, G. Bone marrow mesenchymal progenitor cells inhibit lymphocyte proliferation by activation of the programmed death 1 pathway. *Eur. J. Immunol.* **2005**, *35*, 1482–1490. [CrossRef] [PubMed]

576. Di Nicola, M.; Carlo-Stella, C.; Magni, M.; Milanesi, M.; Longoni, P.D.; Matteucci, P.; Grisanti, S.; Gianni, A.M. Human bone marrow stromal cells suppress T-lymphocyte proliferation induced by cellular or nonspecific mitogenic stimuli. *Blood* **2002**, *99*, 3838–3843. [CrossRef] [PubMed]
577. Whiteside, T.L. The tumor microenvironment and its role in promoting tumor growth. *Oncogene* **2008**, *27*, 5904–5912. [CrossRef]
578. Caires, H.R.; Barros da Silva, P.; Barbosa, M.A.; Almeida, C.R. A co-culture system with three different primary human cell populations reveals that biomaterials and MSC modulate macrophage-driven fibroblast recruitment. *J. Tissue Eng. Regen. Med.* **2018**, *12*, e1433–e1440. [CrossRef]
579. Almand, B.; Clark, J.I.; Nikitina, E.; van Beynen, J.; English, N.R.; Knight, S.C.; Carbone, D.P.; Gabrilovich, D.I. Increased production of immature myeloid cells in cancer patients: A mechanism of immunosuppression in cancer. *J. Immunol.* **2001**, *166*, 678–689. [CrossRef]
580. Leonard, W.; Dufait, I.; Schwarze, J.K.; Law, K.; Engels, B.; Jiang, H.; Van den Berge, D.; Gevaert, T.; Storme, G.; Verovski, V.; et al. Myeloid-derived suppressor cells reveal radioprotective properties through arginase-induced l-arginine depletion. *Radiother. Oncol.* **2016**, *119*, 291–299. [CrossRef]
581. Ochoa, A.C.; Zea, A.H.; Hernandez, C.; Rodriguez, P.C. Arginase, prostaglandins, and myeloid-derived suppressor cells in renal cell carcinoma. *Clin. Cancer Res.* **2007**, *13*, 721s–726s. [CrossRef]
582. Serafini, P.; Borrello, I.; Bronte, V. Myeloid suppressor cells in cancer: Recruitment, phenotype, properties, and mechanisms of immune suppression. *Semin. Cancer Biol.* **2006**, *16*, 53–65. [CrossRef]
583. Munn, D.H.; Mellor, A.L. Indoleamine 2,3-dioxygenase and tumor-induced tolerance. *J. Clin. Investig.* **2007**, *117*, 1147–1154. [CrossRef]
584. Loukinova, E.; Dong, G.; Enamorado-Ayalya, I.; Thomas, G.R.; Chen, Z.; Schreiber, H.; Van Waes, C. Growth regulated oncogene-alpha expression by murine squamous cell carcinoma promotes tumor growth, metastasis, leukocyte infiltration and angiogenesis by a host CXC receptor-2 dependent mechanism. *Oncogene* **2000**, *19*, 3477–3486. [CrossRef] [PubMed]
585. Sakaguchi, S.; Miyara, M.; Costantino, C.M.; Hafler, D.A. FOXP3+ regulatory T cells in the human immune system. *Nat. Rev. Immunol.* **2010**, *10*, 490–500. [CrossRef] [PubMed]
586. Bergmann, C.; Strauss, L.; Zeidler, R.; Lang, S.; Whiteside, T.L. Expansion of human T regulatory type 1 cells in the microenvironment of cyclooxygenase 2 overexpressing head and neck squamous cell carcinoma. *Cancer Res.* **2007**, *67*, 8865–8873. [CrossRef] [PubMed]
587. Colombo, M.P.; Piconese, S. Regulatory-T-cell inhibition versus depletion: The right choice in cancer immunotherapy. *Nat. Rev. Cancer* **2007**, *7*, 880–887. [CrossRef] [PubMed]
588. Arden, K.C. FOXO animal models reveal a variety of diverse roles for FOXO transcription factors. *Oncogene* **2008**, *27*, 2345–2350. [CrossRef]
589. Li, C.; Jiang, P.; Wei, S.; Xu, X.; Wang, J. Regulatory T cells in tumor microenvironment: New mechanisms, potential therapeutic strategies and future prospects. *Mol. Cancer* **2020**, *19*, 116. [CrossRef]
590. Kochetkova, I.; Golden, S.; Holderness, K.; Callis, G.; Pascual, D.W. IL-35 stimulation of CD39+ regulatory T cells confers protection against collagen II-induced arthritis via the production of IL-10. *J. Immunol.* **2010**, *184*, 7144–7153. [CrossRef]
591. Kitahata, Y.; Shinkai, M.; Kido, T. Guidance and nursing of a patient with acute myocardial infarction and senile dementia: A case study. *Kango Gijutsu* **1988**, *34*, 1052–1056.
592. Ihara, F.; Sakurai, D.; Takami, M.; Kamata, T.; Kunii, N.; Yamasaki, K.; Iinuma, T.; Nakayama, T.; Motohashi, S.; Okamoto, Y. Regulatory T cells induce CD4(-) NKT cell anergy and suppress NKT cell cytotoxic function. *Cancer Immunol. Immunother.* **2019**, *68*, 1935–1947. [CrossRef]
593. Spolski, R.; Li, P.; Leonard, W.J. Biology and regulation of IL-2: From molecular mechanisms to human therapy. *Nat. Rev. Immunol.* **2018**, *18*, 648–659. [CrossRef]
594. Ohta, A.; Kini, R.; Ohta, A.; Subramanian, M.; Madasu, M.; Sitkovsky, M. The development and immunosuppressive functions of CD4(+) CD25(+) FoxP3(+) regulatory T cells are under influence of the adenosine-A2A adenosine receptor pathway. *Front. Immunol.* **2012**, *3*, 190. [CrossRef] [PubMed]
595. Raimondi, G.; Turner, M.S.; Thomson, A.W.; Morel, P.A. Naturally occurring regulatory T cells: Recent insights in health and disease. *Crit. Rev. Immunol.* **2007**, *27*, 61–95. [CrossRef] [PubMed]
596. Roncarolo, M.G.; Gregori, S.; Battaglia, M.; Bacchetta, R.; Fleischhauer, K.; Levings, M.K. Interleukin-10-secreting type 1 regulatory T cells in rodents and humans. *Immunol. Rev.* **2006**, *212*, 28–50. [CrossRef] [PubMed]
597. Baratelli, F.; Lin, Y.; Zhu, L.; Yang, S.C.; Heuze-Vourc'h, N.; Zeng, G.; Reckamp, K.; Dohadwala, M.; Sharma, S.; Dubinett, S.M. Prostaglandin E2 induces FOXP3 gene expression and T regulatory cell function in human CD4+ T cells. *J. Immunol.* **2005**, *175*, 1483–1490. [CrossRef] [PubMed]
598. Brown, N.F.; Carter, T.J.; Ottaviani, D.; Mulholland, P. Harnessing the immune system in glioblastoma. *Br. J. Cancer* **2018**, *119*, 1171–1181. [CrossRef]
599. Abedalthagafi, M.; Barakeh, D.; Foshay, K.M. Immunogenetics of glioblastoma: The future of personalized patient management. *NPJ Precis. Oncol.* **2018**, *2*, 27. [CrossRef] [PubMed]
600. Liang, J.; Piao, Y.; Holmes, L.; Fuller, G.N.; Henry, V.; Tiao, N.; de Groot, J.F. Neutrophils promote the malignant glioma phenotype through S100A4. *Clin. Cancer Res.* **2014**, *20*, 187–198. [CrossRef]

601. Calabrese, C.; Poppleton, H.; Kocak, M.; Hogg, T.L.; Fuller, C.; Hamner, B.; Oh, E.Y.; Gaber, M.W.; Finklestein, D.; Allen, M.; et al. A perivascular niche for brain tumor stem cells. *Cancer Cell* **2007**, *11*, 69–82. [CrossRef]
602. Cui, Y.H.; Suh, Y.; Lee, H.J.; Yoo, K.C.; Uddin, N.; Jeong, Y.J.; Lee, J.S.; Hwang, S.G.; Nam, S.Y.; Kim, M.J.; et al. Radiation promotes invasiveness of non-small-cell lung cancer cells through granulocyte-colony-stimulating factor. *Oncogene* **2015**, *34*, 5372–5382. [CrossRef]

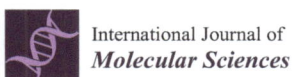

Article

Radiation-Induced Bystander Effect Mediated by Exosomes Involves the Replication Stress in Recipient Cells

Mateusz Smolarz [1], Łukasz Skoczylas [1], Marta Gawin [1], Monika Krzyżowska [1], Monika Pietrowska [1,*] and Piotr Widłak [2,*]

[1] Maria Skłodowska-Curie National Research Institute of Oncology, 44-102 Gliwice, Poland; mateusz.smolarz@io.gliwice.pl (M.S.); lukasz.skoczylas@io.gliwice.pl (Ł.S.); marta.gawin@io.gliwice.pl (M.G.); monikaxx41@interia.pl (M.K.)
[2] Clinical Research Support Centre, Medical University of Gdańsk, 80-210 Gdańsk, Poland
* Correspondence: monika.pietrowska@io.gliwice.pl (M.P.); piotr.widlak@gumed.edu.pl (P.W.); Tel.: +48-32-278-9627 (M.P.); +48-58-349-2767 (P.W.)

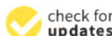

Citation: Smolarz, M.; Skoczylas, Ł.; Gawin, M.; Krzyżowska, M.; Pietrowska, M.; Widłak, P. Radiation-Induced Bystander Effect Mediated by Exosomes Involves the Replication Stress in Recipient Cells. *Int. J. Mol. Sci.* **2022**, *23*, 4169. https://doi.org/10.3390/ijms23084169

Academic Editor: François Chevalier

Received: 8 March 2022
Accepted: 7 April 2022
Published: 10 April 2022

Publisher's Note: MDPI stays neutral with regard to jurisdictional claims in published maps and institutional affiliations.

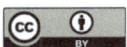

Copyright: © 2022 by the authors. Licensee MDPI, Basel, Switzerland. This article is an open access article distributed under the terms and conditions of the Creative Commons Attribution (CC BY) license (https:// creativecommons.org/licenses/by/ 4.0/).

Abstract: Exosomes released by irradiated cells mediate the radiation-induced bystander effect, which is manifested by DNA breaks detected in recipient cells; yet, the specific mechanism responsible for the generation of chromosome lesions remains unclear. In this study, naive FaDu head and neck cancer cells were stimulated with exosomes released by irradiated (a single 2 Gy dose) or mock-irradiated cells. Maximum accumulation of gamma H2A.X foci, a marker of DNA breaks, was detected after one hour of stimulation with exosomes from irradiated donors, the level of which was comparable to the one observed in directly irradiated cells (a weaker wave of the gamma H2A.X foci accumulation was also noted after 23 h of stimulation). Exosomes from irradiated cells, but not from control ones, activated two stress-induced protein kinases: ATM and ATR. Noteworthy is that while direct irradiation activated only ATM, both ATM and ATR were activated by two factors known to induce the replication stress: hydroxyurea and camptothecin (with subsequent phosphorylation of gamma H2A.X). One hour of stimulation with exosomes from irradiated cells suppressed DNA synthesis in recipient cells and resulted in the subsequent nuclear accumulation of RNA:DNA hybrids, which is an indicator of impaired replication. Interestingly, the abovementioned effects were observed before a substantial internalization of exosomes, which may suggest a receptor-mediated mechanism. It was observed that after one hour of stimulation with exosomes from irradiated donors, phosphorylation of several nuclear proteins, including replication factors and regulators of heterochromatin remodeling as well as components of multiple intracellular signaling pathways increased. Hence, we concluded that the bystander effect mediated by exosomes released from irradiated cells involves the replication stress in recipient cells.

Keywords: bystander effect; exosomes; ionizing radiation; non-targeted effects of radiation; replication stress

1. Introduction

The radiation-induced bystander effect (RIBE) is a phenomenon in which non-irradiated cells exhibit several molecular and cellular features typical for a response to ionizing radiation. Such effects, which include changes in gene and protein expression, proliferation, genetic instability, and cell death, are the results of different signals received from nearby (or distant) directly irradiated cells. Clastogenic effects, including DNA strand breaks, chromosome aberrations, and mutations, are the most characteristic features of RIBE. Therefore, it is postulated that local irradiation (e.g., during radiotherapy) may cause systemic cytotoxic and genotoxic damages outside of the radiation field and can even lead to carcinogenic effects beyond the therapy field. Although there is no generally accepted direct evidence yet, it has been suggested that RIBE (and other potential "non-targeted" effects of radiation) may putatively interfere with the results of radiation therapy [1–3]. There are several different classes of signals involved in the RIBE. Many "soluble" factors released by irradiated cells to the cell culture media were proposed, including cytokines, chemokines, and other inflammation mediators, as well as reactive oxygen species (ROS), nitric oxide (NO), and different miRNA species [4–6]. More recently, extracellular vesicles have also been implicated in this signaling mechanism.

All types of cells released into the extracellular environment different membrane-enclosed vesicles (i.e., extracellular vesicles (EVs)), which appear as key mediators of intercellular communication. Exosomes are the smallest EVs (30–150 nm), which derive from the inward budding of the endosomal membrane to form the multivesicular body that fuses with the plasma membrane to release exosomes to the extracellular space. The cargo of exosomes consists of selected molecules located inside these vesicles or associated with their membrane, which specifically reflects the phenotypic state of donor/parent cells [7–9]. The important role of exosomes and other EVs in multiple biological processes initiated a large number of studies focused on their structure and function, which enabled the discovery of different classes of these vesicles with different biogenesis. Therefore, for practical purposes, exosomes and other classes of virus-sized vesicles (<200 nm) are collectively termed small EVs (sEVs) [10]. Endosome-derived exosomes and other classes of sEVs are well-known mediators of cellular response to different types of stress [11,12]. It has been documented that exosomes released by irradiated cells are involved in different aspects of the systemic response to ionizing radiation. It is noteworthy that both cytotoxic/genotoxic and cytoprotective effects were reported in the context of exosome-mediated RIBE. For example, exosomes released by irradiated cells increased levels of chromosomal aberrations and genetic instability in recipient breast cancer cells [13] as well as reduced viability, caused calcium influx, and stimulated production of reactive oxygen species in recipient keratinocytes [14]. On the other hand, exosomes released by irradiated head and neck cancer cells were shown to stimulate DNA repair and enhance the survival of recipient cells subjected to irradiation after exosome uptake [15]. Hence, different effects mediated by exosomes released from irradiated cells could be observed in recipient cells, which putatively depend on the cell context. Moreover, though phenotypic effects associated with such exosomes are readily observed in different experimental models, the molecular mechanism underlying their action remains unclear. Here, we addressed molecular and cellular mechanisms mediated by exosomes released from irradiated cells and found that exosomes induced acute replication stress in recipients, which may have different consequences depending on a specific cellular context.

2. Results

The total population of sEVs was isolated by size-exclusion chromatography (SEC) from the cell culture media 24 h after irradiation with a single 2 Gy dose or after sham irradiation of FaDu cells (cell line derived from human head and neck carcinoma). The response of FaDu cells to different doses of radiation has previously been analyzed in studies focused on radiation-induced changes in molecular components (i.e., proteins and miRNA) of released exosomes [16,17], which revealed the full viability of cells irradiated with 2 Gy at the time of vesicle collection [17]. Purified vesicles were characterized according to the MISEV2018 guidelines [10]. The morphology and size of the vesicles released either from irradiated cells (Ex_2Gy) or sham-irradiated ones (Ex_0Gy) were analyzed by transmission electron microscopy and dynamic light scattering, which revealed an average vesicle size in the range of 50–100 nm in both cases (Figure 1A,B). The analyzed fraction of vesicles contained typical exosome biomarkers, including CD9 and CD63 (Figure 1C); hence, for simplicity, small EVs present in the studied material are called exosomes hereinafter. We found that irradiated cells released markedly more vesicles, and the amounts of total exosome proteins (TEPs) produced by the same number of cells were at least five-fold higher in the case of Ex_2Gy (which is also shown in Figure 1C). Both types of purified exosomes (i.e., Ex_2Gy and Ex_0Gy) were added to the culture of the naive FaDu cells;

the proportion of vesicles and target cells assumed 10-fold excess of (hypothetical) donor cells over recipient cells. To compare the rate of exosome internalization, differently labeled Ex_2Gy and Ex_0Gy were added simultaneously to the culture media. Then, the kinetics of the uptake of a specific dye by cells were analyzed by fluorescence microscopy. We observed that internalization of exosome membrane-bound dye started after 30 min of co-incubation with cells and that internalization of Ex_2Gy-specific dye was 2-3-fold faster than Ex_0Gy-specific dye (Figure 1D; relative uptake of both types of vesicles was normalized regarding their saturation levels after 6 h of co-incubation).

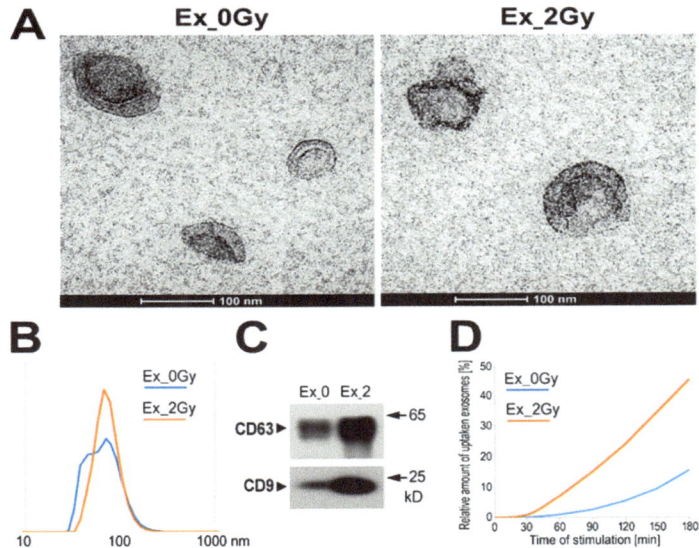

Figure 1. Characteristics of exosomes: TEM imaging of vesicles (**A**); size of vesicles assessed by DLS measurement (**B**); and the presence of exosome markers (**C**) in total sEVs released by mock-irradiated FaDu cells (Ex_0Gy) and cells irradiated with 2 Gy dose (Ex_2Gy); (**D**) relative amounts of internalized vesicles based on the accumulation of exosome membrane-bound dyes (expressed as a percentage of a dye level noted after 6 h of co-incubation).

To address a hypothetical RIBE activated in exosome-stimulated cells, we analyzed the presence of the so-called γH2A.X foci in nuclei of recipient cells, a generally accepted marker of DNA strand breaks which, in the case of radiation-induced DNA double-stranded breaks, showed dose dependence [18]. We found that the levels of γH2A.X foci in the nuclei of cells directly irradiated with a 2 Gy dose (1 h after irradiation) and nuclei of Ex_2Gy-stimulated cells (after 1 h of incubation) were comparably high. In marked contrast, generally low levels of γH2A.X foci in nuclei of Ex_0Gy-stimulated cells were similar to that in the naive untreated control cells (Figure 2A), which indicated that exosomes released by irradiated cells induced RIBE in the naive, non-irradiated cells. The highest level of Ex_2Gy-induced γH2A.X foci was noted after 1 h of co-incubation; then, it gradually decreased, and the levels of γH2A.X foci in cells stimulated with Ex_2Gy were similar to the background level in control cells after 6–8 h of co-incubation. However, another wave of γH2A.X foci was noted after 23 h of stimulation with Ex_2Gy; the latter effect was weaker (Figure 2B), and we further focused on the early effect. The number of γH2A.X foci was significantly higher in cells stimulated with Ex_2Gy than in control naive cells or cells stimulated with Ex_0Gy, both after 1 and 3 h of stimulation ($p > 0.001$ and $p > 0.05$, respectively; Figure 2C). Furthermore, a similar difference between exosomes released by irradiated and mock-irradiated cells was observed when the amounts of Ex_2Gy and Ex_0Gy were standardized according to the actual TEP (Figure 2D), which indicated that the specific effect of exosomes released by irradiated cells was associated with their "quality", not quantity.

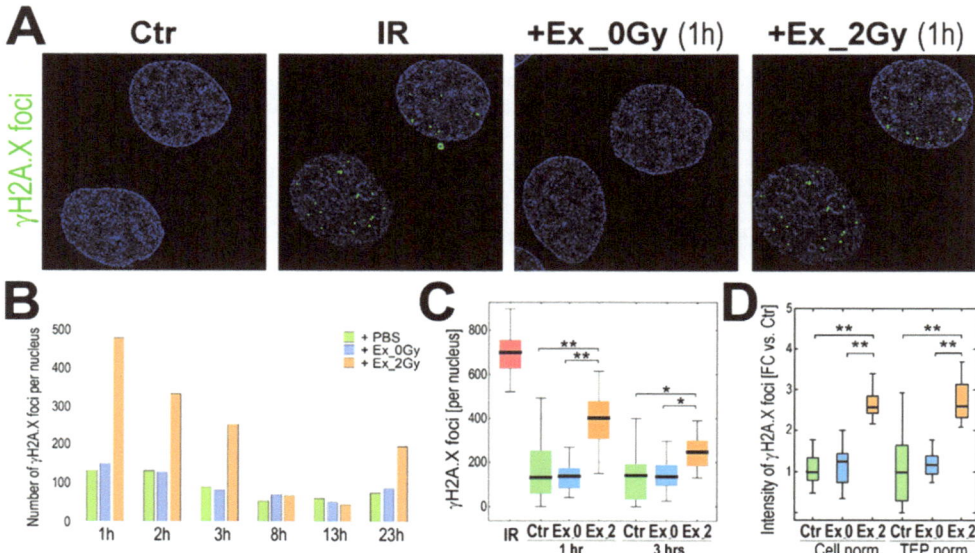

Figure 2. Induction of γH2A.X foci by exosomes from irradiated cells. (**A**) Visualization of γH2A.X foci in FaDu cells co-incubated (1 h) with exosomes released by sham-irradiated (Ex_0Gy) or irradiated (Ex_2Gy) cells; untreated cells (PBS control, Ctr) or cells directly irradiated with 2Gy (IR) were used as controls. (**B**) The number γH2A.X foci after different times of co-incubation with exosomes (1–23 h). (**C**) The number γH2A.X foci after 1 and 3 h of co-incubation with exosomes; directly irradiated cells (IR) were analyzed 1 h after irradiation. (**D**) The relative intensity of γH2A.X foci after 1 h of co-incubation; the number of Ex_0Gy and Ex_2Gy exosomes were normalized according to the number of donor cells (Cell norm.) or according to the total exosome proteins (TEP norm.); the nucleus-integrated intensity was expressed as a fold-change versus PBS-treated controls (FC vs. Ctr). Box plots show the median, minimum, maximum, and lower and upper quartiles; statistically significant differences between groups are represented by asterisks: * $p < 0.05$ and ** $p < 0.001$ (only differences between Ctr and exosome-stimulated cells are shown for clarity).

To search for mechanisms induced by exosomes released by irradiated cells, several molecular features were addressed in the recipient cells. The phosphorylation of H2A.X at Ser-139 could be catalyzed by a few phosphoinositide 3-kinase-related protein kinases including two stress-activated kinases: ATM, activated by radiation-induced double-stranded DNA breaks [19], and ATR, activated in response to single-stranded DNA breaks and during the replication stress [20]. Activation of both protein kinases was analyzed in our experimental model by addressing their active phospho-forms: P-ATM at Ser-1981 and P-ATR at Thr-1989 after one hour of stimulation. We found that stimulation with Ex_2Gy but not with Ex_0Gy resulted in the activation of both ATM and ATR. Of note was that direct irradiation (with 2 Gy) activated primarily ATM (1 h after irradiation). In marked contrast, two factors that are known to induce the replication stress, hydroxyurea (HU) and Topoisomerase I inhibitor camptothecin (CPT), activated both ATM and ATR. All types of stimuli that activated ATM and/or ATR (i.e., Ex_2Gy, IR, HU, and CPT) resulted in phosphorylation of H2A.X at Ser-139 and p53 at Ser-15 (Figure 3A). Hence, one could conclude that stimulation of recipient cells with exosomes released by irradiated cells might induce effects similar to factors known to induce the replication stress.

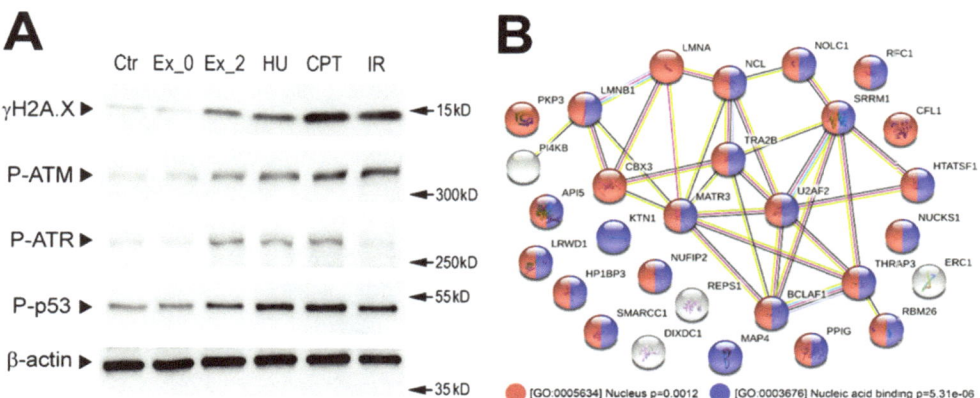

Figure 3. Exosome-stimulated changes in the phosphoproteome of the recipient cells. (**A**) Phosphorylation of selected DNA damage-related proteins analyzed by Western blotting. FaDu cells were stimulated with exosomes released by sham-irradiated (Ex_0Gy) or irradiated (Ex_2Gy) cells, hydroxyurea (HU), and camptothecin (CPT) or directly irradiated with 2 Gy (IR); β-actin was used as a loading control (raw Western blot images are available in Figure S1). (**B**) Network of putative interactions between proteins phosphorylation which was induced in FaDu cells after one hour of stimulation with Ex_2Gy vesicles; color-coded are the proteins associated with two selected GO terms: nuclear localization and nucleic acid binding function (p-value refers to the significance of the term overrepresentation).

To further address molecular changes induced by exosomes from irradiated cells, we analyzed changes in the whole phosphoproteome of recipient cells after 1 h of stimulation with exosomes using a shotgun LC-MS approach. The performed analysis revealed 36 phosphopeptides that were significantly upregulated, specifically in cells stimulated with exosomes from irradiated cells (phosphopeptides corresponding to phosphoproteins analyzed in Figure 3A were not identified due to the shortcomings of the untargeted approach). Proteins corresponding to phosphopeptides that were detected in this untargeted approach (Supplementary materials File Table S1) are presented in Figure 3B. In general, upregulated phosphopeptides corresponded to proteins that had nuclear localization (GO:0005634) and nucleic acid binding functions (GO:0003676). Nuclear proteins whose phosphorylation was induced by exosomes from irradiated cells included replication factors (RFC1, RLWD1) and regulators of heterochromatin remodeling (HP1BP3, CBX3, SMARCC1, NCL) as well as components of the nuclear lamina (LMNB1 and LMNA) and nuclear matrix (MATR3, SRRM1). Moreover, proteins whose phosphorylation was specific for cells stimulated with Ex_2Gy included phosphatidylinositol 4-kinase beta (PI4KB, P-Ser-511), a protein involved in the PIP-mediated intracellular signaling network [21], and plakophilin-3 (PKP3, P-Ser-238), a desmosome protein involved in different signaling pathways [22].

To verify directly the hypothesis that exosomes from irradiated cells affect DNA replication in recipient cells, the labeled analog of thymidine was added to cells pre-stimulated (1 h) with exosomes (Ex_2Gy or Ex_0Gy) and classical inducers of the replication stress (HU or CPT), and then the foci of newly replicated DNA were visualized by fluorescence microscopy (Figure 4A). Pre-incubation with HU or CPT almost totally inhibited DNA replication. Most interestingly, however, stimulation with Ex_2Gy (but not with Ex_0Gy) also markedly reduced the number of the active replication sites (though the response was more heterogeneous in the cell population). To further address the observed phenomenon, we searched for the presence of RNA:DNA hybrids, the appearance of which is frequently associated with the malfunction of the replication process [23]. We found that after 3 h of stimulation with exosomes, Ex_2Gy in particular, RNA:DNA hybrids were abundant in the nuclei of recipient cells. The nuclear areas occupied by such structures were comparable in cells incubated with HU and stimulated with Ex_2Gy (Figure 4B), which additionally indicated that exosomes released by irradiated cells induced mechanisms resembling the replication stress in the naive recipient cells.

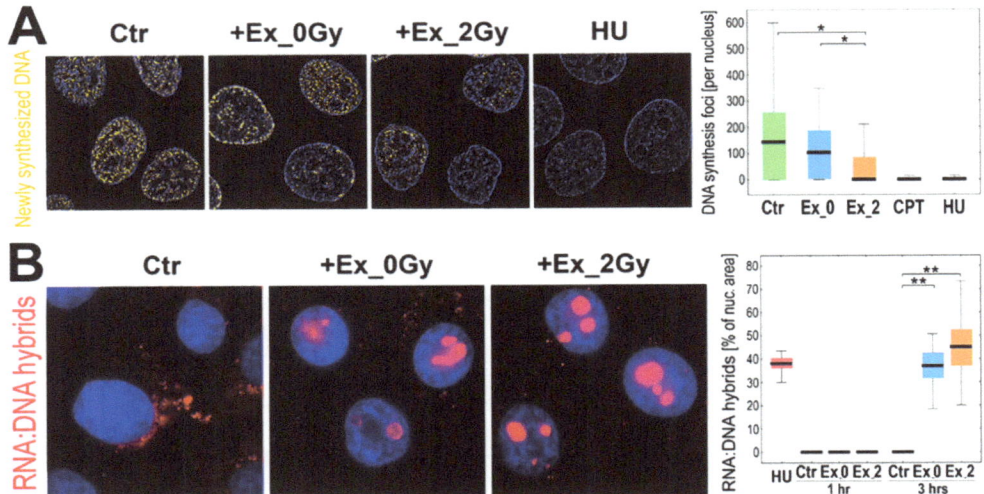

Figure 4. Inhibition of DNA replication by exosomes from irradiated cells. (A) Foci of newly replicated DNA initiated in FaDu cells after one-hour of incubation with exosomes released by sham-irradiated (Ex_0Gy) or irradiated (Ex_2Gy) cells or with HU or CPT. (B) Visualization of RNA:DNA hybrids in nuclei of FaDu cells incubated for 3 h with Ex_0Gy or Ex_2Gy vesicles; the graph shows the relative occupancy of RNA:DNA hybrids in the nuclei cells incubated with exosomes (1 or 3 h) or HU (1 h). Box plots show the median, minimum, maximum, and lower and upper quartiles; statistically significant differences between groups are represented by asterisks: * $p < 0.05$ and ** $p < 0.001$ (only differences between Ctr and exosome-stimulated cells are shown for clarity).

3. Discussion

The plethora of phenomena induced in non-irradiated cells by signals from irradiated ones has been known under the collective term of the non-targeted effects of radiation or radiation-induced bystander effect. Several independent mechanisms involved in radiation-induced non-targeted effects exist including two major types of signaling: (1) direct cell-to-cell communication between irradiated and non-irradiated cells through gap junctions; (2) paracrine/endocrine signaling via "soluble" factors secreted by the irradiated cells into the surroundings [4]. In the recent decade, an interesting mediator of these effects was proposed: exosomes and other classes of membrane-enclosed vesicles released by cells into the extracellular space. Several works documented that exosomes from irradiated cells could increase the viability and (radio) resistance of target cells [24–26], partly by stimulation of DNA repair in recipients [15], while in other experimental models, exosomes from irradiated cells were clastogenic [27] and stimulated cell death [28]. However, although exosome-mediated mechanisms of the systemic response to radiation may have important clinical implications, many aspects of their action remain unknown. Here, we showed that early exosome-mediated radiation-induced non-targeted effects, observed within one hour of the bystander cell stimulation, included the replication stress in the recipient cell.

Due to the limitations of cytogenetic methods used for the assessment of RIBE, exosome-mediated effects were usually observed in long-term assays [13,14,27,29]. A few exceptions included studies where exosome-mediated RIBE was assessed using molecular tests enabling observation of earlier effects, which could be represented by the report of Arioshi and coworkers, who observed increased accumulation of γH2A.X foci and 53BP1 foci after 24 h of stimulation with exosomes from irradiated cells [30]. However, in other experimental models, where less-defined "soluble" components of conditioned media were tested, the formation of γH2A.X foci and other molecular changes were observed, even after a few minutes of stimulation (with their maximum after 30–60 min) [5]. Such early changes are reported here for the first time in the context of exosome-mediated mechanisms, where a high level of γH2A.X foci accumulated after 60 min of stimulation. Although the second (weaker) wave of γH2A.X foci accumulation was observed after approximately 24 h of stimulation, which corresponded to the effects observed by others, the latter effect was putatively associated with distinct mechanisms induced in recipient cells. Interestingly, molecular changes induced in recipient cells by exosomes from irradiated cells were observed before a substantial number of exosomes were internalized. We started to observe labeled membranes of exosomes inside the target cells after 30 min of co-incubation, while after 60 min of co-incubation, very few exosomes were visible inside the cells (below 5% of the "saturation" level). Moreover, the level of internalized exosomes did not correlate with the extent of changes observed in the recipient cells. This suggested that early exosome-mediated mechanisms of RIBE depended on ligand–receptor interactions between vesicles and the target cells, while the specific molecular cargo delivered to the recipient cells after the exosome uptake could be involved in later events. Hence, it is important to note that phosphatidylinositol 4-kinase beta (PI4KB), a component of the PIP-mediated intracellular signaling network associated with the regulation of cell division [21] and viral replication [31], was rapidly phosphorylated specifically in cells stimulated by exosomes from irradiated cells.

The generally accepted model assumes that RIBE signals upregulate the generation of reactive oxygen species (ROS) in the targeted cell, which via generation of DNA damage, likely in conjunction with DNA replication and transcription, initiate the DNA damage response (DDR) in the bystander cell. This DDR involves the activation of ATM/ATR-dependent signaling cascades, which aside from participation in the repair of DNA strand breaks, activates Chk1 and Chk2 checkpoint kinases. The activation of checkpoint kinases stops the progression of the cell cycle, which may have either cytoprotective or cytotoxic consequences depending on the cell context [4]. Data presented in this report fit this general model. Reactive oxygen species and ROS-induced DNA damage are known activators of replication stress [32,33]. Incorrect DNA structures that form during the replications stress are recognized by the ATR/ATRIP complexes, which activate further cellular response [3,34]. Here, we observed that early molecular effects induced by exosomes from irradiated cells included activation of both ATM and ATR, which resembled the patterns of ATM/ATR activation observed in cells treated with hydroxyurea and inhibitor of Topo I, i.e., canonical inducers of the replication stress. Indeed, both exosomes from irradiated cells and inducers of the replication stress triggered the suppression of DNA synthesis and subsequent nuclear accumulation of RNA:DNA hybrids. Moreover, the majority of early changes induced by exosomes from irradiated cells in the cellular phosphoproteome involved nuclear proteins associated with replication and the maintenance of chromatin structure. Interestingly, this includes nuclear lamins, which were recently linked to the management of replicative stress [32]. Hence, our data indicated collectively that activation of the replication stress is a key element of the cellular response induced in the recipient cells by exosomes released by irradiated cells. Moreover, proteins phosphorylated specifically in response to exosomes from irradiated cells also included components of desmosome (plakophilin) and cytoskeleton (dixin and MAP4) involved in cell adhesion and migration. This is important to note because previous studies reported that exosomes from irradiated cells increased the motility of recipient cells [35,36].

Hypothetically, three potential explanations for changes induced in bystander cells by vesicles released from irradiated but not from unexposed donor cells could be offered: (i) larger amounts of vesicles released by irradiated donors; (ii) more efficient uptake of vesicles from irradiated donors; (iii) differences in molecular cargo between exosomes from irradiated and non-irradiated cells. Several previous reports [15,25,37], including the current study, documented higher amounts of exosomes recovered from irradiated cells. However, we showed here that if cells were exposed to an equal total exosome protein load, the induction of γH2A.X remained significantly higher after the stimulation with vesicles from irradiated cells, which indicated that the differences between exosomes from irradiated and non-irradiated donors were mostly qualitative, not only quantitative. It has been reported that radiation affects the cellular uptake of exosomes: irradiation can enhance the uptake of exosomes by affected cells [15,38], and exosomes from irradiated cells could be taken faster by recipient cells [35]; the latter effect was observed also in our study. However, as discussed above, the early effect of exosomes seemed to be independent of their uptake into the target cell. Finally, numerous papers showed that radiation globally changed the protein and RNA content of released exosomes [16,17,36,39,40], and functional changes in bystander cells could be attributed to protein and RNA (mRNA, miRNA, and lncRNA) cargo delivered by exosomes [24,26,27,36]. More recently, mitochondrial DNA transferred by exosomes was proposed as another signal involved in the RIBE [30]. Importantly, however, our data discussed above suggested that ligand-receptor interactions were important for early effects induced in a target cell by exosomes released by irradiated donors. Hence, radiation-upregulated proteins that putatively localize in exosome membranes are of particular interest. In this context, it is important to note that about half of proteins characteristic for exosomes released by irradiated FaDu cells were associated with the GO term "membranes" [16]. Similarly, the third part of proteins, the level of which increased after irradiation in exosomes released by another head and neck cancer cell line UM-SCC6, was associated with the GO term "plasma membrane" including RAC1 and RAC2 membrane-associated small GTPases that augment the production of ROS by NADPH oxidase [40]. Therefore, the potential role of radiation-upregulated proteins with actual exosome membrane localization in DDR signaling (the generation of ROS in particular) is an interesting subject of future studies.

4. Materials and Methods

4.1. Cell Model

The FaDu cell line (HTB-43) was purchased from ATCC (as a component of the Head and Neck Cancer Panel; TCP-1012); these cells were originally derived from human squamous cell carcinoma located in the hypopharynx (HPV negative). Cells were grown in a modified MEM medium with a final concentration of non-heat-inactivated FBS (Thermo Fisher Scientific, Waltham, MA, USA; 10270106) of 10% (v/v) as described in detail elsewhere [17]. The medium was replaced 3 times per week, and cells were incubated at 37 °C, in air with 5% CO_2. At the time of the experiments, cells were between passages 10 and 15. Cells were irradiated with a single dose of 2 Gy at a dose rate of 1 Gy/min using 6 MeV photons and a linear accelerator (True Beam, Varian, Palo Alto, CA, USA). To analyze the effects of exosomes, naive cells were incubated with sEVs purified from cell culture media (details below) on a cell imaging cover glass (Eppendorf, Hamburg, Germany; 0030742036) coated with poly-L-lysine (Merck, Darmstadt, Germany; P4832) before seeding the cells. The ratio of vesicles to recipient cells was calculated based on the number of sEV-releasing cells (donor cells to recipient cells ratio of 10:1). Recipient cells were incubated with sEVs in a fresh medium containing 5% (v/v) Gibco exosome-depleted FBS (Thermo Fisher Scientific, Waltham, MA, USA; A2720801). Moreover, when indicated, cells were incubated with hydroxyurea or camptothecin at a final concentration of 2 mM and 2.5 µM, respectively.

4.2. Purification and Characterization of sEVs

For vesicle isolation, FaDu cells were grown in T175 flasks (Greiner BioOne, Kremsmünster, Austria; 660175) in a modified MEM with a final concentration of non-heat-inactivated FBS (Thermo Fisher Scientific, Waltham, MA, USA; 10270106) of 10% (v/v). The standard culture medium was replaced with a fresh one containing 5% (v/v) Gibco

Exosome-Depleted FBS (Thermo Fisher Scientific, Waltham, MA, USA; A2720801). Then, cells were irradiated (or sham-irradiated) and the cell culture medium was harvested 24 h later. Forty milliliters of medium (corresponding to approximately 2.7×10^7 cells) were centrifuged sequentially at 200× g (10 min), 2000× g (10 min), and 10,000× g (30 min) to remove cellular debris and then filtered with a 0.22 µm filter (Merck, Darmstadt, Germany; SLGP033RB) to remove large EVs (including putative apoptotic bodies or microvesicles). The filtered medium was concentrated to 1 mL using a Vivacell100 ultrafiltration unit (Sartorius, Göttingen, Germany; VC1042) and then loaded onto an Econo-Pac 10DG column (BioRad, Hercules, CA, USA; 732-2010) filled with 10 mL of Sepharose CL-2B (GE Healthcare, Chicago, IL, USA; 17014001) at a length of 6 cm. The column was left until dripping ceased (void volume); then, 1 mL fractions were eluted by loading stepwise 1 mL of PBS; sEVs of interest were eluted in fraction 4 (F4). For further analyses, 1 mL of fraction F4 was concentrated to approximately 50 µL using Vivaspin500 ultrafiltration tubes (Sartorius, Göttingen, Germany; VS0102). Exosome markers (CD9, CD63) were analyzed by Western blot as described in detail elsewhere [41]. The size distribution profile of EVs was estimated by the dynamic light scattering (DLS) measurement using a Zetasizer Nano-ZS90 instrument (Malvern Instruments, Malvern, UK) as described in detail elsewhere [41]. To assess the morphology of the vesicles, transmission electron microscopy (TEM) analysis was performed according to the protocol provided by Thery et al. [42] as described in detail elsewhere [41].

4.3. Western Blot Analysis

Whole-cell lysates were prepared in the RIPA buffer (50 mM Tris-HCl, pH 8.0, 150 mM NaCl, 1.0% NP-40, 0.5% sodium deoxycholate, and 0.1% sodium dodecyl sulfate) enriched with protease (Roche, Mannheim, Germany; 11836153001) and phosphatase (Roche, Mannheim, Germany; 04906845001) inhibitors. The concentration of proteins in the analyzed samples was assessed using the Pierce™ BCA Protein Assay kit (Thermo Fisher Scientific, Waltham, MA, USA; 23225) according to the manufacturer's instructions. Proteins samples (15 µg) were mixed with the loading buffer to a final concentration of 2% (v/v) SDS, 0.1% (v/v) bromophenol blue, 10% (v/v) glycerol, and 100 mM DTT, then denatured for 5 min at 95 °C and separated by 12% SDS–polyacrylamide gel electrophoresis followed by wet transfer onto nitrocellulose membranes (Thermo Fisher Scientific, Waltham, MA, USA; 88018). Membranes were blocked for 1 h in 5% non-fatty milk and 0.1% Tween in PBS, and then the primary antibodies were added for 16 h incubation at 4 °C: anti-P-Ser15-p53 (Cell Signaling Technology, Danvers, MA, USA, 9284S; 1:1250), anti-P-Ser139-H2A.X (Cell Signaling Technology, 9718S; 1:1000), anti-P-Ser1981-ATM (Cell Signaling Technology, 5883S; 1:1250), anti-P-Thr1989-ATR (Thermo Fisher, PA-5-77873; 1:1000), and anti-β-Actin (Cell Signaling Technology, 4967S; 1:1000). After triplicate washes, a secondary antibody conjugated with HRP was added for 1 h at 23 °C. Chemiluminescence detection of bands was performed with WesternBright Sirius HRP substrate (Advansta, San Jose, CA, USA, K-12043-D10) according to the manufacturer's instructions.

4.4. Immunocytochemistry and Fluorescence Microscopy

Cells co-incubated with sEVs were washed three times with PBS and fixed with 4% formaldehyde solution in PBS for 20 min. After three washes with PBS, cells were permeabilized in 0.1% Triton X-100/0.1× citrate buffer for 5 min on ice and washed three times with PBS. Non-specific binding of antibody was blocked with a 3% BSA solution in PBS for 30 min at 23 °C. The preparations were incubated with the primary antibodies anti-P-Ser139-H2A.X (Cell Signaling Technology, Danvers, MA, USA, 9718S; 1:400) or anti-DNA-RNA hybrid S9.6 (Kerafast, Boston, MA, USA, ENH001; 1:100) in 3% BSA/PBS for 1 h and then with the secondary antibody conjugated with FITC (2% BSA/PBS) for 1 h in the dark at 23 °C. In order to identify newly replicated DNA after stimulation of sEV cells, incubation was performed for 30 min with a thymine analog EdU (5-ethynyl-2'-deoxyuridine; Thermo Fisher Scientific, Waltham, MA, USA; C10339) at a final concentration of 10 µM. Then, the cells were washed three times with PBS and fixed with 4% formaldehyde in PBS for 20 min. Nuclei were counterstained with DAPI, and the preparations were examined using the ELYRA 7 system (Carl Zeiss, Oberkochen, Germany) at a magnification of 63×. To visualize exosome uptake, purified vesicles were stained with PKH26 (Ex_0Gy) or with PKH67 (Ex_2Gy) (Merck, Darmstadt, Germany; MINI26 and MINI67, respectively) according to the manufacturer's procedure. Then, the excess dye was removed using Exospin 3 kDa columns (Thermo Fisher Scientific, Waltham, MA, USA; 4484449). The stained vesicles (both types simultaneously) were added to the FaDu cells and a 24 h real-time observation was performed using the ELYRA 7 system at a magnification of 20×.

4.5. Protein Identification by LC-MS/MS

Whole-cell lysates in the RIPA buffer were prepared for mass spectrometry-based shotgun global phosphoproteomic analysis according to Supplementary Protocol P1 given in the Supplementary Materials. Enrichment of phosphopeptides was realized using titanium dioxide according to the protocol of Borisova et al. [43] with modifications. Peptides were analyzed using the Dionex UltiMate 3000 RSLC nanoLC System coupled with the Q Exactive Plus Orbitrap mass spectrometer (Thermo Fisher Scientific). The spectrometer was operated in data-dependent MS/MS mode with survey scans acquired at the resolution of 70,000 at m/z 50 in the MS mode, and 17,500 at m/z 200 in the MS2 mode. Based on the Swiss-Prot human database, peptide and fragment ion masses were used for protein identification with a precision tolerance of 10 ppm and 0.02 Da, respectively. A protein was considered as positively identified if at least one specific peptide was detected, and the peptide score met the significance threshold FDR = 0.01. Protein abundances were determined in Proteome Discoverer by using the Precursor Ions Area detector mode, which uses an average intensity of the three most intensive peptides for a given protein, normalized to the total ion current (TIC). A detailed description of the implemented protocol is provided in Supplementary Protocol P2. The obtained data were deposited to the ProteomeXchange Consortium [44] via the PRIDE [45] partner repository with the data set identifier PXD032143.

4.6. Statistical and Bioinformatics Analyses

The significance of the differences between the analyzed groups was assessed using the Kruskal–Wallis test followed by Dunn's post hoc test for pairwise comparisons; $p < 0.05$ was found to be statistically significant. To assess the effects of exosome stimulation on phosphoproteome of the recipient cells, nine ratios between 3 technical replicas of pairwise compared samples (Ex_0Gy vs. Ex_2Gy) were established, and their global distributions were modeled by Gaussian mixture allowing for quantification of differences between the compared samples [46]. The major components located around the ratio 1.0 were considered as the model of the "not changed" feature, while thresholds for "changed" features were set at 1.710. A feature was considered upregulated (or downregulated) when the median fold-change ratio for all combinations of replicas exceeded the abovementioned thresholds. The String-db knowledgebase [47] was used to predict potential interactions between selected proteins (accessed on 25 January 2022).

Supplementary Materials: The following supporting information can be downloaded at: https://www.mdpi.com/article/10.3390/ijms23084169/s1.

Author Contributions: Conceptualization, P.W. and M.P.; investigation, M.S., Ł.S., M.G., M.K. and M.P.; data curation, M.P.; methodology, M.S., M.G. and P.W.; writing—original draft preparation, P.W.; writing—review and editing, M.S., M.G., M.P. and P.W.; funding acquisition, P.W. and M.P. All authors have read and agreed to the published version of the manuscript.

Funding: This research was financed by the National Science Centre (Poland) as a part of a Preludium-Bis grant (no. 2020/39/O/NZ4/02838).

Institutional Review Board Statement: Not applicable.

Informed Consent Statement: Not applicable.

Data Availability Statement: The mass spectrometry proteomics data were deposited at the ProteomeXchange Consortium with the data set identifier: PXD032143.

Acknowledgments: The authors would like to acknowledge Agata Kurczyk for help with statistical analyses, colleagues from the Department of Radiotherapy, NRIO Gliwice, for help and assistance with the irradiation of cells, and Michael D. Story, UT Southwestern Medical Center in Dallas, for his support and helpful discussion.

Conflicts of Interest: The authors declare no conflict of interest. The funders had no role in the design of the study; in the collection, analyses, or interpretation of data; in the writing of the manuscript, or in the decision to publish the results.

References

1. Mothersill, C.; Seymour, C.B. Radiation-induced bystander effects—Implications for cancer. *Nat. Rev. Cancer* **2004**, *4*, 158–164. [CrossRef] [PubMed]
2. Mothersill, C.; Seymour, C.B. Radiation-induced non-targeted effects: Some open questions. *Radiat. Prot. Dosim.* **2015**, *166*, 125–130. [CrossRef] [PubMed]
3. Cortez, D.; Guntuku, S.; Qin, J.; Elledge, S. ATR and ATRIP: Partners in Checkpoint Signaling. *Science* **2001**, *294*, 1713–1716. [CrossRef]
4. Klammer, H.; Mladenov, E.; Li, F.; Iliakis, G. Bystander effects as manifestation of intercellular communication of DNA damage and of the cellular oxidative status. *Cancer Lett.* **2015**, *356*, 58–71. [CrossRef] [PubMed]
5. Wang, H.; Yu, K.N.; Hou, J.; Liu, Q.; Han, W. Radiation-induced bystander effect: Early process and rapid assessment. *Cancer Lett.* **2015**, *356*, 137–144. [CrossRef] [PubMed]
6. Sprung, C.N.; Ivashkevich, A.; Forrester, H.B.; Redon, C.E.; Georgakilas, A.; Martin, O.A. Oxidative DNA damage caused by inflammation may link to stress-induced non-targeted effects. *Cancer Lett.* **2015**, *356*, 72–81. [CrossRef] [PubMed]
7. Pegte, D.; Gould, S. Exosomes. *Annu. Rev. Biochem.* **2019**, *88*, 487–514. [CrossRef]
8. Jeppesen, D.; Fenix, A.; Franklin, J.; Higginbotham, J.; Zhang, Q.; Zimmerman, L.; Liebler, D.; Ping, J.; Liu, Q.; Evans, R.; et al. Reassessment of Exosome Composition. *Cell* **2019**, *177*, 428–445. [CrossRef]
9. Kalluri, R.; LeBleu, V.S. The biology, function, and biomedical applications of exosomes. *Science* **2020**, *367*, eaau6977. [CrossRef]
10. Théry, C.; Witwer, K.; Aikawa, E.; Alcaraz, M.; Anderson, J.; Andriantsitohaina, R.; Antoniou, A.; Arab, T.; Archer, F.; Atkin-Smith, G.; et al. Minimal information for studies of extracellular vesicles 2018 (MISEV2018), a position statement of the International Society for Extracellular Vesicles and update of the MISEV2014 guidelines. *J. Extracell. Vesicles* **2018**, *7*, 1535750. [CrossRef]
11. Jelonek, K.; Widlak, P.; Pietrowska, M. The Influence of Ionizing Radiation on Exosome Composition, Secretion and Intercellular Communication. *Protein Pept. Lett.* **2016**, *23*, 656–663. [CrossRef] [PubMed]
12. Abramowicz, A.; Widłak, P.; Pietrowska, M. Different Types of Cellular Stress Affect the Proteome Composition of Small Extracellular Vesicles: A Mini-Review. *Proteomes* **2019**, *7*, 23. [CrossRef] [PubMed]
13. Al-Mayah, A.; Irons, S.; Pink, R.; Carter, D.; Kadhim, M. Possible role of exosomes containing RNA in mediating nontargeted effect of ionizing radiation. *Radiat. Res.* **2012**, *177*, 539–545. [CrossRef] [PubMed]
14. Jella, K.; Rani, S.; O'Driscoll, L.; McClean, B.; Byrne, H.; Lyng, F. Exosomes are involved in mediating radiation-induced bystander signaling in human keratinocyte cells. *Radiat. Res.* **2014**, *181*, 138–145. [CrossRef]
15. Mutschelknaus, L.; Peters, C.; Winkler, K.; Yentrapalli, R.; Heider, T.; Atkinson, M.; Moertl, S. Exosomes Derived from Squamous Head and Neck Cancer Promote Cell Survival after Ionizing Radiation. *PLoS ONE* **2016**, *11*, e0152213. [CrossRef]
16. Jelonek, K.; Wojakowska, A.; Marczak, L.; Muer, A.; Tinhofer-Keilholz, I.; Lysek-Gladysinska, M.; Widlak, P.; Pietrowska, M. Ionizing radiation affects protein composition of exosomes secreted in vitro from head and neck squamous cell carcinoma. *Acta Biochim. Pol.* **2015**, *62*, 265–272. [CrossRef]
17. Abramowicz, A.; Łabaj, W.; Mika, J.; Szołtysek, K.; Ślęzak-Prochazka, I.; Mielańczyk, Ł.; Story, M.D.; Pietrowska, M.; Polański, A.; Widłak, P. MicroRNA Profile of Exosomes and Parental Cells is Differently Affected by Ionizing Radiation. *Radiat. Res.* **2020**, *194*, 133–142. [CrossRef]
18. Mah, L.J.; El-Osta, A.; Karagiannis, T. gammaH2AX: A sensitive molecular marker of DNA damage and repair. *Leukemia* **2010**, *24*, 679–686. [CrossRef]
19. Kastan, M.; Lim, D. The many substrates and functions of ATM. *Nat. Rev. Mol. Cell Biol.* **2000**, *1*, 179–186. [CrossRef]
20. Ward, I.; Chen, J. Histone H2AX is phosphorylated in an ATR-dependent manner in response to replicational stress. *J. Biol. Chem.* **2001**, *276*, 47759–47762. [CrossRef]
21. Heilmeyer, L.J.; Vereb, G.J.; Vereb, G.; Kakuk, A.; Szivák, I. Mammalian phosphatidylinositol 4-kinases. *IUBMB Life* **2003**, *55*, 59–65. [CrossRef] [PubMed]
22. Bass-Zubek, A.; Godsel, L.; Delmar, M.; Green, K. Plakophilins: Multifunctional scaffolds for adhesion and signaling. *Curr. Opin. Cell Biol.* **2009**, *21*, 708–716. [CrossRef] [PubMed]
23. Barroso, S.; Herrera-Moyano, E.; Muñoz, S.; García-Rubio, M.; Gómez-González, B.; Aguilera, A. The DNA damage response acts as a safeguard against harmful DNA-RNA hybrids of different origins. *EMBO Rep.* **2019**, *20*, e47250. [CrossRef] [PubMed]

24. Tang, Y.; Cui, Y.; Li, Z.; Jiao, Z.; Zhang, Y.; He, Y.; Chen, G.; Zhou, Q.; Wang, W.; Zhou, X.; et al. Radiation-induced miR-208a increases the proliferation and radioresistance by targeting p21 in human lung cancer cells. *J. Exp. Clin. Cancer Res.* **2016**, *35*, 7. [CrossRef]
25. Mrowczynski, O.D.; Madhankumar, A.B.; Sundstrom, J.M.; Zhao, Y.; Kawasawa, Y.I.; Slagle-Webb, B.; Mau, C.; Payne, R.A.; Rizk, E.B.; Zacharia, B.; et al. Exosomes impact survival to radiation exposure in cell line models of nervous system cancer. *Oncotarget* **2018**, *9*, 36083–36101. [CrossRef]
26. Dai, X.; Liao, K.; Zhuang, Z.; Chen, B.; Zhou, Z.; Zhou, S.; Lin, G.; Zhang, F.; Lin, Y.; Miao, Y.; et al. AHIF promotes glioblastoma progression and radioresistance via exosomes. *Int. J. Oncol.* **2019**, *54*, 261–270. [CrossRef]
27. Al-Mayah, A.; Bright, S.; Bowler, D.; Slijepcevic, P.; Goodwin, E.; Kadhim, M. Exosome-Mediated Telomere Instability in Human Breast Epithelial Cancer Cells after X Irradiation. *Radiat. Res.* **2017**, *187*, 98–106. [CrossRef]
28. de Araujo Farias, V.; O'Valle, F.; Serrano-Saenz, S.; Anderson, P.; Andrés, E.; López-Peñalver, J.; Tovar, I.; Nieto, A.; Santos, A.; Martín, F.; et al. Exosomes derived from mesenchymal stem cells enhance radiotherapy-induced cell death in tumor and metastatic tumor foci. *Mol. Cancer* **2018**, *17*, 122. [CrossRef]
29. Al-Mayah, A.; Bright, S.; Chapman, K.; Irons, S.; Luo, P.; Carter, D.; Goodwin, E.; Kadhim, M. The non-targeted effects of radiation are perpetuated by exosomes. *Mutat. Res.* **2015**, *772*, 38–45. [CrossRef]
30. Ariyoshi, K.; Miur, T.; Kasai, K.; Fujishima, Y.; Nakata, A.; Yoshida, M. Radiation-Induced Bystander Effect is Mediated by Mitochondrial DNA in Exosome-Like Vesicles. *Sci. Rep.* **2019**, *9*, 9103. [CrossRef]
31. Delang, L.; Paeshuyse, J.; Neyts, J. The role of phosphatidylinositol 4-kinases and phosphatidylinositol 4-phosphate during viral replication. *Biochem. Pharmacol.* **2012**, *84*, 1400–1408. [CrossRef] [PubMed]
32. Willaume, S.; Rass, E.; Fontanilla-Ramirez, P.; Moussa, A.; Wanschoor, P.; Bertrand, P. Link between Replicative Stress, Lamin Proteins, and Inflammation. *Genes* **2021**, *12*, 552. [CrossRef] [PubMed]
33. Nagini, S.; Thiyagarajan, P.; Rao, K. *Interplay between Reactive Oxygen Species and Key Players in the DNA Damage Response Signaling Network*; Springer: Berlin/Heidelberg, Germany, 2022; Volume 1, pp. 1005–1022.
34. Zou, L.; Elledge, S. Sensing DNA damage through ATRIP recognition of RPA-ssDNA complexes. *Science* **2003**, *300*, 1542–1548. [CrossRef] [PubMed]
35. Arscott, W.T.; Tandle, A.T.; Zhao, S.; Shabason, J.E.; Gordon, I.K.; Schlaff, C.D.; Zhang, G.; Tofilon, P.J.; Camphausen, K.A. Ionizing radiation and glioblastoma exosomes: Implications in tumor biology and cell migration. *Transl. Oncol.* **2013**, *6*, 638–648. [CrossRef]
36. Mutschelknaus, L.; Azimzadeh, O.; Heider, T.; Winkler, K.; Vetter, M.; Kell, R.; Tapio, S.; Merl-Pham, J.; Huber, S.M.; Edalat, L.; et al. Radiation alters the cargo of exosomes released from squamous head and neck cancer cells to promote migration of recipient cells. *Sci. Rep.* **2017**, *7*, 12423. [CrossRef]
37. Lehmann, B.D.; Paine, M.S.; Brooks, A.; McCubrey, J.A.; Renegar, R.H.; Wang, R.; Terrian, D.M. Senescence-associated exosome release from human prostate cancer cells. *Cancer Res.* **2008**, *68*, 7864–7871. [CrossRef]
38. Hazawa, M.; Tomiyama, K.; Saotome-Nakamura, A.; Obara, C.; Yasuda, T.; Gotoh, T.; Tanaka, I.; Yakumaru, H.; Ishihara, H.; Tajima, K. Radiation increases the cellular uptake of exosomes through CD29/CD81 complex formation. *Biochem. Biophys. Res. Commun.* **2014**, *446*, 1165–1171. [CrossRef]
39. Yentrapalli, R.; Merl-Pham, J.; Azimzadeh, O.; Mutschelknaus, L.; Peters, C.; Hauck, S.M.; Atkinson, M.J.; Tapio, S.; Moertl, S. Quantitative changes in the protein and miRNA cargo of plasma exosome-like vesicles after exposure to ionizing radiation. *Int. J. Radiat. Biol.* **2017**, *93*, 569–580. [CrossRef]
40. Abramowicz, A.; Wojakowska, A.; Marczak, L.; Lysek-Gladysinska, M.; Smolarz, M.; Story, M.D.; Polanska, J.; Widlak, P.; Pietrowska, M. Ionizing radiation affects the composition of the proteome of extracellular vesicles released by head-and-neck cancer cells in vitro. *J. Radiat. Res.* **2019**, *60*, 289–297. [CrossRef]
41. Smolarz, M.; Pietrowska, M.; Matysiak, N.; Mielańczyk, Ł.; Widłak, P. Proteome Profiling of Exosomes Purified from a Small Amount of Human Serum: The Problem of Co-Purified Serum Components. *Proteomes* **2019**, *7*, 18. [CrossRef]
42. Théry, C.; Amigorena, S.; Raposo, G.; Clayton, A. Isolation and characterization of exosomes from cell culture supernatants and biological fluids. *Curr. Protoc. Cell Biol.* **2006**, *3*, 3–22. [CrossRef] [PubMed]
43. Borisova, M.; Wagner, S.; Beli, P. Mass Spectrometry-Based Proteomics for Quantifying DNA Damage-Induced Phosphorylation. *ATM Kinase Methods Protoc.* **2017**, *1599*, 215–227. [CrossRef]
44. Perez-Riverol, Y.; Bai, J.; Bandla, C.; García-Seisdedos, D.; Hewapathirana, S.; Kamatchinathan, S.; Kundu, D.; Prakash, A.; Frericks-Zipper, A.; Eisenacher, M.; et al. The PRIDE database resources in 2022: A hub for mass spectrometry-based proteomics evidences. *Nucleic Acids Res.* **2022**, *50*, D543–D552. [CrossRef] [PubMed]
45. Deutsch, E.; Bandeira, N.; Sharma, V.; Perez-Riverol, Y.; Carver, J.; Kundu, D.; García-Seisdedos, D.; Jarnuczak, A.; Hewapathirana, S.; Pullman, B.; et al. The ProteomeXchange consortium in 2020: Enabling 'big data' approaches in proteomics. *Nucleic Acids Res.* **2020**, *48*, D1145–D1152. [CrossRef]
46. Marczyk, M.; Jaksik, R.; Polanski, A.; Polanska, J. Adaptive filtering of microarray gene expression data based on Gaussian mixture decomposition. *BMC Bioinform.* **2013**, *14*, 101. [CrossRef]
47. Szklarczyk, D.; Gable, A.L.; Lyon, D.; Junge, A.; Wyder, S.; Huerta-Cepas, J.; Simonovic, M.; Doncheva, N.T.; Morris, J.H.; Bork, P. STRING v11: Protein-protein association networks with increased coverage, supporting functional discovery in genome-wide experimental datasets. *Nucleic Acids Res.* **2019**, *47*, D607–D613. [CrossRef]

MDPI AG
Grosspeteranlage 5
4052 Basel
Switzerland
Tel.: +41 61 683 77 34

International Journal of Molecular Sciences Editorial Office
E-mail: ijms@mdpi.com
www.mdpi.com/journal/ijms

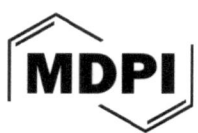

Disclaimer/Publisher's Note: The title and front matter of this reprint are at the discretion of the Guest Editor. The publisher is not responsible for their content or any associated concerns. The statements, opinions and data contained in all individual articles are solely those of the individual Editor and contributors and not of MDPI. MDPI disclaims responsibility for any injury to people or property resulting from any ideas, methods, instructions or products referred to in the content.